Illustrated Pediatric Dentistry (Part 3)

Edited by

Satyawan Damle
Former Professor of Pediatric Dentistry,
Dean Nair Hospital Dental College,
Mumbai, India

Former Vice Chancellor,
Maharishi Markandeshwar University,
Mullana, Ambala, India

Ritesh Kalaskar
Department of Pedodontic and Preventive Dentistry,
Government Dental College & Hospital, Nagpur,
India

&

Dhanashree Sakhare
Founder, Lavanika Dental Academy
Melbourne
Australia

Illustrated Pediatric Dentistry (Part 3)

Editors: Satyawan Damle, Ritesh Kalaskar and Dhanashree Sakhare

ISBN (Online): 978-981-5080-80-3

ISBN (Print): 978-981-5080-81-0

ISBN (Paperback): 978-981-5080-82-7

First published in 2023.

Bentham Science Publishers Pte. Ltd.
80 Robinson Road #02-00
Singapore 068898
Singapore
Email: subscriptions@benthamscience.net

CONTENTS

FOREWORD 1

It is my great pleasure to pen down a foreword for this tremendous book on Pediatric Dentistry for a legend and doyen of the subject, a mentor and guide to the brightest of minds in the field of dentistry.

Rising from the fundamentals, comprehensive in-built, contemporary and authoritative in construct and approach, and hands-on to the core, ***Illustrated Pediatric Dentistry*** is a wonderful work engineered by some of the best-known academics in this noble realm. The chief author, ***Professor Satyawan Damle***, is a colossus among giants, having been a celebrated teacher, distinguished leader, and dynamic policymaker at several dental institutions and universities, including the most prized, the University of Mumbai.

Prof. Satyawan Damle is the rare blend of a gifted clinician and a carved-out academic guru whose intellect has emerged with decades of practice. It is no secret that the degree of acquisition of knowledge by students is one of the measures of the effectiveness of a medical curriculum; and with Pediatric Dentistry being one of the crucial epicentres of growth, it has the potential to make momentous advancements in the evolutionary trajectory of oral and general health.

His co-editors ***Ritesh Kalaskar***, and ***Dhanashree Sakhare*** are examples excellence in their arena. The work reflects their collective understanding of where pediatric dentistry stands today, what have been the treasures and well-kept secrets of the past, and where this tree of knowledge finds fruition today pawing way for the future.

Embedding best care practices of all times, ***Illustrated Pediatric Dentistry*** is a comprehensive yet concise work, which fulfills the essentials of the pediatric dentistry curriculum both for graduates and postgraduates across all universities.

Walking you through the nitty-gritties of preventive, curative and restorative childhood dentistry, be it the behavioral challenges, cariology, endodontics, traumatology, para-surgical themes such as the use of conscious sedation and general anaesthesia at that age, and the management of medically compromised children, the work is a tree of knowledge, nurtured with experiential learning, and carries wonderful blossoms of practical wisdom.

Let us savour and celebrate the chef-d'oeuvre. Indeed, ***Illustrated Pediatric Dentistry*** is a must-read and must-assimilate work for each one of us. Students, practitioners and teachers of Pediatric dentistry will cherish it as a treasured possession on their shelves. I congratulate Prof. Damle and Bentham Science, Singapore, for publishing this irreplaceable tome.

Prof. (Dr.) Mahesh Verma
Vice Chancellor
Guru Gobind Singh
Indraprastha University,
New Delhi,
India

FOREWORD 2

I am delighted to write this foreword for a Book of Illustrated Pediatric Dentistry authored by Professor Satyawan Damle and other academicians. Prof. Satyawan Damle is a well-known researcher and academician with over 44 years of clinical and teaching experience in Dentistry. Besides the several posts and hats he wore in the various roles he played for the profession, he is also a recipient of several awards and recognitions, including the Lifetime Achievement Awards, Outstanding Public Servant Awards, and Research Awards and Fellowships. He is an active member of the Indian Council of Medical Research. Despite his extraordinary achievements as a Pediatric dentist, researcher, and academician, Prof Satyawan Damle will always be known as the longest-serving chief editor of Indexed journals. For almost 35 years. He dedicated himself to overseeing the publication of the highest-quality peer-reviewed studies and opinion pieces on child dental health.

Prof. Damle is actively involved in writing several books on Pediatric Dentistry and Dentistry, which is the testimony of his in-depth knowledge of the subject. The Book of Illustrated Pediatric Dentistry is their new venture initiated by him. I am confident that this book will be accepted by students and faculty involved in teaching Pediatric Dentistry. His work as a teacher, researcher, innovator, visionary and extraordinary academician made him a legend. His role as a mentor and friend made him a role model to those of us who know him and worked with him. His legacy persists not only in academics but also as an able administrator, as he proved his mettle as the Dean of a dental school, Director of Medical Education, Joint Municipal.

Commissioner of Mumbai and, ultimately, the Vice Chancellor of a University. Prof. Damle has worked conscientiously and untiringly to present an unmatched educational endeavour. The topics in this book display clear and succinct clinical expertise and the capability of imparting updated education and information to Oral Health Professionals. The entire volume of this book deals with ultramodern and current state-of-the-art techniques. I take this opportunity to congratulate Prof. Satyawan Damle and his team of contributors - Ritesh Kalaskar and Dhanashree Sakhare for having published this Textbook for Bentham Sciences.

Dr. Ashok Dhoble
Honarary Secretary General
Indian Dental Association H.O.
Mumbai, Maharashtra 400025,
India

PREFACE

It is imperative to have an established approach to handling Children's oral diseases. **'Illustrated Pediatric Dentistry'** is an unpretentious endeavour to integrate the latest developments and up-to-date reviews in the field of Pediatric dentistry by distinguished writers. The book intends to allow students to understand the conceptions of Pediatric dentistry and create a spur to discover the subject by advance reading. Several illustrations, descriptions and graphic drawings have been included to attract the students and make the subject simple to comprehend. A healthy mouth is a gateway to a healthy body and the best time to inculcate healthy habits is through childhood. Prevention of the initiation of oral diseases and training appropriate oral hygiene methods are commenced best throughout the formative years of the child. With a substantial percentage of the worldwide population being in the Pediatric age group, it is imperious to have a scientific approach to behaviour management, prevention and treatment modalities in the dental office, as Pediatric dentistry is a fast-growing division of dental disciplines that lays the basis for the impending dental health of the populace.

The book has been divided into several sections. The sections on child psychology and the emotional development of children are important to learn the basics of various behaviour management strategies. The section on dental caries sensitizes the reader towards the most common dental disorder that is seen in children, and preventive procedures aimed towards lessening dental caries are the necessity of the hour. While an endeavour has been made to include the growth and development of the facial structures and dentition and along with their disturbances and the interceptive and preventive procedures to monitor the erupting teeth.

Pediatric Operative techniques, including endodontics and management of teeth with immature apices affected due to Dental caries and traumatic injuries have been given prominence. Innovations in the field of Pediatric Dentistry are transpiring amazingly fast, and it is crucial to stay up to date with the latest materials, equipment and techniques to deliver the highest quality of care to our little patients.

The New Book cannot be successfully compiled without the collective contribution regarding meticulous reviews of the manuscript to keep pace with the latest innovative novelties. The credit for introducing a New Textbook goes to the contributors for their engrossment, devotion and dedication in presenting a manuscript after applying prudent and well-adjudged scrutiny and analytical approach and have excelled in exploring things to the ultimate.

Accumulation of information and its cogent management would not have been conceivable without the efforts of the contributors who have painstakingly submitted their manuscripts to shape this gargantuan task and introduce this book in the service of Pediatric dentistry.

Satyawan Damle
Former Vice-Chancellor,
Maharishi Markandeshwar University,
Mullana (Ambala), India

Ritesh Kalaskar
Department of Pedodontic and Preventive Dentistry
Government Dental College & Hospital, Nagpur
India

Dhanashree Sakhare
Founder,
Lavanika Dental Academy,
Melbourne
Australia

ACKNOWLEDGEMENTS

We do not find such appropriate words to praise the unique nature of Dr. Mahesh Verma, Vice Chancellor of Guru Gobind Singh Indraprastha University, New Delhi, who himself being a great resolute and connoisseur of dentistry occupying an illustrious position with an eminent background in dentistry, has spared his valuable time from his busy schedule to inscribe the foreword for the Textbook of" Illustrated Pediatric Dentistry." We take it as inventiveness and encouragement rather than a morale-boosting for us to uphold and keep up our determination to satisfy our hunger for academics for the advantage of budding dental professionals.

We also do not find such befitting words to laud the unique nature of Dr. Ashok Dhoble Hon, General Secretary Indian, Dental Association Head Office, who himself is a great advocate and connoisseur of dentistry occupying a distinguished position with an illustrious background in dentistry has spared his precious time from his busy schedule to write the foreword for the Textbook of Illustrated Pediatric Dentistry. I take it as an inspiration and encouragement rather than a morale-boosting for us to uphold and keep up our determination to satisfy our hunger for academics for the advantage of budding dental professionals.

We are also indebted and beholden to the contributors for their altruistic and substantial contribution to make this Textbook of Illustrated Pediatric Dentistry, a great academic endeavour. The contributors are highly competent and knowledgeable clinicians known for their aptitude and capability, which have successfully recognized the most complex and convoluted details of each topic, duly integrating and blending the latest advancements and innovations in Pediatric Dentistry. They are a terrific hard worker and legendary luminaries known for their admirable accomplishments and remarkable involvement in dental education. They have made lots of efforts to lead things to excellence. Credit goes to these patrons and benefactors for the benevolent bequest of their vast knowledge and experience for the betterment of dental education.

We would also like to thank Dr. Priyanka Bhaje, Dr. Parag Kasar, Dr. Sharath Chandra, Dr. Prachi Goyal and Dr. Vidya Iyer for their painstaking efforts and intransigent toil during the editing of this book. They displayed exceptional patients, forbearance, and commitment during the preparation of the book Our dream has come true due to the support of our past and present students. Credit also goes to our family members for their tolerance, Love, and affection.

We would like to appreciate the efforts of Mrs. Humaira Hashmi & Mrs. Fariya Zulfiqar of Bentham Science for giving us an opportunity to pen down our ideas and academic work into reality. We also convey our kind and sincere appreciation to Pascali Pascalis.

Representative of Porter Instrument Business Unit of Parker Hannifin Matrx by Parker and Parker-Porter Product for permitting us to use the company products in our book.

Lastly, we would like to state that fortune favours those who defy complexities and overcome them on their own. We also passionately believe that Man is the architect of his own destiny, and God is on the side of those who toil and perspire to make their providence.

We place our sincerest admiration and gratitude to all those who have delightfully contributed to this cause and for their wishes and devotions made for understanding our dream.

Satyawan Damle
Former Vice-Chancellor,
Maharishi Markandeshwar University,
Mullana (Ambala), India

Ritesh Kalaskar
Department of Pedodontic and Preventive Dentistry
Government Dental College & Hospital, Nagpur
India

&

Dhanashree Sakhare
Founder,
Lavanika Dental Academy,
Melbourne
Australia

List of Contributors

Anil Patil	Department of Pedodontics and Preventive Dentistry, Bharati Vidyapeeth (deemed to be) University Dental College & Hospital, Maharashtra 400614, India
Abdulkadeer M. Jetpurwala	Department of Pediatric Dentistry, Nair Hospital Dental College, Mumbai, India
Anam Mushtaq	Department of Pediatric and Preventive Dentistry, I.T.S. College of Dental Sciences and Research Center, Noida, Uttar Pradesh, India
Dhanashree Sakhare	Founder, Lavanika Dental Academy, Melbourne, Australia
H. Sharath Chandra	Department of Periodontics, SJM Dental College, Chitradurga, Karnataka, India
Harsimran Kaur	Teerthanker Mahaveer Dental College and Research Centre, Moradabad, U.P, India
Heeral Shah	Department of Pediatric and Preventive Dentistry, Sinhgad Dental College and Hospital, Sinhgad Rd, Pune, Maharashtra 411041, India
I. K. Pandit	DAV Dental College, Yamuna Nagar, Haryana 135001, India
Joby Peter	Department of Pediatric and Preventive Dentistry, Annoor Dental College and Hospital, Muvattupuzha, Kerala, India
M.H. Raghunath Reddy	SJM Dental College and Hospital, Chitradurga, Karnataka, India
Mousumi Goswami	Department of Pediatric and Preventive Dentistry, I.T.S. College of Dental Sciences and Research Center, Noida, Uttar Pradesh, India
Nilesh Rathi	Department of Pediatric Dentistry, DY Patil Dental College and Hospital, Pimpri, Pune, India
Nilima Thosar	Department of Pediatric and Preventive Dentistry, Sharad Pawar Dental College, and Hospital, Wardha-442107, Maharashtra, India
Prathamesh P. Nikam	Department of Pedodontics and Preventive Dentistry, Bharati Vidyapeeth (deemed to be) University Dental College & Hospital, Maharashtra 400614, India
Parag D. Kasar	Department of Pediatric Dentistry, Terna Dental College, Navi Mumbai, Maharashtra 400706, India
Palak Jain	Department of Pediatric and Preventive Dentistry, I.T.S. College of Dental Sciences and Research Center, Noida, Uttar Pradesh, India
Priyanka Bhaje	Rungata College of Dental Sciences and Research, Bhilai, Chhattisgarh 490024, India
Rajesh Anegundi	Pediatric Dentistry, SDM College of Dental Sciences, Dharwad, Karnatakan, India
Ritesh Kalaskar	Department of Pediatric Dentistry, Government Dental College and Hospital, Nagpur, India
Rishika Choudhary	Teerthanker Mahaveer Dental College and Research Centre, Moradabad, U.P, India

Ramakrishna Yeluri	Teerthanker Mahaveer Dental College and Research Centre, Moradabad, U.P, India
Satyawan Damle	Department of Pediatric Dentistry, Nair Hospital Dental College, Mumbai, India
Shreya Dasgupta	D. Y. Patil Dental College and Hospital, Pimpri, Pune, India
Shailja Chatterjee	Yamuna Institute of Dental Sciences and Research, Yamuna Nagar, India
S. Srigiri	Department of Pedodontics and Preventive Dentistry, Bharati Vidyapeeth (deemed to be) University Dental College & Hospital, Maharashtra 400614, India
Shivayogi Hugar	Department of Pediatric Dentistry, Kaher's KLE VK Institute of Dental Sciences, Belagavi, Karnataka, India
Vitrat Galhotra	AIIMS Raipur, Chhattisgarh 492099, India
Varinder Goyal	Department of Pediatric and Preventive Dentistry, Guru Nanak Dev Dental College & Research, Institute Bhatinda-Patiala Road, Sunam, Punjab, India
Vidya Iyer	Department of Pediatric and Preventive Dentistry, CSI College of Dental Sciences & Research, Madurai, India
Vishwas Patil	Department of Pediatric and Preventive Dentistry, D. Y. Patil Dental College & Hospital, Sant Tukaram Nagar, Pimpri, Pune, Maharashtra 411018, India
Vishwas Chaugule	Department of Pediatric and Preventive Dentistry, Sinhgad Dental College and Hospital, Sinhgad Rd, Pune, Maharashtra 411041, India

CHAPTER 1

Crown in Pediatric Dentistry

Anil Patil[1,*], **Prathamesh P. Nikam**[1] and **Dhanashree Sakhare**[2]

[1] *Department of Pedodontics and Preventive Dentistry, Bharati Vidyapeeth (deemed to be) University Dental College & Hospital, Maharashtra 400614, India*

[2] *Founder, Lavanika Dental Academy, Melbourne, Australia*

Abstract: The basis for safe permanent teeth in infants and teens is laid during the first years of childhood. Several studies have linked dental caries in children to insufficient diet, unhealthy eating habits, and insufficient toothbrushing habits during the first two years of childhood. The emergence of caries in primary teeth increases the chance of developing caries in permanent teeth. Once a tooth has decayed in young children, the paediatric dentist plays a crucial role to return the tooth to its full functioning potential. The technical advancements in dental products utilized in children over the last few decades are a necessary prerequisite because what was acceptable in the past is not necessarily the safest way to treat young patients nowadays. Several alternatives exist to restore carious teeth in paediatric patients, ranging from stainless steel crowns to aesthetic crowns such as strip crowns and zirconium crowns, which are gaining popularity. This chapter contains a description of the crowns in paediatric dentistry.

Keywords: Stainless steel crowns, Open-faced stainless-steel crown, Polycarbonate, Strip crowns, Pedo jacket, new millennium, Cheng crowns, Kinder crowns, Nu-smile, Dura- crown, Pedo pearls, Zirconia crowns.

INTRODUCTION

Oral wellbeing is a mirror of a person's lifestyle. Dental caries is now one of the most common multifactorial diseases on the planet. In infants, carious lesions begin with the destruction of tooth surface, which may influence aesthetics, self-esteem, mastication, speech, arch length maintenance, and the creation of oral habits, causing disorientation of overall health. So, it is essential to restore the deciduous carious teeth depending on their location, forces delivered to the tooth with various forms of crowns to maintain dental integrity before permanent teeth emerge.

* **Corresponding author Anil Patil:** Department of Pediatric and Preventive Dentistry, Bharati Vidyapeeth (deemed to be) University Dental College & Hospital, Maharashtra 400614, India; E-mail: dranilp0888@gmail.com

The crowns are available into 2 categories [1]

1] Preformed crown and luting cement used for cementation

e.g. Stainless steel with facing, Cheng crowns, Kinder crowns, Nu-smile, Dura-crowns, Whiter bite, Pedo pearls

2] Crown which is bonded to the tooth

e.g. Polycarbonate, Strip crowns, Pedo jacket, new millennium

Stainless steel crown - The Preformed Metal Crown (PMC) most commonly known as the Stainless-steel crown (SSC). It is introduced by Humphrey in 1950 [2]. Stainless steel crown is most commonly used in deciduous dentition than permanent dentition (Tables **1** and **2**).

Classification of Stainless-Steel Crown

Based on Composition

1] Stainless Steel crown (18-8) austenitic type: - 17-19% Chromium, 10-13% Nickel, 67% Iron, 4% Minor elements *e.g.*- Unitek and Rocky Mountain crowns

2] Nickel-Base crowns: -72% Nickel, 14% Chromium, 6-10% Iron, 0.004% Carbon, 0.35% Manganese, 0.2 Silicon *e.g.*- Ion Ni-chro from 3M

3] Tin Based crown

4] Aluminium Based crown

Based on Morphology

1] Uncontoured/ untrimmed crowns – This neither trimmed nor contoured and required lots of adaptation (Fig. **1a**). They are longer in size, and it is time consuming. *e.g.* Unitek and Rocky Mountain crowns.

2] Pretrimmed crowns – It is straight and having non-contoured sides (Fig. **1b**). This crown requires lots of contouring and trimming. It is festooned to follow gingival crest. *e.g.* 3M and Denovo crowns.

3] Precontoured crowns - This crown is festooned and having pre-contoured and pre-trimmed (Fig. **1c**). Manufactures gingival crimp loss due trimming may cause difficulty in adaptation. *e.g.* Ni-chrome crowns and Unitek stainless steel crowns.

Table 1. Indications and contraindications of crowns (Fig. 2).

Indications	Contraindications
1.Extensive decay of primary teeth – when tooth decay includes two or more than two surfaces. 2. Following pulp therapy procedures- Pulp therapy makes tooth brittle and to prevent brittleness or fracture of tooth. 3. As a prevention restoration – Used in high caries index patient 4. Restoration of primary molars affected by localized or generalized developmental problems eg. – Hypoplastic defect 5. Used in a space maintainer or denture 6. Severe bruxism- In this condition tooth surfaces chip off and may cause pulpal exposure. So, to prevent this stainless-steel crown is used.	1. Allergy and sensitivity to nickel 2. Tooth with radicular pathology 3. Physiological tooth mobility or Tooth near to exfoliation 4. Slightly erupted tooth

Table 2. Advantages and Disadvantages of crowns.

Advantages	Disadvantages
1. Their life expectancy is the same as that of a healthy tooth. 2.They give stability to the tooth that may have become brittle after excessive caries removal. 3.The technique sensitivity or the risk of making errors during their application is low. 4. Their long-term cost effectiveness is good. 5. Low clinical failure rate.	1.It looks like metal. 2.It cannot be used when the tooth is slightly erupted.

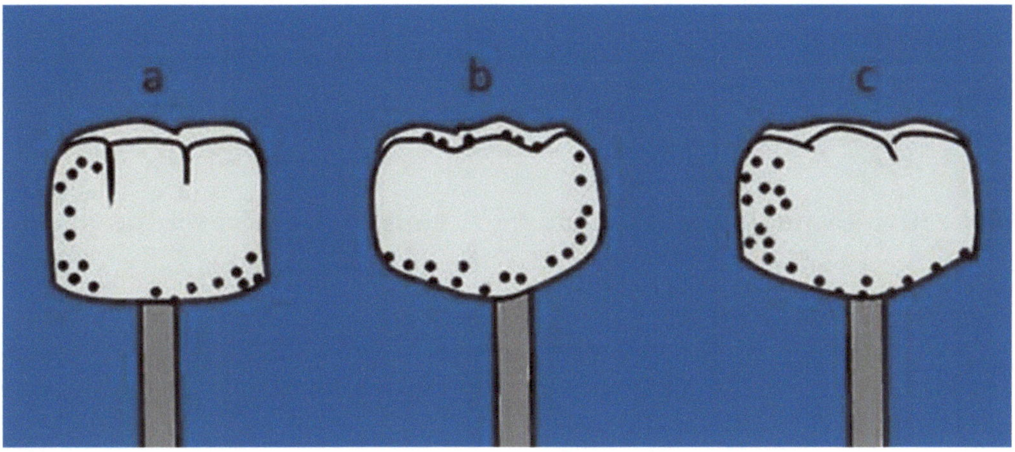

Fig. (1). Types of crowns.
a - Untrimmed crowns b - Pretrimmed crowns c - Precontoured crowns.

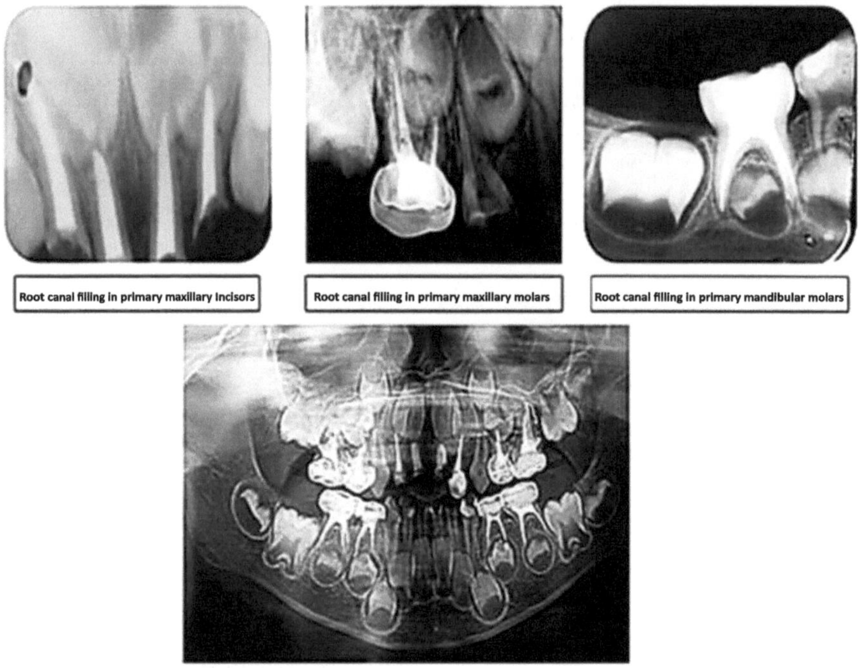

Fig. (2). Indications of crown.

Armamentarium

1] Burs and Stones - Burs no 169L or 69L friction grip shank (F.G.) (Fig. **3a**) Tapered diamond F.G. (Fig. **3b**), Green stones or heatless stone (Fig. **3c**), Rubber wheel.

2] Pliers/Instruments - Ball and socket plier {#112} or Johnson's Contouring pliers {#114 / #134} (Fig. **3d**), Crown crimping plier {#800-417} (Fig. **3e**), Howe plier {#110} (Fig. **3f**), No 137 Gordon plier, Crown removal plier, Crown cutting scissor (Fig. **3g**).

Preoperative Evaluation of Patients for Stainless Steel Crown Restorations [6]

i. Dental Age of the Patient:
   This is recorded by the root development of the underlying tooth. When a primary tooth can be expected to exfoliate within 2 years of restoration, amalgam restoration can be done.
ii. Co-operation of the Patient:
   If the patient is uncooperative, due to younger age or due to negative behaviour, or if the child is stubborn and does not cooperate, first a positive behaviour has to be instilled. If the child is unable to co-operate because of

age (*i.e.*, <3yrs) then a general anaesthesia may have to be considered. In such cases, it is difficult to check the correct occlusion, so it is always better to keep the stainless-steel crown at thc level or slightly below the level of the adjacent tooth, so that the child should not have disturbed occlusion due to premature contact.

iii. Motivation of the Parents:

Parents should be educated regarding the various treatment modalities for their children's carious teeth. They should be motivated for the treatment for their kids at the proper time.

iv. Medically Compromised/Disabled Children:

For children with cardiac problems, prophylactic antibiotics should be administered before tooth reduction. Care should also be taken in treating children with leukaemia and bleeding disorders.

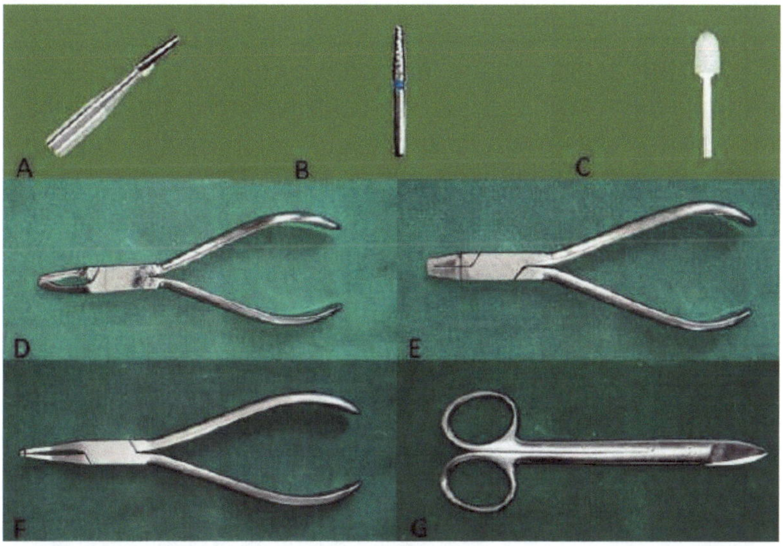

Fig. (3). Armamentarium for stainless steel crown.
A - Burs no 169L, B - Tapered Diamond F.G, C - Green Stone, D - Johnson's Contouring Plier, E - Crown Crimping Plier, F - Howe Plier, G – Crown Cutting Scissor

Clinical Procedure

A] Preoperative evaluation – First take putty or alginate impression of the upper and lower arch of patient to make a diagnostic cast. With the help of diagnostic cast evaluate space between upper central incisor, cusp relationship between two arches, canine relation, extrusion of opposing tooth and mesial drifting of adjacent teeth

B] LA Administration- It reduces the discomfort of patient during subgingival preparation

C] Isolation- Isolation has to be done with help of rubber dam and cotton rolls. Before isolation, check the child's bite pattern. Rubber dam increases work quality as well as improve visibility and efficiency. Rubber dams protect the damage of surrounding tissues.

D] Caries removal- It is removed by large round bur in a slow speed handpiece. After caries removal and pulp therapy, it is filled or built up with GIC cement or Zinc oxyphosphate cement.

E] Crown selection- Crown selection involved following considerations.

- Mesiodistal diameter (Fig. **4**)
- Light resistance to seating
- Proper occlusal height

Before tooth preparation crown size may be selected by using Boley gauge. After tooth preparation crown size selected by trial-and-error procedure. The smallest crown should refer to fit on tooth preparation. While placing the crown friction to be felt when crown slips gingivally.

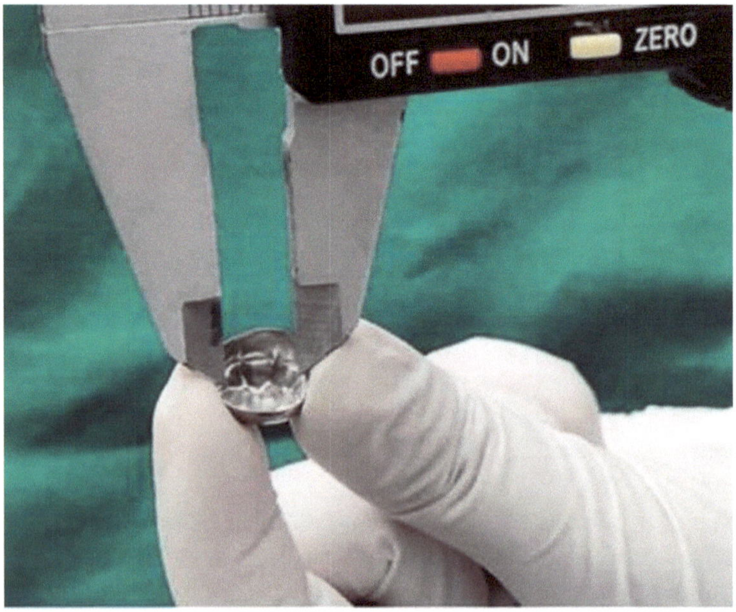

Fig. (4). Measurement of mesiodistal diameter of crown with help of Boley gauge.

F] Tooth preparation-

Purpose of tooth preparation - To gain enough space for crown, to remove complete decay and caries tooth surface, to have sufficient tooth for retention of crown.

Occlusal Reduction

Humphrey in 1950 suggested that the occlusal cusps and all surfaces of tooth should be reduced. In 1966, Rapp advised that when occlusally reduction of tooth was done then gingival margin should be 4mm away from occlusal reduction. In 1968, Mink and Bennett suggested that 1mm of groove has to be made on occlusal surface that will help in a uniform occlusal reduction of 1 to 1.5mm (Fig. **5a,b,c**). After that in 1976, Kennedy recommended that to preserve the tooth structure; bur should follow the anatomy of tooth [6].

Evaluation of Occlusal Reduction

The main aim of evaluation of occlusion is to preserve occlusal anatomy. Main motive of occlusal anatomy preservation is to maintain crown retention and decrease pulp exposure. It is done by visual examination. In 1981, Forrester advised to use wax sheet for evaluation of occlusal reduction.

Proximal Reduction

In second step, tooth preparation starts with interproximal reduction. It is marginal ridge and bur no-69L or 169L should move buccolingually. Proximal reduction should be10 degree converging towards occlusal surface. Proximal preparation should not be over taper. Finishing line of proximal reduction should be feather edge. During preparation, proximal contact with the adjacent teeth should be broken gingivally and buccolingually (Fig. **5c**). Proximal slices converge slightly towards the occlusal and lingual surface, given by Meyers in 1976. The primary principle of the technique for fitting crown is to make the tooth preparation fit the crown form rather than attempt to make the crown fit the tooth preparation. Distal tooth surface reduction is necessary even when there is no growing tooth distally. Failure to follow this recommendation will result in on oversized crown being fitted, which may impede the eruption of first permanent molar [6].

Evaluation of Proximal Reduction

It is done by passing explorer through proximal area and check broken adjacent tooth contact.

Buccal And Lingual Reduction

During buccal and lingual surface reduction, it should be 0.5mm. It is deep enough to be (0.5 – 1mm) into gingival sulcus. Finishing line should be featheredge. Buccal bulge may require reducing in deciduous mandibular 1st molar. All sharp edges should be rounded [8].

Evaluation of Tooth Preparation

The occlusal clearance must be 1.5 to 2mm. Occlusal relationship is established by comparing adjacent marginal ridge heights. All line angles of tooth preparation should be rounded. Excessive gingival blanching should not be seen. Crown should be fitted sub gingival sulcus.

Adaptation of Crown

The adaption of crown is firstly tried on lingual surface of crowns then applying pressure in a buccal direction, so that crown easily fitted on buccal surface into the gingival sulcus (Fig. **5d,e**). Resistance should be felt as the crown pass over the buccal bulge. Mark dotted line on crown surface to cut 1mm below line with scissors. After that, place the crown again, if gingival blanching is seen then remove the crown and retrim the crown surface [4].

The crown adaptation based on Spedding's adaptation principle, and it is given in 1984 [3].

Spedding's adaptation principle-1

The crown must be of correct length and its margins should closely resemble to the tooth. Any point on the tooth occlusal surface to the greatest diameter should be visible clinically and any point on the tooth apical to greatest diameter should be on undercut surface of tooth and should not be visible.

Spedding's adaptation principle-2

The correct contours of buccal and lingual gingival margins of crown should have good adaptation to gingival tissue.

Crown Trimming

If the crown is longer than tooth, the crown margin may interfere complete seating, so in this case crown length may be adjusted by trimming and smoothing with an abrasive stone (Fig. **6a**). Less trimming requires maintaining the retention of the crown [4].

Crown Contouring

The crown is contoured using a ball and socket plier (No-114) at middle third of crown for proper fit of crown (Fig. **6b**). Contouring can be done with No 112 ball and socket plier, No 137 Gordan plier and No 114 Johnson plier. Buccal gingival contour of second primary molar look like smile. Buccal gingival contour of first primary molar resembles like stretched out S shape. Lingual contour of all primary molar form smile like shape. Proximal contour of all primary molar forms frown shape [4].

Crimping of Crown

The crimping of the crown is done using Johnson's contouring plier (No 113) to adapt cervical margins of crown inwards and adapted into undercut area (Fig. **6c,d**). If permanent molar is not erupted properly, little bit care must be taken for adaptation of distal margin of deciduous 2nd molar [4].

Evaluation of Crimping of Crown

It is evaluated using explorer. If margins of crown are open, then recrimping should be done. In 1987, Johnson suggested to check proper crimping of crown by blanching of gingival tissue. Bitewing radiograph technique also useful in evaluation of crimping of crown and it is given by More and Pink in 1973 [4].

Final Trial of Crown Adaptation

Crown should not be able to remove it with finger pressure. If crown is not properly seating and is without gingival blanching, then ledges can be found. If resistance to seating is there with blanching, then crown is wide or there may be tissue interfere.

Crown Finishing and Polishing

After polishing, crown margins should be blunt. If unpolished margin remains on crown it may lead to accumulation of plaque and can cause gingivitis. Rubber wheel helps to smoothen the rough margins of crowns. A large green stone is used to create a knife edge finish around the crown's cervical margin (Fig. **6e**). Bur is rotated counter clockwise at a 45-degree angle. Iron rouge should be used to coat the crown. The final step before cementation is to create a bevelled gingival margin that can be polished.

Cementation of Crown

For cementation of crown GIC is much better than other cement. GIC cements have strengths as compared to zinc phosphate. GIC cement release fluoride as do the silico-phosphate, chelate or bond to tooth structure as the polycarboxylate and are as pulpally compatible as the polycarboxylates. The crown should be one half to two third filled with the cement (Fig. **7**). Dry the tooth and seat the crown completely. Initially bite slowly with increasing pressure. Patient bite will help to seat the crown without distorting it. Cement should flow out from all ends of the crown. Remaining cement can be removed by spoon excavator or explorer. Recheck for excess cement [6].

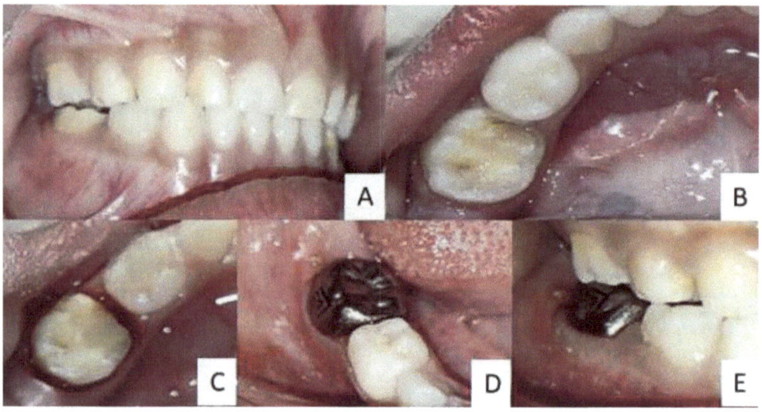

Fig. (5). Tooth preparation of stainless-steel crown.
A – Intra-oral image Showing occlusal reduction of 1 to 1.5mm, **B** – Occlusal view of tooth preparation, **C** – Intra-oral image Showing proximal contact break without touching to adjacent tooth, **D**, **E** – Intra-oral image Showing crown placement in oral cavity.

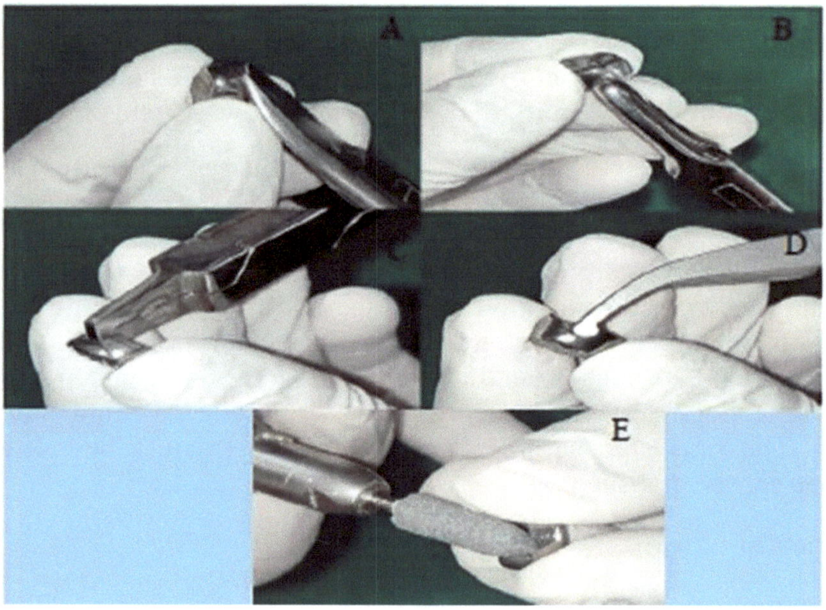

Fig. (6). Adaptation of crown.
A - Crown trimming with scissor, **B** - Crown contouring with Johnson's Contouring plier, **C** - Crown crimping with crimping plier, **D** - Crown crimping with howe plier, **E** - Crown finishing with green stone.

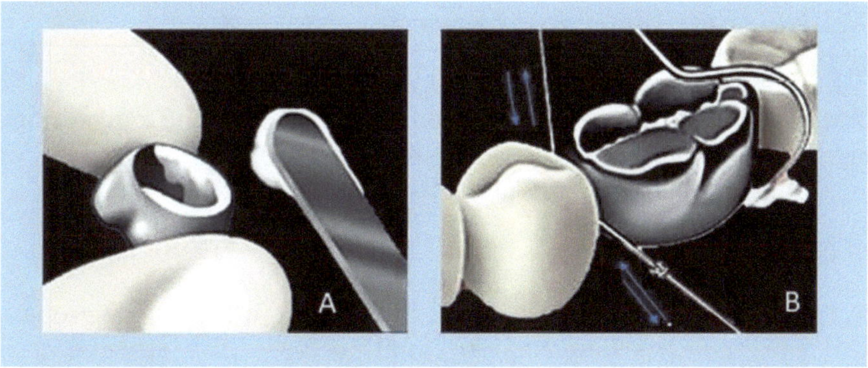

Fig. (7). Cementation of crown.
A – Crown cementation done using luting cement, **B** – Remove excess cement with explore or dental floss.

Clinical Evaluation of Crown Cementation

1. The crown & its margins are smooth & polished properly
2. Properly adapted to the prepared tooth surfaces
3. The proximal contacts are established properly.
4. Crown should be in proper occlusion
5. Crown margins extended 0.5 -1mm into gingival crevice
6. Excess of cement is removed completely

Post-Operative Instructions

Patient should at least avoid sticky foods like caramel, gum, toffees, hard candies, chewing on ice, popcorn kernels and any other hard substances for next 1 hr.

Modifications of Stainless-Steel Crown (Mink and Hill, 1971)

Undersized Tooth or the Oversized Crown:

This mostly occurs in long untreated interproximal caries and space loss due to exfoliation or extraction. The crown circumference is decreased by a V cut made from the gingival surface to the occlusal surface of crown. To make crown circumference smaller the cutting edges are overlapped over one another (Fig. **8a,b,c**). The crown is tried on the tooth preparation and amount of overlapping necessary is marked on the crown surfaces. Overlapping edges of crown close with spot welding machine. Rubber wheel used for polished the surface [5].

Oversized Tooth or the Undersized Crown:

In this V shape cut is made and make 2 separate edges on crown surface. To close that, a piece of 0.004 inches band material place over the cut surface. Then contouring is done and to reduce microscopic deficiency in seal by applying solder on it (Fig. **8d,e,f**). After that, polish the soldered crown [5].

Deep Sub Gingival Caries:

Complete the indicated pulp treatment and then restore the cavity preparation. If subgingival caries occurs between proximal surfaces of tooth, the crown will extend to cover the caries (Fig. **8g**) [5].

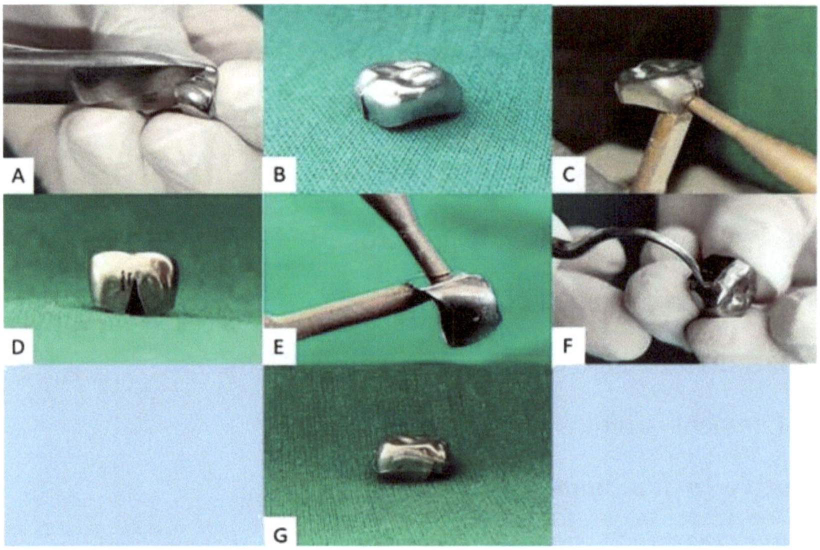

Fig. (8). Modifications of stainless-steel crown.
A, B, C - Modification of stainless-steel crown for undersized tooth or oversized crown
D, E, F - Modification of stainless-steel crown for oversized tooth or undersized crown
G - Modification of stainless-steel crown using adding matrix band to caries side of crown to cover subgingival caries

Complications of Stainless-Steel Crown

The stainless-steel crown is not a cure-all or a miracle wand for treating extensive caries or preventing amalgam loss. When treated wrongly, these crowns can inflict just as much harm as a badly finished amalgam alloy. Some of the most common complications are mentioned below, along with necessary therapies [6].

1. Interproximal ledge: Because of the risk of iatrogenic pulpal exposure, further tooth reduction to remove this ledge should be attempted with caution. If the

ledge is not removed, the crown will be unable to seat, and its borders will tie on the ledge. The interproximal slice is difficult to prepare when the neighbouring tooth is partly erupted, and the contact region is poorly defined. To clear the contact region, extensive subgingival tooth reduction is required; difficulty of access increases the risk of forming a ledge or destroying the erupting tooth, which would be unfortunate if it is the first permanent molar. In such cases, it could be prudent to postpone crowning until the contact areas are properly defined.

2. Poor margins: When a stainless-steel crown is imperfectly adapted, the crown's marginal dignity suffers. Open caries is a rarity around restorations and restorations are seldom precede the formation of caries However, as the anomaly grows, the odds of plaque retention, so does the likelihood of gum disease. On the other hand, it is believed that chronic inflammation and exposure of the supporting tissues may lead to premature tooth enamel loss, although this theory awaits confirmation in the future.
3. Crown tilt: If a full lingual or buccal wall is destroyed by caries or overzealous use of cutting tools, the finished crown can tilt to the deficient hand. This tilting is usually observed on the lingual side of mandibular primary molars due to a lack of tooth support. Prior to crowning, an amalgam alloy or glass-ionomer cement reconstruction is positioned to provide stability and avoid crown tilt (the restoration acting as a core). Crown tilting has no therapeutic importance until it occurs on young permanent molars, where it may result in unfavourable supra-eruption of the opposing tooth.
4. Nickel hypersensitivity: According to research, orthodontic treatment of nickel-containing stainless-steel instruments performed prior to ear piercing seems to decrease the occurrence of nickel hypersensitivity. When compared to skin, higher concentrations of contact allergen may be needed to induce a response from the oral mucosa, but the form, duration, and oral exposure required to trigger this potential remain uncertain (Table **2**).
5. The crown is inhaled or consumed: Fortunately, these mishaps are uncommon, particularly where a rubber dam is used, which we recommend for all children's dentistry. If the rubber dam is not in place, abrupt, unexpected movement can result in inhalation or ingestion of the crown. If this occurs, an attempt at removal should be done as soon as necessary by turning the infant upside down; if this is insufficient, a prescription for an urgent chest X-ray is needed. If the crown is in the bronchi or lung, medical advice and referral will certainly result in a bronchoscope removal attempt. The presence of a cough reflex in a conscious infant decreases the chances of inhalation, though crown ingestion is more possible. Ingestion is less severe, but it must also be diagnosed on a chest radiograph from the absence of the crown. Within 5-10 days, the stainless-steel crown can pass through the alimentary tract without incident. The parent should

take on the unenviable job of tracking down the ejected crown. Taking all practicable measures to avoid crown ingestion or inhalation reduces anguish and tension for the infant, adult, and clinician. As a result, with the rubber dam in place, crown preparing, trimming, and trail fitting can all be done. The interproximal rubber can be sliced, and the ligature withdrawn while a crown is being fitted next to the clamped tooth, revealing the gingival margins. With crown expertise, the operator will cement on the crown with the rubber dam in place, then lift the rubber dam and inspect the occlusion as the cement settles.

Failures in Stainless Steel Crowns can be Caused by a Variety of Factors

1. Inadequate tooth

2. Insufficient crown adaptation and as a result poor retention.

3. Inadequate cementation, resulting in a missing crown or open margins.

4. The pulp treatment failed.

5. Induced ectopic eruption of the permanent first molar.

6. Caries that recurs, especially in the interproximal areas.

7. Abrasion of the crown through the occlusal base.

Considerations for Successful use of Stainless-Steel Crowns

1. Caries removal and, if necessary, effective pulpal therapy

2. Optimal tooth structure reduction for proper crown retention.

3. Lack of damage to adjacent teeth after opening interproximal contacts.

4. Choose a crown that is the right height to keep the arch length.

5. Gingival wellbeing and accurate marginal adaptation

6. Good occlusion for practical purposes.

7. Cementation process that is optimal.

Hall Technique for Stainless Steel Crown

The Hall technique is a way of treating carious primary molars in which decay is sealed under a stainless-steel crown without the use of local anaesthesia, tooth cleaning, or caries removal. The Hall technique is one of the approaches used for biological sealing in primary molar carious lesions. As a result, the bacteria will be isolated from the oral system, and the caries will be rendered inactive. As opposed to traditional treatment modalities used in primary care environments, the Hall technique is regarded as a viable restorative alternative with high acceptability and longevity, as well as a low failure rate for treating carious primary molars. Furthermore, whether given using the Hall technique or conventional training by a paediatric dentist, the survival rate of stainless-steel crowns (SSCs) is considered high. As a result, the Hall procedure can be a useful complement to a clinician's care choices for carious primary molars. However, it can only be seen under limited circumstances [13], (Tables **3** and **4**).

Table 3. Advantages and disadvantages of Hall technique.

Advantages	Disadvantages
1. It is a non-invasive technique that involves the placement of a crown without the use of local anaesthesia, caries excavation, or tooth planning. 2. It is a simple treatment that reduces the child's anxiety. 3. It is thought to be a less painful approach for children. 4. It seals in carious lesions and may be able to avoid or delay the development of caries. 5. It enhances the health of the pulpal tissue. 6. It improves access to dental treatment, reduces the percentage of untreated dental caries, and provides a regeneration that allows for natural tooth exfoliation. 7. It is less costly than standard restorations. 8. The time required to perform the operation is limited if completed in a single visit.	1. Aesthetically unappealing 2. Temporary bite opening 3. The development of caries cannot be determined radiographically or clinically.

Table 4. Indications and contraindications of Hall technique.

Indications	Contraindications
1.Non-cavitated teeth with occlusal caries whether the patient is unable to accept fissure sealant, partial caries removal or tradition restoration. 2. Teeth with proximal caries can be caveated or no-cavitated if the patient is unable to tolerate partial caries removal or traditional reconstruction.	1. Tooth with signs or symptoms of dental inflammation or irreversible pulpitis. 2. Crowns that have been badly damaged by caries and are deemed unsalvageable. 3. Very young children who do not appreciate the treatment or cannot tolerate biting the crown into place without local anaesthesia.

Procedure for Hall Technique

Determine the tooth shape, occlusion, and proximal contact region first. Where there are close contact, orthodontic elastic separators are used for 3-5 days in the mesial and distal contact areas. Crown positioning should take place after sufficient space has been gained. If the marginal ridge of one molar collapses, the adjacent tooth can move to the breakdown region. This complicates the Hall procedure of crown positioning without requiring modifications to the tooth or crown. In this case, reconstruct the marginal ridge and allow the separator to be mounted. Examine the occlusion in relation to the anterior overbite and the buccal connection of the tooth to be crowned with the opposing number. A cotton roll should be placed between the tongue and the tooth before the crown is placed. This protects the patient's airway. Try on various crown sizes to ensure a good match that protects all cusps. Choose the smallest crown size. If the crown is too big, there is a risk that the erupting pathway of permanent first molars would be messed with. Load the crown with GIC luting cement after determining the size and remove any excess cement from the tooth surface. Apply finger pressure to the crown and hold it in place until the cement hardens.

Success criteria of Hall technique crowns according to Innes *et al* (2007) [13].

1. The restorations or crowns are sufficient, and no treatments were necessary.

2. There were no clinical or radiographic symptoms of pulp disease.

3. Exfoliation of the teeth is normal.

Failure criteria of Hall technique crowns according to Innes *et al* (2007) [13].

1. Secondary caries or new caries are developed radiographically or clinically.

2. Repairing a crack or wear that necessitates attention.

3. An abscess or permanent pulpitis that indicates extraction or pulpotomy.

4. Internal root resorption or inter-radicular radiolucency.

5. If the restoration or crown were missing, or if the tooth could not be restored.

Open-Faced Stainless-Steel Crowns

Previously, there were fewer options for stainless steel crowns. Parents preferred prosthesis or extraction of individual teeth for grossly decayed anterior teeth because stainless steel crowns for anterior teeth did not look appealing. As an alternative to preformed metal crowns, open-faced stainless-steel crowns were added (Fig. **9**, Table **5**) (Croll, 1998).

Table 5. Advantages and disadvantages of open-faced stainless-steel crowns

Advantages	Disadvantages
1. It is more aesthetically pleasing than stainless steel crowns, as well as more robust and retentive.	1. Crown placement takes a long time. 2. If there is gingival bleeding or moisture on the crown side, composite cannot bind well.

Tooth Preparation of Open-Faced Stainless-Steel Crowns

Hartmann invented the open-faced stainless-steel crown tooth preparation method in 1983. When the cement has dried, continue expanding the window on the labial surface of the cemented crown with a no. 330 or no.245 bur. The incisal edge of the window should be low and gingivally to the height of the gingival crest when stretching it. The window should extend mesio-distally to the line angles. Following that, 1 mm of cement should be extracted from the sub gingivally. Smoothing the cut margin with a green stone bur. Both the bonding agent and the crown cementation, a glass ionomer lining is used. The resin-based composite should then be applied to the expanded window, and the composite should flow into the undercut and polymerize. For finishing restorations, abrasive discs are used [7].

Polycarbonate Crowns

Polycarbonates are aromatic linear carbonic acid polyesters. Polycarbonate crowns are heat-moulded acrylic resin shells that are self-cured acrylic resin-adapted to teeth. It is moulded as solids by a thermal distortion point of 270 degrees Fahrenheit. They are more visually appealing than stainless steel crowns. The polycarbonate composite is porous and cannot tolerate strong abrasive forces, resulting in regular fracturing and dislodgement (Fig. **10**, Tables **6**, **7**).

Table 6. Indications and contraindications of polycarbonate crowns.

Indications	Contraindications
1. Children with nursing bottle syndrome frequently require full coverage offered by polycarbonate crowns. 2. It is used in Malformed or fractured teeth. 3. Discoloured teeth can be replaced by polycarbonate crowns	1. Tooth with unrestorable conditions

Table 7. Advantages and disadvantages of polycarbonate crown.

Advantages	Disadvantages
1. They are more aesthetically appealing and more robust than composite strip crowns and pre-veneered crowns. 2. Since the manufactured crown is cemented with self-adhesive resin cement rather than bonding, they are not as procedure sensitive as plastic strip crowns. 3. They take the same amount of time to instal as stainless-steel crowns, and plastic strip crowns.	1. They are not recommended for patients who clench their teeth often. 2. A larger amount of tooth reduction is needed during tooth preparation.

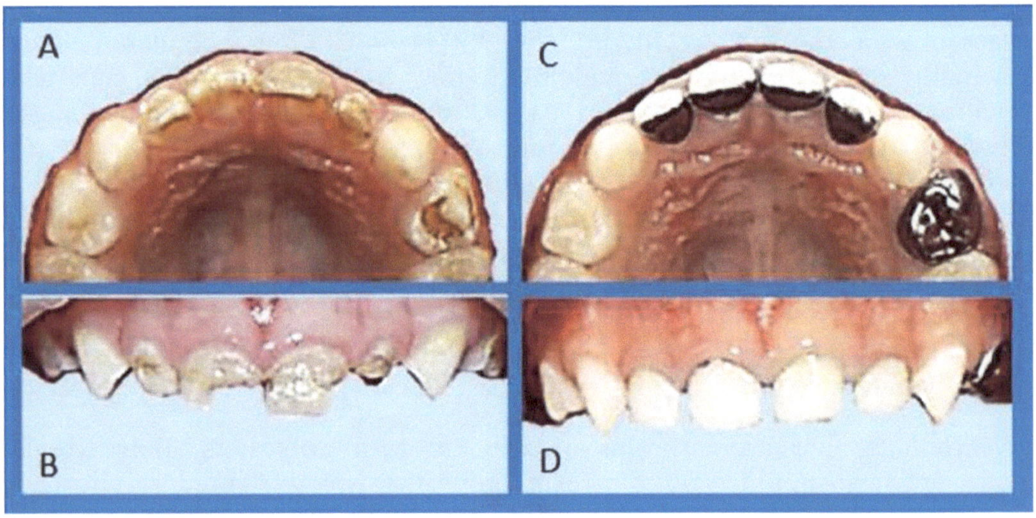

Fig. (9). Open-faced stainless-steel crowns.
A, B – Early childhood caries in primary anterior incisors, **C, D** – Decayed teeth restored with open-faced stainless-steel crown

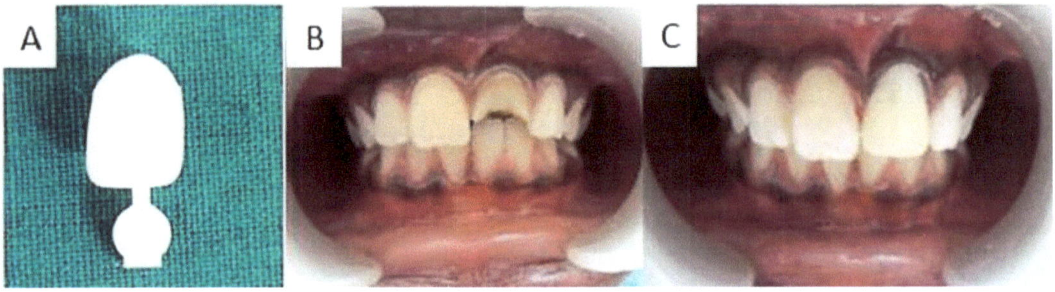

Fig. (10). Polycarbonate crowns.
A - Polycarbonate crown, **B** - fractured incisor due to trauma **C** - Fractured incisor restored with polycarbonate crown

Tooth Preparation of Polycarbonate Crowns

In order to prepare a tooth for a polycarbonate crown, the incisal tip, labial surface, and lingual surface must be reduced (minimum of 2mm) before completing the preparation sub gingivally. Adjacent tooth contact must be interrupted during the interproximal reduction. Any residual decay should be eliminated, as well as any pulp tissue treatment that is needed. Choose a crown that fits comfortably over the prepared tooth and has the proper mesiodistal dimension. Additional tooth reduction will be expected if the crown does not seat without incisal intervention. Then, using a scissor and a sandpaper disc, delete the ID Tab and tab connector from the crown shape. Subgingival crown margins can be used on all crown edges. After seating the crown, verify or estimate the patient's occlusion, then change the margins and occlusion based on dentition. After inspecting and changing, separate the crown from the tooth and crimp all of the crown's gingival edges with a bull nosed crimping pliers [9].

Cementation of Polycarbonate Crown

Rinse the tooth vigorously with a high-speed water spray after cementation. If the tooth has been cleaned, insert gauze on it with hard pressure on the gingival tissues to control any bleeding that could occur when the crown is being filled with self-adhesive resin cement. Self-adhesive resin is used to cover the crown. Seat the crown perfectly and completely. Maintain finger pressure on the crown for 2-3 seconds and light heal the buccal and lingual margins. Using an explorer, scrape out some excess cement. At the end, occlusion is tested and balanced [9].

Strip Crowns

Webber *et al.* first used strip crowns in 1979. Strip crowns are composed of composite-filled celluloid crowns that are bonded to the tooth. Strip crowns are kept in place by dentin and enamel adhesion (Fig. **11a**), (Tables **8, 9**). As a consequence, a lack of tooth structure, the presence of moisture, or haemorrhage all lead to poor retention [9].

Table 8. Indications and contraindications of strip crowns.

Indications	Contraindications
1. It can be used in discoloured, multi surface or extensive caries in primary incisors. 2. Fractured incisors following trauma can be restored with these crowns. 3. In developmental defects like Amelogenesis imperfecta, these crowns can be used.	1. Grossly decayed Tooth with no supporting tooth surfaces

Table 9. Advantages and disadvantages of strip crown.

Advantages	Disadvantages
1. It provides superior aesthetics. 2. The cost of materials is reasonable. 3. The shorter the time needed for placement.	1. It is extremely technique dependent. 2. It is not as rugged or retentive as stainless steel/open faced crowns, pre-veneered crowns, or polycarbonate crowns and should not be used on patients who have bruxism or a deep bite. 3. Adequate moisture management can be impossible to achieve for an uncooperative patient.

Tooth Preparation of Strip Crowns

By positioning the incisal edge of the crown against the incisal edge of the tooth, select a main celluloid crown shape with a mesio-distal incisal diameter equal to the tooth to be restored. Defects can be extracted with a medium to wide circular bur on a slow speed handpiece. If pulp therapy is needed, schedule it now. It was crucial to minimize the interdental area by 0.5 to 1.0 mm. The gingival margin should have a feather edge and the interdental surfaces should be equivalent. Decrease the facial surface by 1mm and the lingual surface by 0.5mm during tooth preparation. All line angles should be rounded. Trim the picked crown with crown and bridge scissors, extracting the collar and gingival excess material. With a bur or explorer, create a small vent hole on the mesial distal edge surface to allow compressed air to escape while the composite-filled crown is seated. The crown should be one millimetre below the gingival margin. Choose the right composite colour. Fill the crown about two-thirds of the way with resin content. After etching the tooth with acid gel for 15 seconds, wash and dry it before applying bonding agent. Place the filled crown shape on top of the tooth. Excess fluid should be separated from the vent hole and gingiva. Rep the operation with the neighbouring teeth. Light cure the substance from both the facial and lingual ways to polymerize it. Cut the substance on the lingual with a composite finishing bur or scalpel to extract the celluloid form. Remove the celluloid form from the tooth. Except for adjusting the occlusion and smoothing the gingival margins, very little finishing is needed. For coating, use flame-shaped and rounded composite finishing burs (Fig. **11b**) [9].

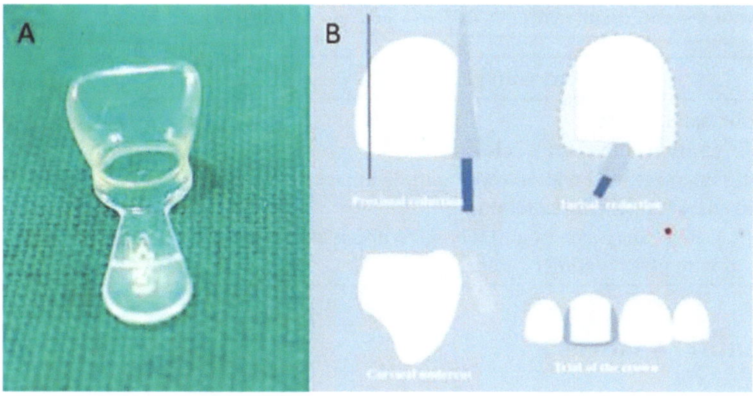

Fig. (11). A - strip crowns, **B** - Tooth Preparation of Strip Crowns.

Pedo Jacket Crowns

The Pedo Jacket is used in the same way as a celluloid crown type, except that the "jacket" is made of a tooth coloured copolyester material that is packed with resin material and left on the tooth after polymerization rather than being stripped like a celluloid crown form (Fig. **12** & Table **10**). There are several issues with this crown. One concern is that these crowns are only available in one colour, which is very white, making matching adjacent, unrestored teeth challenging. Furthermore, since the crowns are made of a copolyester, they cannot be cut or reshaped with a high-speed finishing bur because the material will melt and stick to the bur [10].

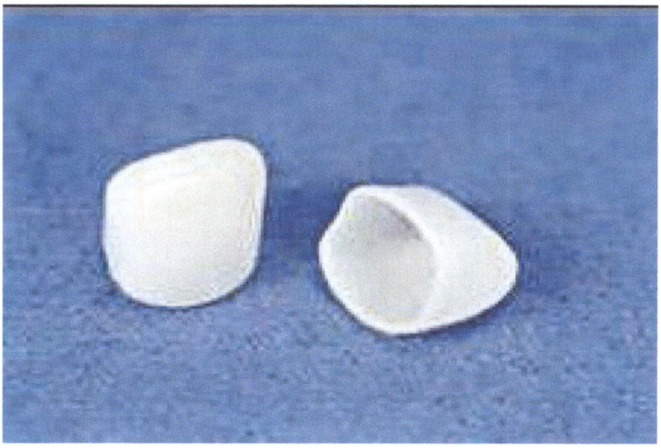

Fig. (12). Pedo jacket crown.

Table 10. Advantages and disadvantages of Pedo jacket crown.

Advantages	Disadvantages
1. It does not split, stain, or crack. 2. Crowns can be easily trimmed with scissors. 3. Thin yet strong interproximal wall allows multiple adjacent restorations with a minimum amount of tooth reduction. 4. Using a plastic primer, they can either be bonded into place with composite resin or cemented with glass ionomer cement.	1. Only one size is available

New Millennium Crowns

This crown resembles the Pedo Jacket and strip crown in shape, but it is made of a laboratory-enhanced composite resin material (Fig. **13**), (Table **11**). The crown shape, like the other two, is packed with resin content and bonded to the tooth. This crown can be very aesthetically pleasing and can be finished and reshaped with a high-speed bur. The crown types, on the other hand, are very fragile and can break or fracture if pressed down into an inadequately reduced preparation. These crown types are also much more costly than the other two [9].

Table 11. Advantages and disadvantages of new millenium crowns.

Advantages	Disadvantages
1. It is highly esthetical and parental satisfaction is high.	1. Technique sensitive and for successful treatment, proper isolation, and achievement of haemostasis is required.

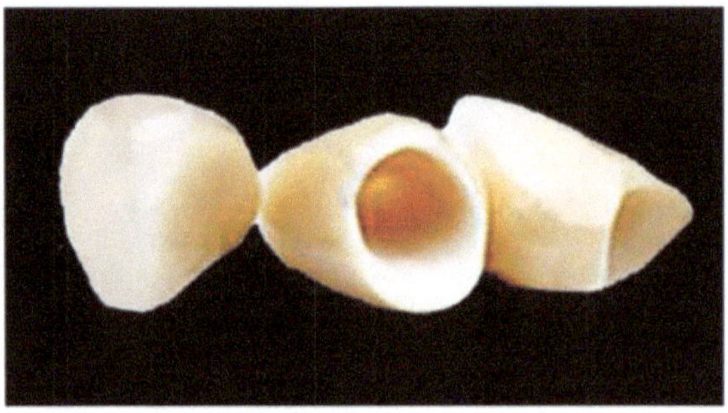

Fig. (13). New millenium crowns.

Pre-Veneered Stainless-Steel Crown

Pre-veneered stainless-steel crowns have the reliability and toughness of traditional stainless-steel crowns with the added benefit of composite resin beauty for a pleasant look (Fig. **14** & Table **12**). A variety of mechanical and chemical bonding processes are used to hold the composite resin on the stainless-steel crown. Although the lingual part of the crown can be modified (crimped), major tooth anatomy must be eliminated in order to match the tooth to the crown rather than the crown to the tooth. There are just a few colour options [9].

Table 12. Advantages and disadvantages of pre-veneered stainless-steel crown.

Advantages	Disadvantages
1. They are aesthetically pleasing 2. They have a comparatively limited operational period. 3. They have the tensile strength of a steel crown. 4. They are less moisture sensitive during placement than composite strip crowns.	1. They are more expensive than stainless steel, strip, and polycarbonate crowns 2. The procedure does not allow for thorough crown recontouring and reshaping. 3. The tooth is tailored to match the crown rather than the crown being adjusted to fit the tooth.

Tooth Preparation of Pre-Veneered Stainless-Steel Crown

The proper crown size is determined by positioning the crown's incisal edge against the incisal edge of the tooth. Preparation of the tooth for this crown is the same as for a regular stainless-steel crown, but more circumferential tooth reduction is needed. Do not put the crown on the prepared tooth by compulsion. A well-fitting crown has a passive fit. The crown should protrude 1mm above the gingival margin. Trimming the gingival surface of the crown with a diamond bur and water spray changes the length of the crown. A no. 137 Gordon plier can be used to subtly crimp the lingual part of the crown. Glass ionomer cement is used to hold the crown over prepared tooth surface. The extra cement is discarded, and the residual cement is left to dry. The incisal edges may be contoured with a finishing disc or point after cementation [8].

Limitations of Pre-Veneered Stainless-Steel Crown

The inclusion of resin results in a thicker SSC than a traditional SSC, necessitating more thorough tooth planning to ensure proper fit and occlusion. The dentist has no control over the colour of the resin, and the provided crowns are often so white that they seem fake in the mouth. Pre-veneered crowns are more costly than regular stainless-steel crowns. Since the bound resin content can disconnect, the labial portion of the margin cannot be crimped. As a result, the uncrimped area would not suit as perfectly as a nonveneered steel crown. Crown shapes that have been attempted in but do not match cannot be sterilised under pressure with high heat so the attached resin coating would be lost. Resin veneer reshaping is often performed to remove the excessively convex nature of these crowns, which requires extra laboratory or clinical time. Difficulty positioning multiple approximating crowns in patients with crowding or room reduction caused by bulk. Resin faced plastic is stiff and brittle, and it is prone to breaking when exposed to high stress [8].

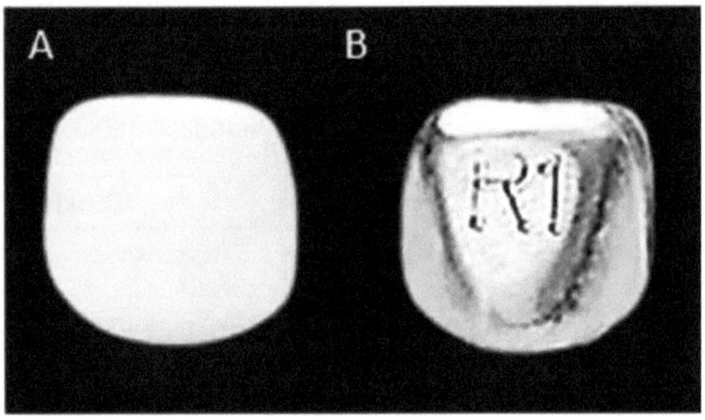

Fig. (14). Pre-veneered stainless-steel crown.
A –Crown showing Veneered surface, **B** –Crown showing stainless steel facing

Nusmile Crowns

It is Specially Formulated Hybrid Composite Substructure. NuSmile Crowns are a time-saving alternative to open-face stainless-steel crowns and the technique-sensitive, less durable composite strip crowns (Table **13**). It is available in 2 Shades for Anterior Crowns (XL and NL) and one shade for Posterior Crowns (XL only) [12].

Table 13. Advantages and disadvantages of Nusmile crown.

Advantages	Disadvantages
1. It requires single appointment 2. It has easy placement technique 3. It reduces operatory time	1. It requires more tooth preparation due to their greater bulk 2. Avoid crimping, so it may be susceptible for fracture, so the tooth is prepared to fit the most appropriate crown

Nusmile crowns anterior teeth - During tooth preparation the incisal length of the tooth reduce by approximately 2mm and break the interproximal contacts. Finishing line should be feather-edge margin.

Nusmile crowns posterior teeth - The tooth should be reduced by approx. 30% of tooth height. It is reduced more on buccal and occlusal aspects (at least 2mm). Do not crimp excessively near the facing. Regular length crowns are the same as regular preformed crowns in length. Short length crowns are 1mm shorter in length and may be appropriate for very young paediatric dental patients. NuSmile's original pedo colour is extra light crowns. Light crowns are marginally yellower than the initial pedo shade and can have a better fit on some single tooth applications.

Cheng Crowns

It was introduced by Peter Cheng in Peter Cheng Orthodontic Laboratory in 1987 (Fig. **15**). Cheng Crowns are biocompatible, autoclavable, and lasts longer than natural enamel. Cheng crowns are the nearest to the real thing in terms of translucency, with no 'black stump' dentin show-through. Cheng crowns Have resin composite facings with welded metal mesh work for mechanical retention (Table **14**) [9].

Table 14. Advantages and disadvantages of Cheng crown.

Advantages	Disadvantages
1. It is completed in single visit and with less patient discomfort 2. The nature of the crowns is stained resistant. 3. It does not cause wear of opposing teeth.	1. It may cause fracture of veneers during crimping 2. It is comparatively expensive than other crowns

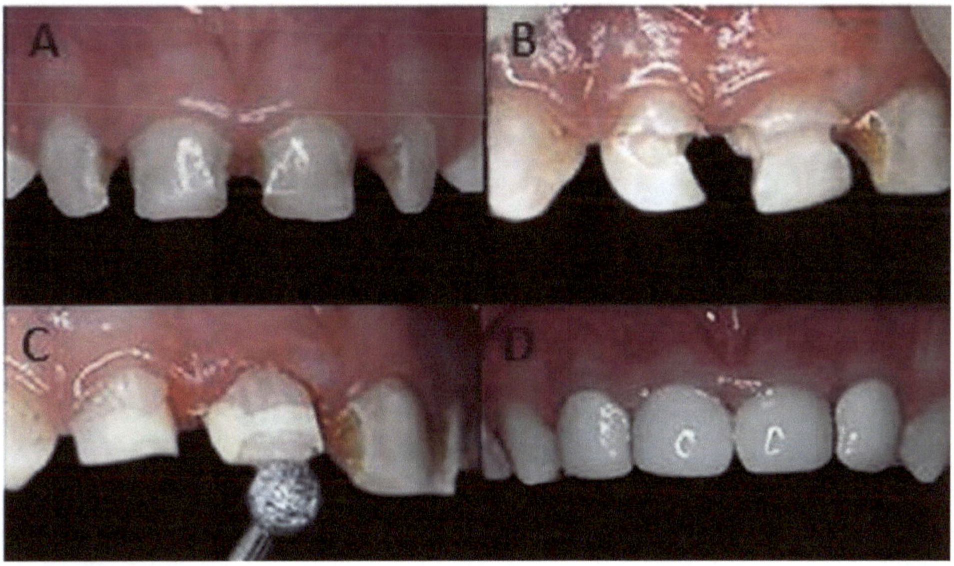

Fig. (15). Cheng crowns.
A – Proximal and smooth surface caries in primary incisors, **B** – Removal of caries, **C** –Caries restoration and tooth preparation done, **D** – Post operative image showing Cheng crowns in place.

Dura Crowns

It is a high-density polyethylene veneered crown with a white face. Crowns can be crimped labially and lingually, cut easily with crown scissors, festooned easily, and have a full-knife tip. This crown may be seated if moisture or haemorrhage suppression is inadequate [8].

Pedo Pearls

Pedo pearls crown having heavy gauge aluminium crowns coated with FDA food grade powder coating and epoxy-resin (Table **15**) [8].

Table 15. Advantages and disadvantages of pedo pearls crown.

Advantages	Disadvantages
1. The crown is in Universal anatomy and used on either side of dental arch. 2. It is easy to cut and crimp, without chipping or peeling. 3. It is non bulky and fits easily on tooth preparation.	1. This crown having less durability and the crowns are soft. 2. Self-cured or dual-cured composite is recommended for repairing.

Kinder Crowns

Kinder crowns were introduced in 1988 (Fig. **16a**). In 1997, Kinder crowns were modified with incisal lock (Fig. **16b**). It is available in natural shades and contour. Kinder crowns come with 2 shades- A] PEDO 1 – It is look like lighter bleached shade B] PEDO 2 – Its colour is natural AI/BI blended.

A B

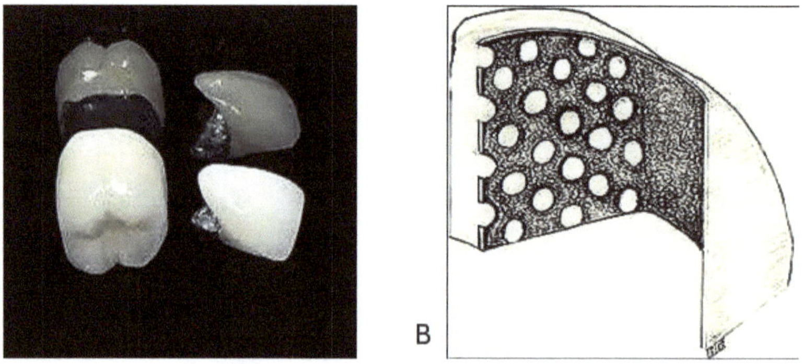

Fig. (16). Kinder crowns. **A** Images of Kinder crown, **B** – Incisal lock system of Kinder crown.

ADVANCES IN FULL COVERAGE RESTORATIONS FOR PRIMARY TEETH

Fibreglass Crowns

Fibreglass crowns are constructed from medical and dental-grade fibre glass and composite resin. Figaro crowns, which are commercially available, are metal-free and have flex-fit technology, which makes for a smoother fit of the crown with limited tooth reduction and has very similar adaptation. Figaro Crowns introduced in 2017. Figaro crowns are the most preformed crowns on the market today, with 2.5 times the compressive strength of stainless steel and zirconia crowns in ball bearing and compression tests. Figaro crowns allow for decorative, grinding, and/or quirky occlusion modifications. Figaro crowns have a wall thickness of 0.5-1 mm, which is comparable to stainless steel and much thinner than most cosmetic crowns. Cementation can also be achieved with type 1 cement, *i.e.*, luting glass ionomer cement, and there is no need to wait for the cement to set for delivery, making the whole procedure very quick and effective. The only disadvantage of this crown is that it cannot be seen on a radiograph. Because of their unmatched benefits, prefabricated Figaro crowns are predicted to be a simple, restorative alternative to conventional composite restorations and strip crowns in the near future [14].

Preformed Zirconia Crown

For several years, zirconia crowns have been used effectively for permanent teeth which provide excellent aesthetics due to their natural look. Zirconia crowns, which were first used in paediatric dentistry in 2010, are a recent addition to the field. They are advised on both the anterior and posterior teeth. They have a remarkable ability to avoid crack progression by transforming from one crystalline phase to another, resulting in a volume rise that blocks the crack and keeps it from propagating. It has shown excellent wear resistance, biocompatibility, and corrosion resistance. Zirconia crown made of polycrystalline ceramic and free of glass. Pediatric zirconia crowns, like stainless steel crowns, are prefabricated in six to seven different sizes for each tooth and are sold in kits. The caries is eliminated before the crowns are set, and the tooth is prepared with occlusal and circumferential reduction to a gingival featheredge. The preparation is then fitted with a correctly sized crown. If the crown does not suit, another size is attempted, or further tooth reduction is performed before the crown is passively seated into the preparation. Zirconia is a polymorph that comes in three varieties: A] Monoclinic - pure zirconia stable at 1107 °C B] Tetraclonic – temperatures over 1107 °C C] Cubic face – temperatures above 2370 °C. The addition of a trace amount of yttria to zirconia to produce high compressive power, crack resistance, corrosion resistance, longevity, and biocompatibility (Table **16**), (Fig. **17a,b,c**) [14]. These are available as: 1] Nusmile Zr 2] Kinder Zr 3] EZ-Pedo 4] Kids-e crown (Fig. **17a**).

Anterior Zirconia Crown Technique

The crown size is determined by the tooth's mesio-distal diameter. In the following step, use wheel bur no. 13 to cut the incisal edge up to 1.5 to 2mm. Build a chamfer margin all around the tooth with chamfer bur no. 21 by reducing up to 0.5-1mm. In the following stage, the chamfer margin is eliminated, and the tooth preparation is extended 2mm sub gingivally without the forming of a ledge.

The angles of both lines should be circular. The crown should be fitted passively. The crown should be washed with water and alcohol before cementation. With the aid of a cotton roll, you can control the bleeding. Cementation is performed with light finger pressure, and excess cement is removed [12].

Table 16. Indications and contraindications of preformed zirconia crown.

Indications	Contraindications
1. Whenever aesthetics required 2. Developmental anomalies such as amelogenesis imperfecta 3. Hypoplastic defects 4. After pulp therapy 5. If patient allergic to nickel	1. Patient with irregular or crowded teeth 2. If sub-gingival soft caries present 3. Orthodontic appliance requires soldering to be done on crown

Posterior Zirconia Crown Technique

Crown size is determined by the tooth's mesio-distal diameter. In the following stage, the occlusal height was reduced to 1.5 to 2mm using wheel bur no 13 and the occlusal surface was flattened. Build a chamfer margin all around the tooth by decreasing it to 0.5-1mm with chamfer bur no 21. In the following stage, the chamfer margin is cut, and the tooth preparation is extended 2mm sub gingivally without the forming of a ledge. All line angles should be round. The crown should be passively fitted. Until cementation, the crown should be washed with water and alcohol. Control the bleeding with a cotton roll. Cementation is completed with light finger pressure, and excess cement is removed [12].

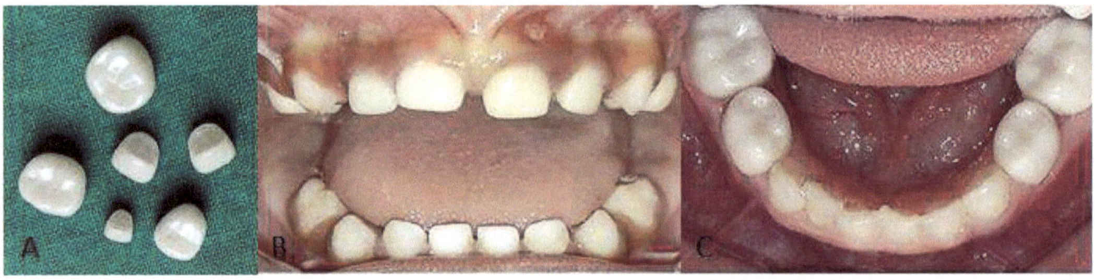

Fig. (17). Preformed zirconia crown, **A** - Kids-e preformed zirconia crown, **B** - Zirconia crowns for primary central and lateral incisor, **C** - Zirconia crowns for 1st and 2nd primary molar.

Disinfection of Crown

Autoclave sterilization is not recommended for pre-veneered stainless-steel crown as their lies the risk of discoloration of facing material. Therefore, chemical sterilization is recommended for these crowns. Zirconium crowns are autoclavable.

CONCLUSION

There are biological consequences to every dental, surgical, and restorative treatment. Restoration of primary teeth with crowns is no exception. The clinician should strive to re-establish, as closely as possible, the natural state when restoring a tooth. That means restoring a tooth to its proper form, function, and purpose in the most biologically acceptable manner. esthetics demands by parents, the child's behaviour, and moisture and haemorrhage control are all variables which affect the decision and ultimate outcome of whatever restorative outcome is chosen. Many options exist to repair carious teeth in pediatric patients as discussed in the chapter from stainless steel crowns to its various modifications to other esthetics crowns like strip crowns and zirconium crowns which are rising in their popularity. Varied primary crowns with composite facings--are evaluated as to their advantages and disadvantages. Alternative esthetics anterior restorations, fixed and removable, are discussed and evaluated in this chapter.

CONSENT FOR PUBLICATION

Not applicable.

CONFLICT OF INTEREST

The authors declare no conflict of interest, financial or otherwise.

ACKNOWLEDGEMENT

Declared none.

REFERENCES

[1] American Academy of Pediatric Dentistry reference manual 2019-2020. Pediatr Dent 2019; 33(6): 340-52.

[2] Abuelniel G, Eltawil S. Clinical and Radiographic Evaluation of Stainless Steel versus Zirconia Crowns on Primary Molars: Randomized Controlled Trial. Egyptian Dental Journal. 2018 Apr 1;64(2-April (Orthodontics, Pediatric & Preventive Dentistry):977-89.

[3] Mosharafian S, Afshar H, Kazemi S, Abazarian N. Comparison of the flexibility of two different stainless steel crowns (3M and MIB) while seating on primary molars. Iranian Journal of Pediatric Dentistry 2019; 15(1): 103-10. [http://dx.doi.org/10.29252/ijpd.15.1.103]

[4] Patel RV, Thikkurissy S, Schwartz SB, Gosnell ES, Sun Q, Cully JL. Preferential Use of Stainless Steel Crowns as a Strategy to Minimize Retreatment of Primary Molars under General Anesthesia. Pediatr Dent 2021; 43(1): 24-7. [PMID: 33662246]

[5] Afshar H, Ghandehari M, Soleimani B. Comparison of marginal circumference of two different pre-crimped stainless steel crowns for primary molars after re-crimping. J Dent (Tehran) 2015; 12(12): 926-31. [PMID: 27559353]

[6] Helder C, Fleagle J, Alimorad L, Cottam M. Postoperative Bleeding Complications after Stainless Steel Crown Placement: A Case Series. J Clin Pediatr Dent 2021; 45(1): 12-4. [http://dx.doi.org/10.17796/1053-4625-45.1.3] [PMID: 33690824]

[7] Kratunova E, O'Connell AC. A randomized clinical trial investigating the performance of two commercially available posterior pediatric preveneered stainless steel crowns: a continuation study. Pediatr Dent 2014; 36(7): 494-8. [PMID: 25514079]

[8] Peña HA, Padilla EE, Martínez-Menchaca HR, *et al.* Aesthetic evaluation of six types of crowns for primary teeth. Revista de Odontopediatría Latinoamericana 2020; 7(1): 6-15.

[9] Shrestha S, Koirala B, Dali M, Birajee G. Anterior Crowns in Pediatric Dentistry: A Review. J Nepal Assoc Pediatr Dent. 2020; 1 (1): 32.;8.

[10] Castro A, Badr SB, El-Badrawy W, Kulkarni G. Clinical performance of pedo jacket crowns in maxillary anterior primary teeth. ASDC J Dent Child 2016; 83(3): 125-31. [PMID: 28327262]

[11] Holsinger DM, Wells MH, Scarbecz M, Donaldson M. Clinical evaluation and parental satisfaction with pediatric zirconia anterior crowns. Pediatr Dent 2016; 38(3): 192-7. [PMID: 27306242]

[12] Abdulhabi BS, Abdullah MM, Alaki SM, Alamoudi NM, Attar MH. Clinical evaluation between zirconia crowns and stainless steel crowns in primary molar teeth. J Pediatr Dent 2017; 5: 21-7.

[13] Altoukhi DH, El-Housseiny AA. Hall technique for carious primary molars: a review of the literature. Dent J 2020; 8(1): 11. [http://dx.doi.org/10.3390/dj8010011] [PMID: 31963463]

[14] Alrashdi M, Ardoin J, Liu AJ. Zirconia crowns for children: A systematic review. Int J Paediatr Dent 2021. [PMID: 33772904]

CHAPTER 2

Prosthetic Management in Pediatric Dentistry

Anil Patil[1,*], **S Srigiri**[1] and **Dhanashree Sakhare**[2]

[1] *Department of Pedodontics and Preventive Dentistry, Bharati Vidyapeeth (deemed to be) University Dental College & Hospital, Maharashtra 400614, India*

[2] *Founder, Lavanika Dental Academy, Melbourne, Australia*

Abstract: Prosthetic management is the healing part of the dentistry which plays a crucial role in rehabilitating the missing or damaged oral and maxillofacial structures. Dental aesthetics is a paramount important aspect in today's society and is faced by many challenges like age, periodontal condition, occlusal adjustments, patient's cooperation *etc.*, to overcome this the dentist should have a thorough knowledge regarding prothesis before the fabrication and delivery. In this chapter, various prosthesis like removable partial denture, fixed partial denture, complete denture, implants, maxillofacial prostheses their types, advantages, disadvantages, indications, contraindications, fabrication *etc.*, have been discussed in detail which will help in successfully understanding and treating the patient to obtain positive treatment outcome.

Keywords: Prosthetic Management, Removable Partial Denture, Fixed Partial Denture, Complete Denture, Implants, Maxillofacial Prosthesis.

INTRODUCTION

While treating children whose dentition fails to develop normally prosthetic treatment plays a crucial role. Prosthetic replacement for young children is frequently indicated in the existence of congenitally absent teeth in cases like cleft palate, ectodermal dysplasia *etc.*, A prosthetic rehabilitation offers a functional and aesthetic outcome that will allow the child a scenario close to normal lifestyle, without destroying the self-esteem or psychological development [1] (Table **1**).

* **Corresponding author Anil Patil:** Department of Pedodontics and Preventive Dentistry, Bharati Vidyapeeth (deemed to be) University Dental College & Hospital, Maharashtra 400614, India; E-mail: dranilp0888@gmail.com

Satyawan Damle, Ritesh Kalaskar & Dhanashree Sakhare (Eds.)

Table 1. Sequelae of missing primary teeth.

Missing primary incisors or molars results in deleterious oral habits that might cause forward or lateral tongue thrusting, respectively.
Early loss can cause resorption of the alveolar ridge, tooth migration, and impaired occlusion, which eventually effect the mastication, speech, and aesthetics.
Immature loss of tooth could lead to disproportionate growth of orofacial structures.
Congenitally missing anterior teeth or missing teeth due to trauma may cause psychological disturbance in children [3].

Terminology

A prosthesis is an artificial replacement of part of the human anatomy restoring form, function, and esthetics (GPT-9) [2].

Dental prosthesis is an artificial replacement (prosthesis) of one or more teeth (up to the entire dentition in either arch) or associated dental/alveolar structures (GPT-9) [2].

Important Considerations During Prosthetic Treatment in Children

Proper diagnosis and treatment strategy are important before starting any dental procedures on pediatric patients. It involves thorough history, intraoral examination, extraoral examination and radiographic examination.

Prosthetic Treatment Option in Children

Based on the defect type, various methods of prosthetic management can be planned.

1. Removable prosthesis
    a. Complete denture
    b. Partial denture
    c. Overdenture
    d. Immediate denture
2. Fixed partial denture
    a. Conventional fixed partial denture
    b. Resin bonded fixed partial denture
3. Implant prosthesis
4. Maxillofacial prosthesis

Removable Partial Dentures (RPD)

Removable partial denture is a removable denture that replaces some teeth in a partially edentulous arch; the removable partial denture can be readily inserted and removed from the mouth by the patient (GPT-9) [2], Fig. (**1**).

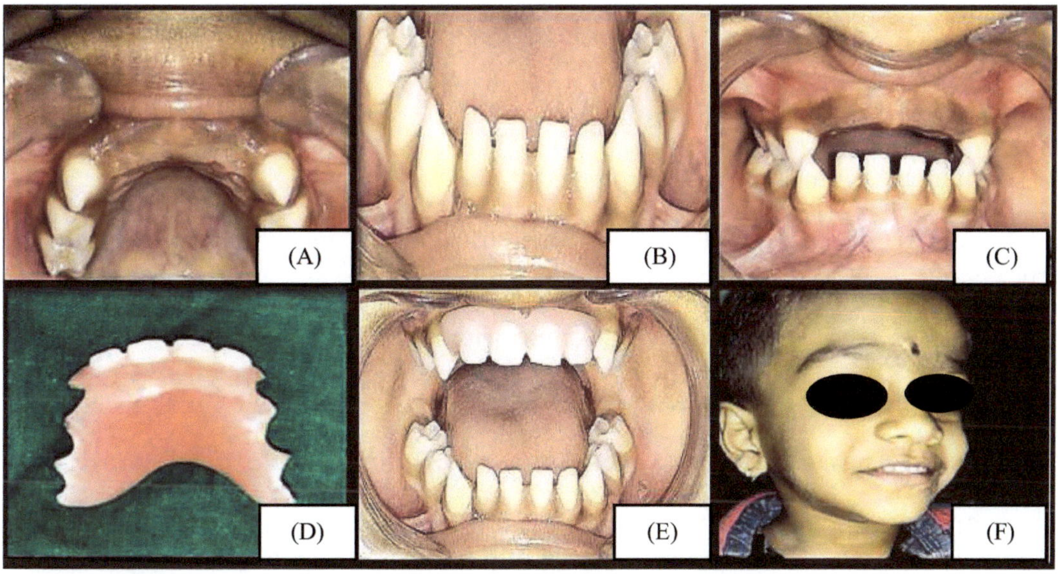

Fig. (1). Removable partial denture **(A – F)**: A –Intraoral image showing missing anterior in maxillary arch, **B** – Mandibular arch, **C** Intraoral view showing occlusion, **D** RPD for maxillary anterior teeth, **E** RPD in place, **F** Post insertion extraoral image of child.

Indications and contraindications of RPD are enumerated in Table **2**.

Table 2. Indications and contraindications of RPD.

Indications	Contraindications
Premature loss of primary molars, requiring space maintenance.	When FPD can be planned.
Radiographic evaluation confirms that the time period between the primary teeth lost and the eruption of succedaneous teeth is greater than six months.	In substituting a smaller number of anterior teeth where aesthetics is a main concern.
Removable partial dentures are frequently indicated in children who have lost their teeth as a sequalae of trauma.	Disabled patients who cannot maintain RPD.
Congenital conditions requiring prosthesis. E.g., partial anodontia in ectodermal dysplasia.	In children with uncooperative behaviour.
Compromised periodontal support of remaining teeth.	-
To obtain cross arch stabilization.	-

(Table 2) cont.....

Indications	Contraindications
Long edentulous span.	-
Indicated for individuals whose health condition contraindicates the lengthy and physical trying appointments often associated with FPD construction.	-

Objectives

1. To restore the speech and mastication.

2. To maintain optimum tooth eruption.

3. To allow maxillofacial growth, which requires periodic adjustment and processing.

4. To re-establish occlusal - articular equilibrium.

5. To prevent damage to the dental follicles [4].

Considerations with Respect to Maxillary and Mandibular Partial Dentures

There are various modifications in RPD for both maxillary and mandibular arch (Table **3**). For maxillary removable partial denture, full palatal coverage with the acrylic base should be offered. When buccal or labial flanges are provided, they should be comparatively short. For the mandibular partial dentures, an acrylic base is helpful in most situations, if prolonged use is anticipated, it is best to use metal framework or a wrought lingual bar. It is advisable to place lingual bar 2mm below the soft tissue, accordingly it will accommodate the growth variations in the arch when succedaneous teeth start erupting. If extended period is anticipated, occlusal rests with permanent molars are advised.

Table 3. Types of removable partial dentures.

Maxillary Dentures	Mandibular Dentures
1. Acrylic.	1. Acrylic.
2. Acrylic with wrought wire clasps.	2. Acrylic with wrought wire clasps.
3. Acrylic with cast metal clasps.	3. Acrylic with lingual bar and wrought wire clasps.
4. Acrylic saddles with cast metal framework	4. Acrylic with cast metal clasps containing occlusal rests.
-	5. Wrought wire clasps soldered to a lingual bar with acrylic saddles.
-	6. Cast metal framework and clasps with acrylic saddles.

Various Parts of RPD

1. The denture base.

2. Retentive Clasps.

3. Artificial teeth.

Fabrication of RPD (Fig. 2)

Clinical Procedure

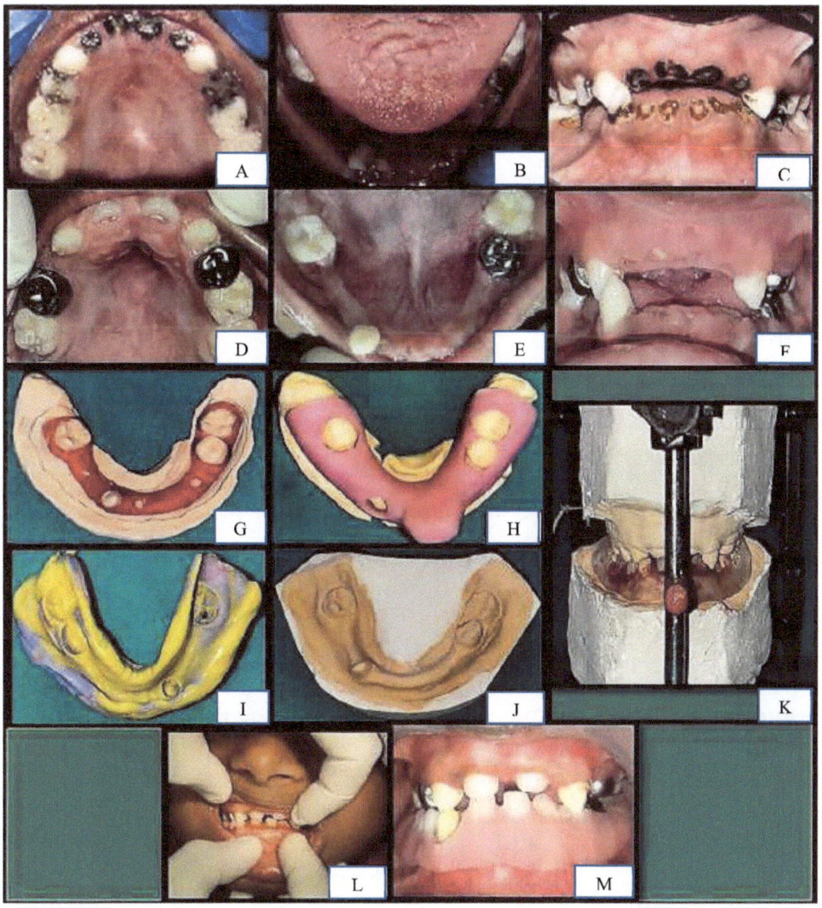

Fig. (2). Removable partial denture **(A- M)**: **A** Pre-operative image of maxillary arch showing grossly decayed teeth, **B** Pre-operative image of mandibular arch, **C** Pre-operative intraoral image showing occlusion, **D** Intra-operative image of maxillary arch, **E** Intra-operative image of mandibular arch after healing of extraction sockets, **F** – Intra - operative image showing occlusion, **G** - Spacer adaptation, **H** Custom tray fabrication, **I** Final impression, **J** Master cast, **K** Jaw relation record, **L** Try – in of occlusal rim with teeth arrangement, **M** Removable partial denture in place.

Before taking impression of oral cavity oral prophylaxis is carried out. Select the appropriate impression trays. Impression of maxillary and mandibular jaw is taken using alginate impression material. Impressions should present the peripheral areas and should accurately capture the teeth and soft tissues. Bite registration is obtained by making the patient bite in centric occlusion on softened bite registration wax. Young children who tend to approximate their incisors in an edge relationship when asked to close, it might be essential for the dentist to demonstrate the child how to occlude the dentition in accurate position. Primary cast is fabricated on which custom try is prepared. Thereafter record base with occlusal rims prepared and casts are articulated. Teeth arrangement is done followed by denture acrylization and finishing and polishing.

Advantages and disadvantage of RPD are described in Table **4**.

Table 4. Advantages and disadvantage of RPD in children.

Advantages	Disadvantages
Economic	Patient's cooperation is essential.
Easy to fabricate.	Due to palatal coverage in the upper denture, it might be uncomfortable to the child.
It is useful as a space maintainer.	Breakage of appliance/ prosthesis can cause injury to soft tissue.
Easy to reframe or reline during the period of jaw development.	Unhygienic use of prosthesis can cause alveolar bone resorption.
Oral hygiene can be well maintained.	Accidental aspiration of the appliance [4, 5].
Improves mastication and phonetics.	

Complete Denture

Complete denture is a fixed or removable dental prosthesis that replaces the entire dentition and associated structures of the maxillae or mandible (GPT - 9) [2].

Complete Denture Rehabilitation in Ectodermal Dysplasia Patients

There are situations which lead to anodontia in patients and warrant the necessity of complete denture rehabilitation in paediatric dentistry. The most magnificent and commonly encountered condition is ectodermal dysplasia.

Ectodermal dysplasia (ED) syndrome is a X-linked hypohidrotic dysplasia, also known as Christ - Siemens - Touraine syndrome [4].

Clinical Signs

Freire-Maia demarcated the ED as any syndrome that displays at least two of the following features:

1. Trichodysplasia (abnormal hair),

2. Abnormal dentition,

3. Onchodysplasia (abnormal nails), and

4. Dyshidrosis (abnormal or missing sweat glands).

Clinical Stages for Denture Construction

Proper history of patients is taken, followed by intraoral and radiographic assessment of patient. Primary impressions of maxillary and mandibular jaw are taken using alginate impression material. Impressions are boxed by wax to preserve periphery created by muscles. Wax rims are constructed on the casts. Centric relation records are registered using occlusal rims with check bite procedure. Face bow transfer done. To permit freedom to centric position, teeth inclines are decreased, and central fosse are enlarged in anterior and lateral direction. Teeth setting and balancing done followed by denture acrylization and finishing and polishing [5].

Overdenture

Overdenture is defined as any removable dental prosthesis that covers and rests on one or more remaining natural teeth, the roots of natural teeth, and/or dental implants (GPT- 9) [2].

Congenital abnormalities or trauma can cause loss of multiple teeth and resulting interarch relationship does not allow a conventional removable denture to re-establish proper occlusion with opposing teeth. This situation demands fabrication of prosthesis which overlays dentition so that suitable function and facial esthetics would be established.

Overdentures offer a good retentive option and are used when teeth are present for support. They help to preserve alveolar bone compared with complete denture. The retained dentition is called ad abutments and are treated to receive the overdenture. The abutments usually require intentional endodontics as the coronal structure is reduced to receive the denture.

Detailed description of advantages and disadvantages of overdentures are given in Table **5**

Table 5. Advantages and disadvantages of overdenture.

Advantages	Disadvantages
Preserves bone as abutments are retained. Improves aesthetics and proprioception.	It requires more clinical settings thus greater cooperation from the child.
Easy to construct and is much conservative.	It is more expensive than conventional prosthesis, as abutments have to be treated.
Masticatory efficiency, swallowing, speech, and aesthetics are highly improved.	-
It provides good stability and support compared to complete dentures.	-

Complications

- Abutment teeth prone to decay.
- Patient acceptance is important.
- Recall of 6 months to assess the need of reline, rebase, or refit.

Overlay Denture

According to Brewer and Fenton, "An overlay denture is a complete or partial removable denture fabricated over retained teeth or roots that are not prepared with a coping to interface with the denture" [6]. In addition to the following advantages (Fig. **3**) of overlay denture, it also does not require specialised tooth preparation as seen with overdenture.

Fixed Partial Denture (FPD)

Fixed partial denture (FPD) can be defined as any dental prosthesis that is luted, screwed, or mechanically attached or otherwise securely retained to natural teeth, tooth roots, and/or dental implants/abutments that furnish the primary support for the dental prosthesis and restoring teeth in a partially edentulous arch; it cannot be removed by the patient (GPT - 9) [2].

Various Types of FPD

1. Porcelain fused to metal fixed partial denture.

2. All metal fixed partial denture.

3. All ceramic fixed partial denture.

4. Resin bonded fixed partial denture. (Maryland bridge)

5. Cantilever fixed partial denture

Advantages of overlay dentures

1. Improved mastication and esthetics.

2. Alveolar bone is conserved by retaining the teeth.

3. Improved proprioception compared with complete denture because of retained dentition.

4. In comparison with an overdenture, overlay denture is economical, needs less chairside time, and does not involve any specialized tooth preparation.

5. Has excellent retention and stability.

6. Positive psychological aid to the child [6].

Fig. (3). Advantages of overlay dentures.

FPD with rigid connectors are usually avoided in young, actively growing children because they could restrict jaw growth, specially if the prosthesis crosses the midline. Band-retained partial dentures are gaining popularity and are well tolerated by the patients and shown to have improved retention and stability (Fig. **4**).

Indications and contraindications of FPD are shown in Table **6**.

Table 6. Indications and contraindications of FPD.

Indications	Contraindications
Endodontically treated teeth.	Age of patient - (very young or advanced age).
Congenitally abnormal or missing teeth.	Extreme bone loss in the place of missing teeth.
For maintaining appropriate function and aesthetics.	Edentulous ridge with severe soft tissue defect.
If the supporting teeth are periodontally healthy.	-
Span of edentulism is short.	-

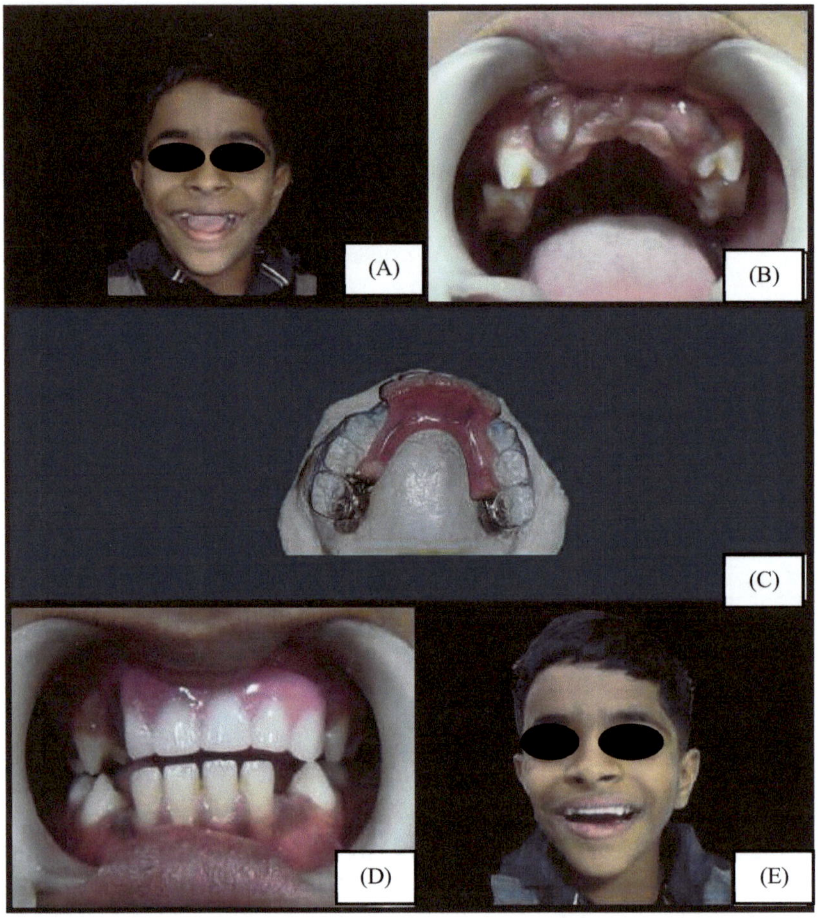

Fig. (4). Fixed partial denture (**A** – **E**): **A** – Preoperative extraoral images of patient, **B** – Intraoral images of patient, **C** - Fixed partial denture, **D** - Fixed partial denture in place, **E** – Extraoral images of patient with Fixed partial denture in place.

Components of FPD (Fig. 5)

- *Retainer*
- *Connector*
- *Pontic*

Resin Bonded Fixed Partial Denture

The resin-bonded fixed partial denture is a conventional restoration first used in 1973 by Rochette. This prosthesis might be reserved for a young patient as the tooth preparation is minimal reducing pulpal injury. However, case selection is extremely important.

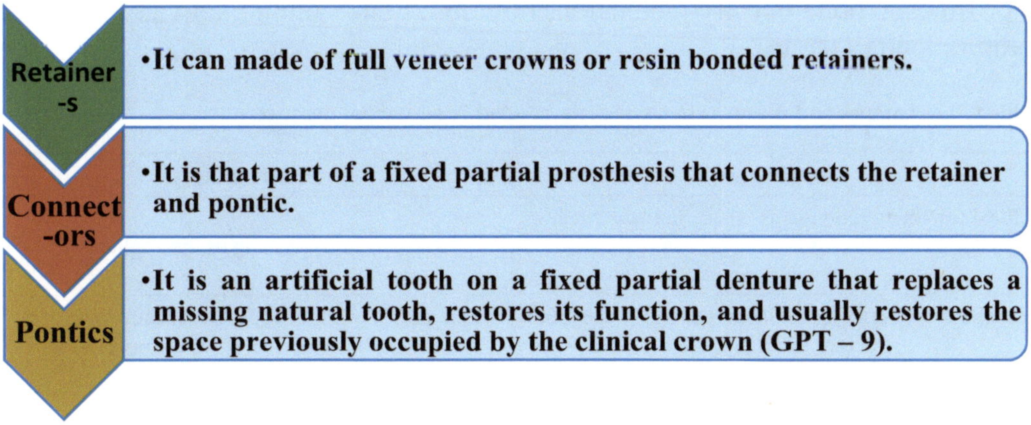

Fig. (5). Components of FPD.

Detailed description of indication and contraindications of Resin bonded fixed partial dentures are given in Table 7.

Table 7. Indications and contraindications of resin bonded fixed partial denture.

Indications	Contraindications
Vital, immobile, and minimally treated abutment teeth.	Patients with affected enamel like enamel hypoplasia as bonding is poor.
Brief edentulous period, and negligible dynamic occlusal interaction on the abutment teeth.	Replacement of posterior teeth.
Most common indication is congenitally missing single anterior teeth, e.g., lateral incisor.	Replacement in people with abnormal muscle activity. It is not advised in a child with crowding in the abutment teeth.
In defect-free abutments, in situations with only one missing tooth, an incisor or premolar	It is contradicted as a substitute in missing anterior teeth with deep vertical overlap.
Missing mandibular incisors.	-
Edentulous ridge with moderate resorption and no major soft tissue defects [7].	-

Advantages and disadvantages of Resin bonded fixed partial dentures are given in Table 8.

Implants in Pediatric Dentistry

Dental implant rehabilitation is a widely recognized treatment modality for restoring aesthetic and masticatory function in partially or completely edentulous patients. While planning for dental implants the treatment should consider the sort of prosthesis, bone density, occlusion, function, bone volume, and any medically compromising factors.

Table 8. Advantages and disadvantages of resin bonded fixed partial denture.

Advantages	Disadvantages
Ideal for young individuals whose immature teeth have larger pulp, as it requires minimal tooth preparation.	Frequent debonding of the appliance.
Excellent aesthetics as the labial portion of the tooth structure is not prepared.	Laboratory techniques for fabrication have to be identical for a perfect fit of the restoration.
No Local anaesthesia will be required as the preparation is minimal.	It may cause greyish discoloration of the abutment tooth.
Cost effective than all - ceramic or metal ceramic restoration.	The prosthesis cannot be maintained if the supporting abutment has an enormous carious lesion.

Definition

Dental Implant

'A dental implant is a device which is surgically placed into the jawbone to replace one or several lost teeth.'

Osseointegration

Zarb and Albrekts (1991) defined osseointegration as – 'A process whereby clinically asymptomatic rigid fixation of alloplastic materials is achieved and maintained in bone during functional loading.'

Brånemark and Skalak originally noted that an oral implant may be called Osseointegrated if "it provides a stable and apparently immobile support of a prosthesis under functional loads without pain, inflammation, or loosening".

Types of Implants

Dental implants are grouped into three major categories:

1. Subperiosteal implants

2. Transosseous implants

3. Endosseous implants

Endosteal implants may be further grouped into plate form and root form.

Subperiosteal Implants

A subperiosteal implant lie over the surface of the bone below the periosteum, with posts traversing the mucosal tissue. These are used when the bone is insufficient or else in the prevalence of anatomical structures that contradict the usage of endosseous implants.

Transosseous Implants

A transosseous mandibular bone plate penetrate through the lower margin of the mandible, emerging through the alveolar ridge and oral mucosa to anchor a prosthesis. They engage two cortical plates and underlying intermediate medullary bone.

Endosseous Implants

An endosseous implant is fixed along the maxilla or mandible and penetrate through the mucosa overlaying the edentulous ridge. They involve a single cortical plate together with medullary bone. These implants are frequently indicated to secure either single crowns, fixed bridges or to hold the removable prosthesis.

Based on their shape endosseous implants are further subdivided into:

i. Plate form (blades)
ii. Root form

Plate form endosseous implants are flatter and can be used in cases with insufficient bone width and adequate bone depth. However, it is associated with disadvantages such as difficulty in preparing precision slots for blade placement and failure of blade leads to damage to a larger portion of jaw.

Root form endosseous implants are either cylindrical or conical in shape and have the adaptability to several intraoral sites, homogenously detailed implant site preparation, and a low rate of adverse effects.

Classification

Pediatric Patient Classification

Group 1: Missing a single permanent tooth

Implant placement should be delayed until completion of alveolar development and eruption of all permanent teeth. Implants placed early may get submerged due to growth of the surrounding bone, requiring a longer sized prosthesis and compromising implant success.

Group 2: Oligodontia

The growth of the alveolar process is impaired; hence the chances of the implant being submerged is low. Implant can be placed as soon as the patient understands the importance of the treatment and can satisfactorily maintain oral hygiene.

Group 3: Acquired Anodontia

Teeth lost due to tumour resection or trauma and the defect reconstructed with bone graft. Implants can be placed as soon as it is appropriate from the psychosocial standpoint.

There are two principal concerns when placing the implants during growth in children [8]:

i. First, when the implants exist during the periods of facial growth, there are chances of implant becoming embedded, repositioned, or displaced as the jaw matures.
ii. Secondly, the significance of implant on the growth. Design modifications should be merged into such prosthesis to allow compensation in the growth changes.

Indications and Contraindications of Implant (Table 9)

Table 9. Indications and contraindications of implants.

Indications	Contraindications
Inability to provide a removable or complete denture prosthesis.	Uncontrolled metabolic disease and patients with abnormal bone metabolism.
Requirement for long-span fixed dental prosthesis and with unfavourable prognosis.	Patient who has undergone previous irradiation of the implant site.
Uncertain number and site of possible natural tooth abutments.	Inadequate patient motivation i.e., patients with poor oral hygiene.
Loss of single tooth, which would demand a minimally prepared dentition for fixed prosthesis.	Failure to restore using a prosthesis.

Advantages and Disadvantages of Implants (Table 10)

Table 10. Advantages and disadvantages of implants.

Advantages	Disadvantages
Less risk for caries, endodontics, restoration, and tooth fracture, unretained prosthesis.	Increased treatment time.
No need to prepare adjacent teeth.	Possible hard and soft tissue grafting.
Improved oral hygiene conditions.	-
Improved aesthetics, phonetics, occlusion in most cases.	-
Maintains hard and soft tissue bone at site.	-
Decreases adjacent tooth loss.	-

Stages of Implant Placement (Fig. 6)

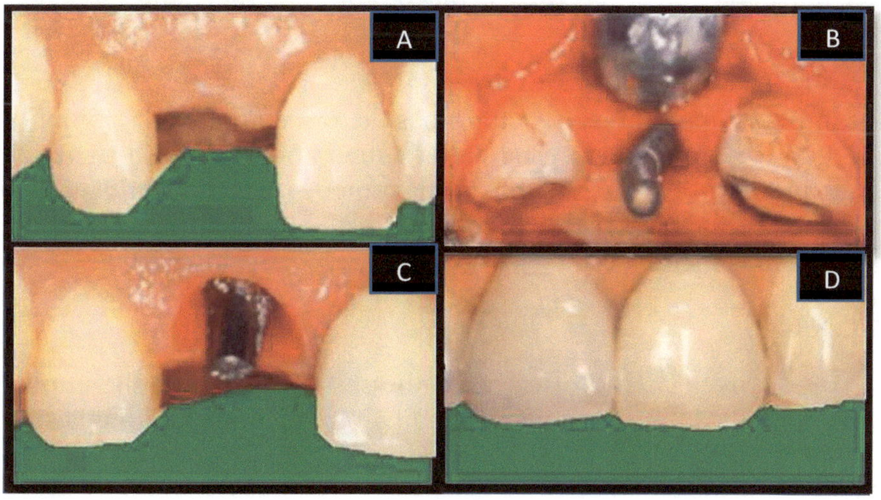

Fig. (6). – Stages of implant placement (A – D): A – Preoperative image of patient, B – Surgical phase, C – Implant abutment in place, D – Implant supported prosthesis.

The placement of the implants is done in stages as shown below:

Patient Preparation

A well-documented report of patient's medical history, findings of clinical examination and expectations of the patient and parents should be maintained. Bone quality and quantity is judged and prepared if inadequate and an appropriate implant system is chosen.

Surgical Stage

Stage I surgery – Implant placement

An incision is completed on the alveolar ridge 0.5cm beyond the mesio-distal width of the implant and a mucoperiosteal flap is raised.

The implant position is prepared through the bone using drills along with copious irrigation, osteotomes or bone expanders to obtain an appropriately sized implant.

The implants are seated under compression by screwing/tapping with a mallet and the flap is sutured to cover the implant completely.

Stage II surgery - Exposure/externalization of implant

After waiting for osseointegration (4-6 months approximately) the second stage surgery is performed. The implant is then exposed through the mucosa using a punch incision and a gingival former is placed for gingival healing.

Impression Stage

This stage is very important, as it determines the orientation and inclination of the prosthesis as it is prepared on a cast outside the patient's mouth. After adequate gingival healing (2 - 4 weeks), the gingival former is detached, and an impression analogue is placed to transfer the alignment of the implant to the cast. A rubber-based impression is then taken.

Prosthetic Stage

An appropriate prosthesis is fabricated on the cast and fixed on the implants with the help of screws or luting cements depending on the type of implants system.

Mini Implant

Mini implant is a dental implant that is fabricated with a reduced diameter (less than 3.0 mm) and shorter in length with the same biocompatible material as compared with standard dental implants (GPT - 9) [2].

Orthodontic implants were first manufactured in the 1990s by alteration of implant designs, making them shorter (*e.g.*, 4–6 mm length) and wider (*e.g.*, 3 mm diameter). However, they retained the key prerequisite for osseointegration. In contrast, orthodontic miniplates and mini implants (miniscrews) are obtained from bone fixation mechanism, and primarily depend on mechanical retention rather than osseointegration.

Clinical Indications for Mini Implants

Based on case application and form of anchorage Mini implant can be grouped into following:

Routine Cases

- Cases which require high anchorage, such as retraction of protruding upper incisors or for the correction of centreline.
- Adolescents and adults who would not respond with other anchorage options.
- In conditions where there might be unfavourable extrusive tooth movements. (Causing an anterior open bite or vertical excess).

Complex Cases

- Conditions with limited conventional biomechanics, for example intrusion of molar to correct an anterior openbite.
- Where dental anchorage is inadequate by a limited amount of anchor teeth (due to tooth loss or hypodontia) or periodontal support.

Apart from this, there are various criteria for mini-implant body and neck dimensions with respect to insertion site and directions.

Components (Fig. 7)

1. Head

2. Neck and

3. Body

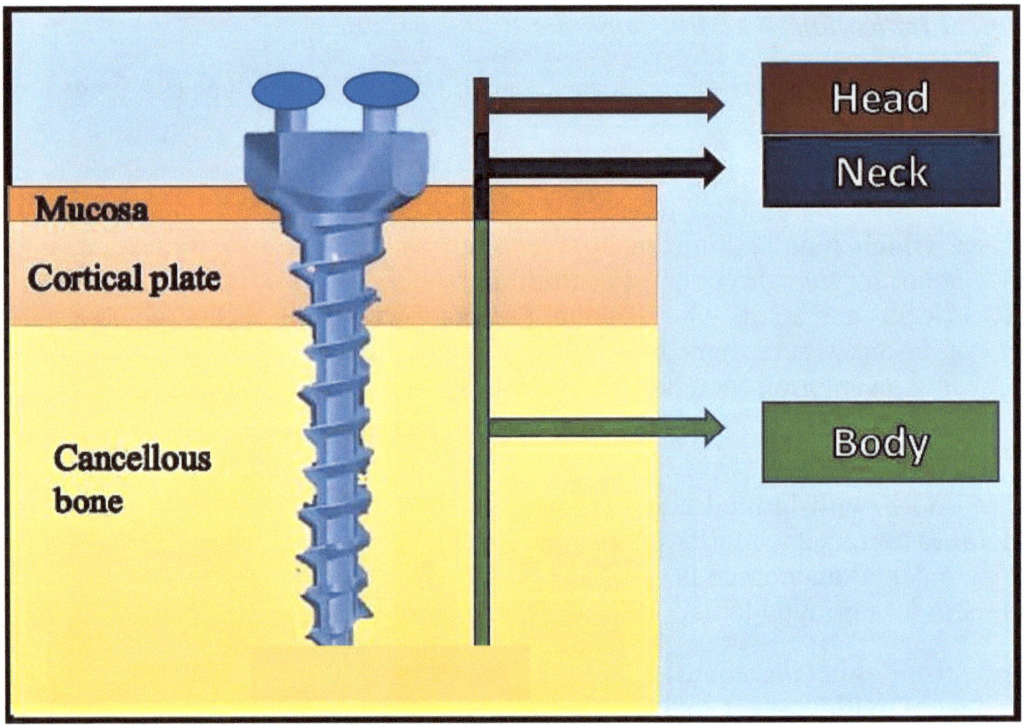

Fig. (7). The three sections of a mini-implant: the head superficial to the tissues, the neck passing through the mucosa, and the body within the cortical and cancellous bone.

Implant Materials

Frequently used materials can be divided into three categories:

- Biotolerant (stainless steel, chromium–cobalt alloy)
- Bioinert (titanium, carbon), and
- Bioactive (hydroxyapatite, ceramic oxidized aluminium).

Because of the characteristics of titanium's (no allergic and immunologic reactions), it is an ideal material and is widely used.

Driving Methods of Mini Implants

The mode of placement of a screw into the bone depends upon the type of screw chosen.

Self-tapping

It is concerned with pre – drilling. Here a tunnel is first drilled into the bone using a pilot drill and then implant is penetrated into the tunnel. It is indicated in case of long treatment schedule. This method is used when we use small diameter miniscrew. The tips are blunt, smooth, and rounded. The threads of screw are thick, rounded, and blunt. They may cause complications like thermal damage, root damage, and drill fractures due to pre-drilling [9, 10].

Self-drilling

It is drill free. Here, the implant itself act as a drill and it is directly introduced into bone. This method can be employed when we want to use larger diameter (more than 1.5 mm) miniscrew. The tips sharp, hooked and pointed. The threads are thin and pointed. Self-drilling involves lesser time and thermal damage. In high-density bone or dense cortical bone, this system is less beneficial, as gaining satisfactory primary stability require an extreme pressure in those sites. So, the chances of microfracture are higher [9, 10].

Selection of mini implant are given in Table **11**.

Table 11. Selection of optimum mini-implant body and neck dimensions with planned insertion site and directions.

Maxillary Mini-implant Selection	Mandibular Mini-implant Selection
1. Interproximal site? • Yes → 1.5 mm body diameter • No → 2.0 mm body diameter	1. Interproximal site? • Yes →1.5 mm body diameter • No → 2.0 mm body diameter
2. Antero-posterior position? • Anterior to canine → 6 mm body length for perpendicular insertion angle / 9 mm for oblique insertion and/or if alveolar depth sufficient • Posterior to canine → 9 mm body length	2. Antero-posterior position? • Anterior to canine → 6 mm body length • Posterior to canine → 6 mm body length for perpendicular insertion angle / 9 mm for oblique insertion
3. Transverse position? • Buccal → short neck length • Palatal or edentulous site →long neck length If mucosa > 2 mm thickness and incomplete body insertion expected → 2.0 mm body diameter	3. Alveolar position? • Buccal → short neck length • Edentulous or retromolar site → long neck length. If mucosa > 2 mm thickness and incomplete body insertion expected→2.0 mm body diameter
4. Adolescent patient? • Yes → consider larger body size for increased stability i.e., 2.0 mm diameter or 9 mm length if there is sufficient interproximal space and alveolar width, respectively • No → standard (adult) size selections, although 1.5 mm diameter may be sufficient when multiple mini-implants linked in mid-palate site	4. Adolescent patient? • Yes → consider larger body size for increased stability i.e., 2.0 mm diameter or 9 mm length if there is sufficient interproximal space and alveolar width, respectively • No → standard (adult) size selections

Mini-implant Insertion Steps

After proper case selection, all necessary records and working models are obtained. Insertion site and timing should be evaluated, followed by appropriate selection of mini-implant dimensions is done. Anaesthesia is given and patient is asked to gargle chlorhexidine mouthwash for one minute. Soft tissue removal is performed if site is in thick or loose mucosa. Cortex is perforated and mini-implant is slowly inserted in screwdriver rotation. If torque is high, then pause for 10–20 seconds or partially derotate. Percuss adjacent teeth to gauge implant–root proximity and take a radiograph or reinsert implant in case of proximity with the root [11].

Maxillofacial Prosthesis

Maxillofacial prosthetics is the art and science of anatomic, functional, or cosmetic reconstruction by means of non-living substitutes of those regions in the maxilla, mandible and face that are missing or defective because of surgical intervention, trauma, pathology or development or congenital malformation.

Classification of Maxillofacial Prosthesi73 (Table 12)

Table 12. Classification of Maxillofacial Prosthesis.

Classification	
Intraoral prosthesis	**Extraoral prosthesis**
1. Maxillary Defect a) Hard Palate Surgical Obturator, Interim Obturator, Definitive Obturator b) Soft Palate Speech Appliance, Meatus Obturator, Palatal Lift Prosthesis	1. Orbital
2. Mandibular defect Mandibular Resection Prosthesis	2. Nasal
3. Glossectomy Tongue Prosthesis, Palatal Augmentation.	3. Auricular
4. Splints/Stents Surgical Splints, Bite Splints, TMJ Appliance.	4.Mid-Facial

Need for Maxillofacial Prosthesis:

- Restore the aesthetics or appearance of the patient.
- Restore the form and function.
- Protect the tissues.
- Therapeutics or healing effect.
- Psychological therapy.

Obturator

Obturator is a maxillofacial prosthesis used to close a congenital or acquired tissue opening, primarily of the hard palate and/or contiguous alveolar/soft tissue structures (GPT-9) [2].

An obturator is a disc or plate, natural or artificial, which closes an opening or defect of the maxilla as a result of a cleft palate or partial or total removal of maxilla for a tumour mass (Chalina 1971).

Functions of Obturator

- It is useful in feeding.
- It helps in maintaining surgical site hygienic.
- Enhances recovery of traumatized tissues.
- Aids to redesign and recreate palatal contour.
- Recovers speech or makes speech possible.
- Can be used to guide the position of lip and cheek.
- Helps to regain patient's cosmetic appearance.
- Decreases the flow of nasal exudates into mouth.
- Used as stent to hold and maintain dressings or packs.

Obturators can be used for congenital and acquired defects [12].

For congenital defects, a plate type prosthesis to assist in feeding, or palatal lift prosthesis or an overlay denture can be fabricated.

For acquired defects a surgical, interim, or definitive obturator are fabricated.

Types of obturators (Fig. 8)

- Feeding
- Surgical
- Speech
- Functional

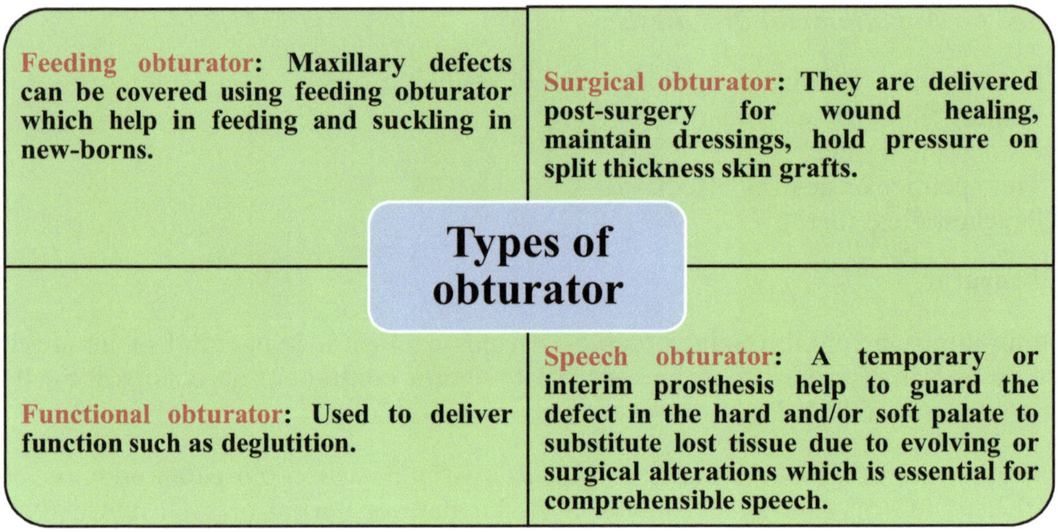

Fig. (8). Types of obturators.

Feeding Obturator

Feeding prosthesis is a prosthesis indicated for newborns with cleft palates to permit normal sucking and feeding (GPT – 9) [2].

The utmost congenital deformities involving oro-facial region are clefts of the lip and palate. These clefts may be syndromic or non-syndromic. The feeding plate is a passive maxillary prosthetic device that aid to re-establish the palatal cleft and helps to create satisfactory negative pressure which permit adequate sucking of milk.

Clinical Features of Cleft Palate which Necessitate Importance of Feeding Plate

The oro-nasal communication reduces the capacity to provide appropriate negative pressure which is required for suckling. To compensate, the baby squeezes the milk by pressing the nipple between the tongue and the hard palate, but this pressure is inadequate if cleft is wide, and the nipple gets trapped within the defect. Nasal regurgitation of food in cleft patients complicate the feeding process. The excessive air intake that demands frequent burping and choking. Feeding time is long and fatigues both the baby and mother. The obturator restores the separation between the oral and nasal cavities and helps to overcome above problems (Fig. **9**).

Advantages

1. It is a cost effective and simple to fabricate.

2. It provides a rigid platform, against which the child can press the nipple and get proper feeding thus reducing feeding time.

3. It diminishes the chance of choking.

4. It decreases nasal regurgitation thus inhibiting nasopharyngeal and ear infections.

5. It helps to place the tongue far from the cleft area in its correct position, by this it may cause spontaneous growth of palatal shelves towards each other, thus aiding in pre-surgical naso-alveolar moulding.

6. It greatly improves the final outcome after surgical treatment and also limits the number of surgeries.

7. It results in better speech and aesthetics, thus providing a positive psychological impact on the parents.

Fig. (9). Advantages of feeding obturator.

Fabrication of Feeding Obturator

Modelling plastic impression compound is obtained to make the primary impression of the maxillary arch. The impression material is held using two fingers, and the compound is adapted to the maxilla with the help of fingers. The impression is attempted when the infant is completely conscious deprived of any anaesthesia or pre-medication. The infant's face is held towards the floor to avoid aspiration in the incident of vomiting and suffocation because of airway obstruction. Primary casts are fabricated. Cleft area is revised with wax to mimic the contour and then a custom acrylic tray is prepared. In the next appointment a secondary impression is made using the custom tray. Master cast is made by using dental stone. Then undercuts are blocked and lubricated with petroleum jelly. Feeding obturator is then processed with heat polymerizing acrylic resin material. Final obturator is trimmed and polished. Parents need to be instructed regarding placement and removal of the appliance and its daily cleaning. A regular follow up of the child patient should be scheduled after 24 hours, 1 week and monthly. During the regular follow up, a record of neonate weight gain should be kept (Fig. **10**).

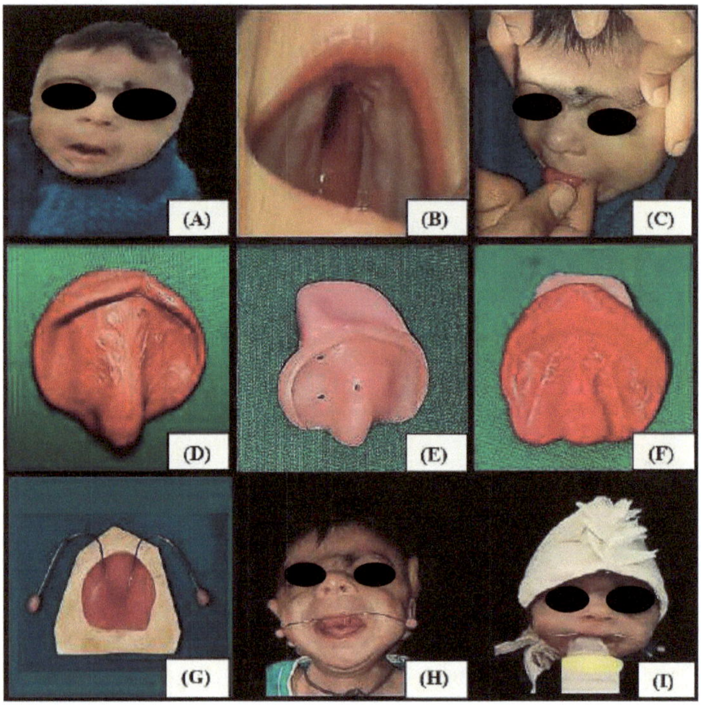

Fig. (10). Feeding obturator (A-I): A - Extraoral image of the child, B - intraoral image showing cleft palate, C – Taking primary impression, D - Primary impression, E - Special tray, F – Final impression, G - Feeding obturator, H - Feeding obturator in place, I - Follow up after 30 days with no problem in feeding.

CONCLUSION

Childhood and adolescence represent a period of intense growth and development of orofacial system. In such placid period, alternative of missing teeth is of vital clinical importance, and array of materials and restoration strategy options exist to ensure that proper chewing, aesthetics, and intonation is achieved. Adequate prosthetic restoration in children or adolescents must not in any way hinder proper development of jawbones, dental arches, and permanent teeth. Dental prosthetic appliances in Pediatric dentistry must be planned with respect to the special conditions that led to tooth loss or damage. Multi-disciplinary approach is needed, under constant supervision of pediatric dentist, as well as regular check-ups with clinical and radiographical examinations The use of partial acrylic prosthesis is an interesting and practical alternative that provides a quick, easy, acceptable, and economical solution to this functional and esthetics oral rehabilitation in patients with pronounced edentulism. It helps to normalize the function of masticatory and perioral muscles consequently the growth pattern of basal bones and gives psychological boost to the self-image of the child. But one must remember that any form of restoration or prosthesis should provide dentition confirming with the age of the patient.

CONSENT FOR PUBLICATION

Not applicable.

CONFLICT OF INTEREST

The authors declare no conflict of interest, financial or otherwise.

ACKNOWLEDGEMENT

Declared none.

REFERENCES

[1] Trivedi BD, Bhatia R. Complete and removable partial prosthesis for a child with hypohidrotic ectodermal dysplasia. Int J Clin Pediatr Dent 2013; 6(1): 71-4. [http://dx.doi.org/10.5005/jp-journals-10005-1192] [PMID: 25206194]

[2] Morgano SM, VanBlarcom CW, Ferro KJ, Bartlett DW. The history of the glossary of prosthodontic terms. J Prosthet Dent 2018; 119(3): 311-2. [http://dx.doi.org/10.1016/j.prosdent.2017.10.001] [PMID: 29475757]

[3] Ali Hassan S, Bhateja S, Arora G, Prathyusha F. Prosthesis in pediatric dentistry. IP Journal of Paediatrics and Nursing Science 2020; 3(3): 64-7. [http://dx.doi.org/10.18231/j.ijpns.2020.014]

[4] Dimova-Gabrovska M, Dimitrova D, Mitronin V. Removable prosthetic treatment in children - literature review. Journal of IMAB - Annual Proceeding (Scientific Papers) 2018; 24(3): 2172-6.

[5] Teixeira Marques NC, Gurgel CV, Fernandes AP, *et al.* Prosthetic rehabilitation in children: an alternative clinical technique. Case Rep Dent 2013; 2013: 1-5. [http://dx.doi.org/10.1155/2013/512951] [PMID: 24175103]

[6] Rupesh S, Joseph E, Rupesh S, Mathew J. Complete overlay denture for pedodontic patient with severe dentinogenesis imperfecta. Int J Clin Pediatr Dent 2017; 10(4): 394-8. [http://dx.doi.org/10.5005/jp-journals-10005-1472] [PMID: 29403236]

[7] Abu-Hussein M, Watted N, Abdulgani A, Kontoes N. Prosthodontic-orthodontic treatment plan with two-unit cantilevered resin-bonded fixed partial denture. IOSR-JDMS 2015; 14(12): 131-6.

[8] Mishra SK, Chowdhary N, Chowdhary R. Dental implants in growing children. J Indian Soc Pedod Prev Dent 2013; 31(1): 3-9. [http://dx.doi.org/10.4103/0970-4388.112392] [PMID: 23727735]

[9] Bajaj R, Shenoy U, Banerjee S, Hazare A, Karia H, Atulkar M. Implants in orthodontics-a brief review. International journal oforal health and medical research 2017; 3(5): 92-7.

[10] Nosouhian S, Rismanchian M, Sabzian R, Shadmehr E, Badrian H, Davoudi A. A mini-review on the effect of mini-implants on contemporary orthodontic science. J Int Oral Health 2015; 7(1) (Suppl. 1): 83-7. [PMID: 26225113]

[11] de Oliveira NS, Barbosa GLR, Lanza LD, Pretti H. Prosthetic rehabilitation of child victim of avulsion of anterior teeth with orthodontic mini-implant. Case Rep Dent 2017; 2017: 1-4. [http://dx.doi.org/10.1155/2017/8905965] [PMID: 29093976]

[12] Gupta A, Verma A, Dubey T, Thakur S. Maxillofacial prosthetics Part I: A Review. Int J Adv Res (Indore) 2017; 5(9): 31-40. [http://dx.doi.org/10.21474/IJAR01/5504]

CHAPTER 3

Diseases of Pulp and Periradicular Tissues

Shivayogi Hugar[1,*], **Dhanashree Sakhare**[2] and **H. Sharath Chandra**[3]

[1] *Department of Pediatric Dentistry, Kaher's KLE VK Institute of Dental Sciences, Belagavi, Karnataka, India*

[2] *Founder, Lavanika Dental Academy, Melbourne, Australia*

[3] *Department of Periodontics, SJM Dental College, Chitradurga, Karnataka, India*

Abstract: The Dental pulp has remained a diagnostic enigma to the dental surgeon. While some dental pulps would react inadvertently even to the slightest injury, at other times highly resistant pulp tissue has regenerative properties even after extensive damage has been noted. However, most of the time clinicians can make a uniform decision about the status of the dental pulp with the help of clinical signs and symptoms and make a patient-centric treatment plan that can provide pain relief and restore the form and function of the tooth. A distinction needs to be made between acute and chronic inflammatory conditions of the pulp and between the reversibility or irreversibility of the pulpal changes so that appropriate vital or non-vital pulp therapies can be selected.

It is also important to distinguish between inflammatory conditions and degenerative conditions of the pulp. While inflammation almost always requires intervention, changes like degenerative calcific changes may require observation and occasional intervention.

Keywords: Degenerative Pulpal Disease, Pulp Diseases, Pulp Inflammation.

INTRODUCTION

The dental pulp is sensitive to external factors such as microbial infection from dental caries and or mechanical/chemical irritations during dental procedures. Dental tissue behaves differently than other connective tissues. It is unique in the way that its soft tissues which are the pulp and pulp-dentin complex are enclosed within mineralized hard tissues of the tooth namely enamel, dentin, and cementum, and are supplied by a rich neurovascular network that regulates various inflammatory mediators. Inflammatory signals may progress to rapid

* **Corresponding Author Shivayogi Hugar:** Department of Pediatric Dentistry, Kaher's K L E VK Institute of Dental Sciences, Belagavi Karnataka; E-mail: dr.hugarsm@gmail.com

Satyawan Damle, Ritesh Kalaskar & Dhanashree Sakhare (Eds.)

degeneration and necrosis, and such events could inflict serious damage to tissues in the body. One of the sequelae of dental caries is inflammation of pulp and pulpal diseases when the carious lesion involves the pulpal tissue.

Causes of Pulp Disease

Following are the common etiological factors for pulp pathology. Many classifications of etiologies have been proposed by a couple of authors. The classification of etiology of pulpal diseases has been given as follows:

1. Physical damage
    a. Mechanical
        i. Trauma
            1. Trauma from dental and non-dental origin
            2. Rapid orthodontic movements
            3. Iatrogenic pulp exposure during cavity preparation
            4. Abfraction
            5. Crack Tooth Syndrome
        ii. Pathologic wear
            1. Attrition
            2. Abrasion
            3. Bruxism (Fig. **1**)
        iii. Barometric changes: Barodontalgia
        iv. Radiation
    b. Thermal
        i. Heat due to cavity preparation
        ii. Inadequate or no use of coolants
        iii. Exothermic heat from the setting of restorative materials
        iv. Finishing and polishing of restorations
        v. Inadequate or absence of base under restoration
    c. Electrical: Galvanism due to dissimilar metals
2. Chemical
    a. Leaching of harmful products from restorative materials
    b. Erosion of teeth
3. Bacterial
    a. Direct invasion of pulp by bacteria due to caries or trauma
    b. Bacterial toxins
    c. Anachoresis
        i. Retrograde bacterial invasion
        ii. Perio-endo lesions
4. Developmental disorders of teeth

   a. Dens invaginatus
   b. Dens evaginatus
   c. Dentinogenisis imperfecta
   d. Amelogenesis imperfecta
   e. Molar Incisor Hypoplasia
5. Iatrogenic
   a. Intentional extirpation of pulp
   b. Electrosurgery
   c. Laser burn
   d. Surgical techniques
      i. Intubation during general anaesthesia
      ii. Enucleation of cysts and tumours
      iii. Placement of Osseo plating screws
      iv. Osteotomies

Classification of Pulpal diseases

Many different classification systems have been proposed for pulp diseases, although most of them are based on histopathological findings. Many authors and clinicians have attempted to correlate the histological conditions of the pulp to the clinical signs and symptoms [3]. A clinician's ability to diagnose accurately is dependent on having a thorough understanding of the disease processes involved as well as the diagnostic procedures and tests being used and their limitations.

Grossmann's Classification [1, 2]

1. Pulpits [inflammatory diseases]

a. Reversible

i. Acute Symptomatic

ii. Chronic asymptomatic

b. Irreversible

i. Acute

• Abnormally responsive to cold

• Abnormally responsive to heat.

ii. Chronic

• Asymptomatic with pulp exposure

• Hyperplasic pulpitis

• Internal resorption

2. Pulp degeneration

a. Calcific

b. Atrophic

c. Fibrous.

3. Pulp Necrosis

Cohens Classification

- Reversible pulpitis
- Irreversible pulpitis
- Asymptomatic irreversible pulpitis
- Hyperplastic pulpits
- Internal resorption
- Symptomatic irreversible pulpitis
- Pulp necrosis

WHO Classification [3, 4]

K04.0 Pulpitis/ Pulpal abscess/Pulp polyp, acute/chronic hyperplastic / ulcerative pulpitis.

K04.1 Necrosed pulp/ pulp gangrene.

K04.2 Pulp degeneration, Denticles/pulp calcification

K04.3 Abnormal hard tissue formation in secondary or irregular dentin.

Seltzer and Bender's Classification [5]

1. Treatable:
    a. Intact uninflamed pulp
    b. Transitional stage
    c. Atrophic pulp
    d. Acute pulpitis
    e. Chronic partial pulpitis without necrosis
2. Untreatable
    a. Chronic partial pulpits with necrosis

b. Chronic total pulpitis
c. Total pulp necrosis

Clinically Normal Pulp

The term 'clinically normal pulp' is used to classify a pulp that has no signs or symptoms to suggest the occurrence of any disease. The term 'clinically' is used, since such a pulp may not be histologically normal and/or may have some degree of fibrosis (scarring) or inflammatory cellular infiltrate because of previous injury or stimuli [5].

Pulpitis

Pulpitis is inflammation of dental pulp tissue. The pulp contains blood vessels, nerves, and connective tissue that is responsible for blood and nutrients to the tooth. Pulpitis is caused due to many reasons but mainly due to bacterial infection which itself is a secondary consequence of caries. It manifests itself in the form of pain.

Reversible Pulpitis [6]

[Focal Reversible Pulpitis/ Initial pulpitis/ Pulpal Hyperemia]

Reversible pulpitis is a mild to moderate inflammatory condition of the pulp caused by a noxious stimulus in which the pulp can return to the un-inflamed state following removal of the stimuli. Due to inflammation, intrapulpal blood flow increases, and hence, it is also referred to as pulp hyperemia. Reversible pulpitis is one of the earliest forms of pulpitis. Mild transient pulpitis is localized chiefly to the pulpal ends of dentinal tubules.

Symptom

It is characterized by a sharp, shooting pain lasting for a moment which will subside soon after the removal of the stimuli and does not occur spontaneously. The increasing unilateral, sharp, stabbing type of pain is intermittent and of immediate onset more often brought by cold air/beverages than hot food stimulus. Sometimes there is difficulty in the localization of the offending tooth.

Signs

Clinically large intra/extra coronal restoration, carious lesion involving the dentin and pin placed close to the pulp or involving the pulp is seen. Severe dentinal involvement due to pathologic wear of the teeth may also lead to reversible pulpal changes.

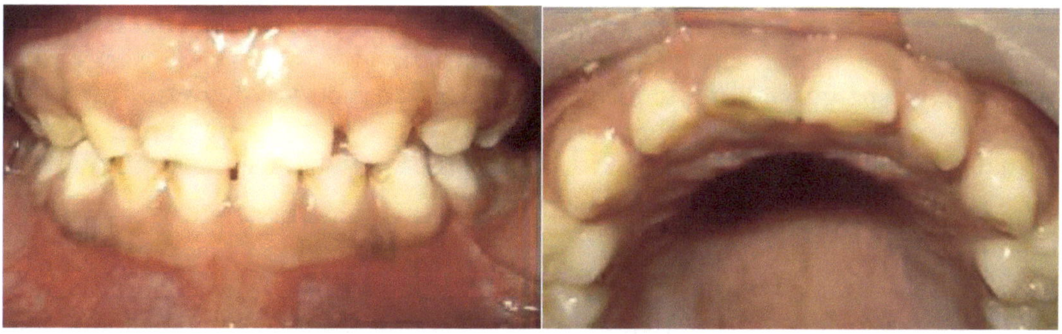

Fig. (1). Bruxism and exposure to dentin due to pathologic wear.

Histopathology

Reversible pulpitis may range from hyperemia to mild to moderate inflammatory changes. Increased blood volume associated with hyperemia increases intra pulpal pressure in the involved area, which may be limited to a segment of the pulp chamber. An increase in intra pulpal pressure is due to an initial ingress of plasma fluid, a minimal WBC infiltration, and erythrocyte extravasation. The pressure created against the odontoblasts and A-δ nerve fibres in the affected peripheral area are not great enough to initiate pain impulses, but their excitatory threshold is lowered. A-δ fibres produce initial, sharp, momentary pain due to their peripheral location, the low threshold of excitability, and greater conductivity. Hyperemia may be accompanied by hypersensitive dentin, but the presence of hypersensitive dentin does not necessarily indicate the presence of hyperemia.

Radiographic Finding

No visible radiographic changes are seen in pulpal hyperemia. Periapical tissue is normal on radiographic examination.

Vitality test

Thermal tests are useful in locating the affected tooth, as reversible pulpitis responds readily to cold. The Electric Pulp Test (EPT) is an excellent corroborating test. The hyperalgesic pulp responds more readily to cold stimulation than the normal adjacent teeth. Electric pulp testing requires minimal current to initiate a positive response, due to the increased excitability of Aδ fibres.

Diagnosis

Sharp pain lasts for a few seconds and disappears when the stimulus is removed. The patient complains of pain with the intake of cold, sweet, or sour food. On intraoral examination, caries/ restorations/ traumatic fractures or traumatic occlusion are evident. The patient sometimes gives a history of past dental treatment. On percussion, no tenderness is observed, and the colour of the tooth seems to be normal as compared to the adjacent tooth. Radiographs show a normal appearance of apical and periodontal tissues with no loss of lamina dura.

Treatment

Removal of noxious stimulus followed by desensitization of the exposed dentin will relieve the pain. The best treatment is prevention, by caries removal and pulp protection by the placement of calcium hydroxide or use of cavity varnish or placement of suitable base in deep carious lesions before insertion of restoration. Periodic review by pulp vitality test should be scheduled at 3-, 6- & 12-months intervals to monitor the pulpal condition.

Prognosis

The prognosis of pulp is favourable if the irritant is removed in the early phases or else it will lead to irreversible pulpitis.

Irreversible Pulpitis

It is a persistent inflammatory condition of the pulp, symptomatic or asymptomatic, and is caused by a noxious stimulus. The pulp has been damaged irreversibly and does not heal even with the removal of the irritant. The pulp will progressively degenerate, causing necrosis and reactive destruction. Pulp death often occurs slowly and without dramatic symptoms. A carious exposure is that point at which infected dentin comes in contact with pulpal soft tissues. This leads to the development of micro abscesses due to the direct access of large numbers of bacteria, bacterial by-products, salivary by-products, and chemicals from ingested foods.

Irreversible pulpitis can be of two types acute and chronic.

Acute irreversible pulpitis occurs as sequelae of reversible pulpitis present as a primary, acute condition and an acute exacerbation of chronic pulpitis. Chronic irreversible pulpitis is seen as inflammation due to long-term, low-grade injury with exposed pulp and can be symptomatic or asymptomatic.

Symptoms

In the early stages usually, pain is caused by the sudden change in temperature, sweet intake, pressure on biting, and suction exerted by the tongue or cheek. In the later stages, pain is more severe; boring, gnawing, or throbbing type. At times, the pain may be mild to severe excruciating. The patient may complain of sharp, piercing, and shooting type of pain. A history of nocturnal pain is also given by the patient. Pain may increase with a change in a position like bending over or lying down due to a change in intra-pulpal pressure. In acute conditions, a paroxysm of pain, due to sudden changes in temperature or pressure may be observed. Spontaneous, persisting pain for several minutes to hours even after removal of stimulus is seen.

Signs

Leathery slough-like material is found on the affected tooth (Fig. **2**). It may also be associated with large intra or extra coronal restorations. When the maxillary posterior teeth are involved, referred pain is usually felt in adjacent teeth or temple regions. Sometimes, the pain may be referred to as the sinuses when an upper posterior tooth is involved. When mandibular posterior teeth are involved, pain may be referred to the ear. Pain relief can be simply achieved by placing a temporary restoration. Tenderness on percussion may be present due to the exudation of acute inflammatory products in the periodontium. The term 'acute pulpitis with acute apical periodontitis' is applicable in this situation.

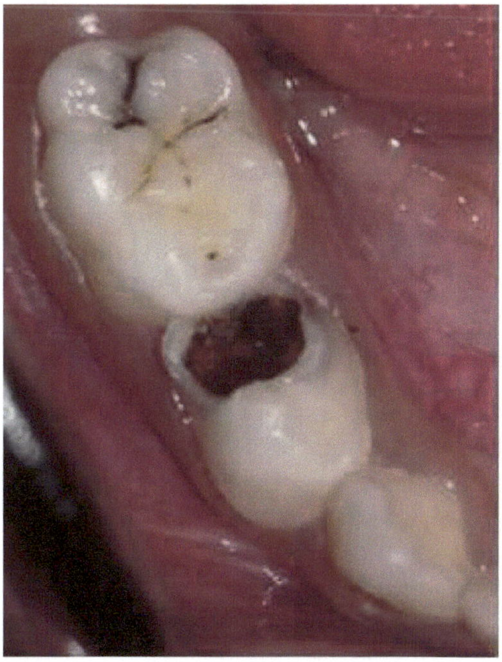

Fig. (2). Leathery dentin extending up to dentin.

Histopathology

Both acute and chronic inflammatory changes are present. Vasodilatation, accumulation of fluid in connective tissue, pavement of PMNLs along blood vessel wall with odontoblastic destruction occurs. If the carious process continues to advance, gradual localized destruction of pulp by PMNLs and formation of micro abscesses takes place which in turn leads to an area of ulceration and is called chronic ulcerative pulpitis. According to Seltzer and Bender, there is a possible mechanism by which a high concentration of antigens in the carious process may induce the formation of immunoglobulins [6]. An antigen-antibody precipitate in presence of complement which attracts PMNL's phagocytosis & cell degeneration stimulates the release of proteases by lysosomes to form an abscess and the pulp eventually ends up in irreversible pulpitis and progresses to necrosis.

Radiographic Examination

A radiograph may disclose an interproximal or occlusal cavity or caries under a filling threatening the integrity of pulp. Coronal radiolucency at the pulp horn showing its destruction, sometimes having no periapical changes, may be seen. In some cases blunting of the pulp, and the horn may be evident.

Vitality Test

Heat will intensify the responses because it has an expansive effect on blood vessels, tissue & gaseous products of proteolysis. Conversely, cold will tend to relieve the pain in advanced stages of pulpitis, because it has a contractile effect on the central or apical functional vascular bed, reducing intrapulpal pressure. Irreversible pulpitis will be associated with a higher threshold value compared to control teeth due to the involvement of C-fibers.

Diagnosis

A deep cavity extending into the pulp or secondary caries under the restoration is seen. A deep cavity extending to the pulp shows a greyish, scum-like layer over the exposed pulp and the surrounding dentin. Deep probing will result in both, haemorrhage and occasionally pus. Pain can be spontaneous which is sharp, piercing, intermittent, or continuous. Pain can be exacerbated by bending down or lying down due to a change in intra pulpal pressure. Usually, a negative response to percussion is present in irreversible pulpitis.

Treatment

Pulpectomy and the placement of an intracanal medicament to function as a disinfectant or obturation followed by root canal treatment is the treatment of choice. Extraction may be considered if the tooth is non-restorable.

Prognosis

Prognosis is favourable if the pulp is extirpated, and the tooth undergoes proper endodontic therapy and restoration. If there is the presence of any peri radicular or furcal radiolucency, the tooth should be radiographically monitored at 3, 6, and 12 months to ascertain the resolution of the lesion.

Chronic Hyperplastic Pulpitis [Pulp Polyp]

Pulp polyp is clinically characterized by the development of reddish cauliflower-like outgrowth of pulp tissue through and around the carious exposure that undergoes a granulomatous transformation. It is covered with epithelium and results from long-standing, low-grade irritation in resistant pulp tissue. It is usually asymptomatic and causes discomfort and bleeding during mastication or tooth brushing. Polypoid tissue is less sensitive than normal pulp and more sensitive than gingival tissue. The lesion may or may not bleed readily and commonly deciduous molars and permanent first molars are involved (Fig. **3**).

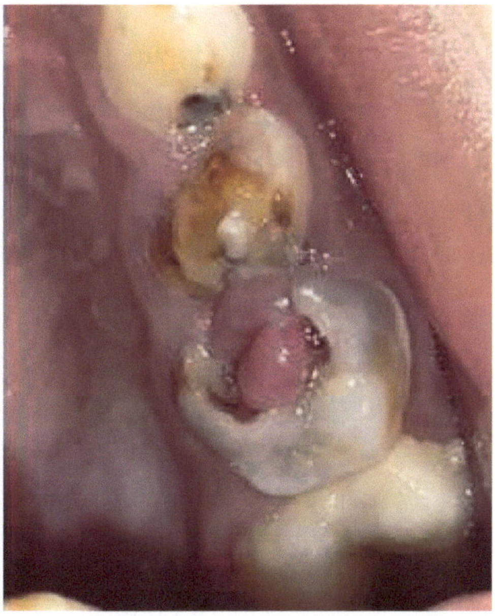

Fig. (3). Chronic Hyperplastic Pulpitis.

Symptoms

It may be asymptomatic, except during mastication or oral hygiene procedure, and may cause discomfort. The patient may complain of a lump in the mouth.

Signs

It is usually seen in children & young adults. Clinically visible polyp within the grossly decayed tooth and extensive carious destruction of coronal tooth tissue is often observed. Careful examination is necessary to differentiate pulp polyps from gingival overgrowths that may grow over the margins of the tooth and encroach on the pulp space.

Histopathology

Histopathologically, budding capillaries, proliferating fibroblasts & inflammatory cells are seen. The presence of granulation tissue, which is young vascular connective tissue containing PMNLs, lymphocytes, plasma cells, and multinucleated giant cells is commonly seen. Collagen fibres are rooted in the deeper tissue of the pulp chamber. Sensory nerve fibres are almost absent near-the surface which is usually covered by stratified squamous epithelium.

Radiographic Examination

The radiograph may disclose a deep carious lesion with extensive involvement of the pulp chamber. Soft tissue shadow of the pulp polyp may be visible when the contrast of the image is adjusted.

Vitality Test

The teeth are responsive to heat and cold but to a lesser degree than the control teeth. Similarly, the tooth will also respond to a higher value on an electric pulp tester.

Diagnosis

The appearance of polyp tissue clinically, characteristic as a fleshy, reddish, or pinkish polypoid tissue, pulpal mass filling most of the pulp chamber and surrounded by a band of carious tooth structure.

Treatment

Elimination of polypoid tissue with a periodontal curette or spoon excavator, followed by extirpation of the pulp, provided the tooth can be endodontically restored. Conventional root canal treatment is the choice of treatment. If the tooth cannot be endodontically restored, then extraction is the treatment of choice.

Prognosis

The prognosis for the tooth is favourable after the endodontic procedure followed by post-obturation restoration.

Internal Resorption

[Pink tooth of Mummery/ Idiopathic Resorption]

Internal resorption is an idiopathic slow or fast progressive resorptive process occurring in the dentin of the pulp chamber or root canals of teeth (Fig. **4**).> Internal resorption was first reported by Bell in the year 1830. Later it was named the pink tooth of Mummery in the year 1920, due to pink discolouration on the crown and is named after the anatomist Mummery [7].

It is often seen that patients give a history of dental trauma or persistent chronic pulpitis. Internal desorption following Ca $(OH)_2$ pulpotomy, cracked tooth, and orthodontic tooth movement may also be the etiological factors for internal resorption [8]. However, its exact cause is still unknown.

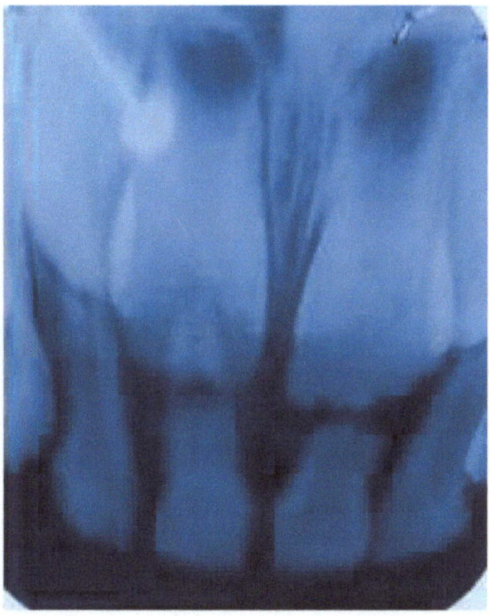

Fig. (4). Internal resorption with 51 and external resorption with 61.

Symptoms

The tooth is asymptomatic and usually may manifest as a pink spot on the crown. The reddish area represents the granulation tissue showing through the resorbed area of the crown.

Signs

The tooth may be associated with excessive mobility and pain on palpation or tenderness on percussion.

Histopathology

Cytological alterations occur in the pulp when odontoclasts form undifferentiated reserve connective tissue cells. Resorptive lacunae may be filled in by osteoid tissue as osteoclastic activity markedly increases. The presence of granulation tissue, multinucleated giant cells, dentinoclasts, and chronic inflammatory cells are evident histologically. These cells show an intense tartrate-resistant to acid phosphatase activity. A pulp cavity of teeth undergoing internal resorption differs markedly from normal pulp tissue and are appeared to be replaced by growing connective tissue or has undergone metaplasia. Histochemical studies have shown that dentine resorbing cells have enzymes like acid phosphates and β-glucuronidase.

Radiographic Feature

A round or oval radiolucent area is evident in the wall of the root canal radiographically. The resorptive lesion may progress extensively to involve the external tooth surface. When internal resorption progresses into the PDL space and perforation of the root occurs, it is difficult to differentiate from external root resorption. In internal resorption, the resorptive defect is usually more extensive on the pulpal wall than on the root surface.

Diagnosis

Internal resorption is usually diagnosed during routine radiographic examination involving either crown or root of the teeth or may be extensive enough to involve both. It is usually a slow, progressive, intermittent process extending over 1-2 years.

Treatment

Extirpation of pulp stops the internal resorptive process. Routine endodontic treatment can be conducted, but in advanced cases, calcium hydroxide paste, or MTA dressing may be advocated. Periodic radiographic observation is required until the defect is repaired which is evident as a calcific barrier in the radiograph. Later the repaired canal is obturated with Thermo-plasticized gutta-percha in permanent teeth. For deciduous teeth, endodontic treatment may be attempted till the lesion is confined within the pulp chamber or root canal space and has not extensively caused resorption. If the lesion is extensive, it is advisable to extract the tooth.

Prognosis

Prognosis is favourable before perforation of root and crown occurs. In the case of perforation, if calcific barrier formation is possible using inert restorative material, then conventional root canal therapy can be considered.

Necrosis of Pulp

Necrosis is the death of the pulp. It may be either partial or total depending on the degree of involvement of the pulp. Usually, the death of pulpal tissue is sequelae of acute or chronic inflammation leading to strangulation of the pulp due to either an increase in the intra-pulpal pressure or an immediate arrest of circulation by a traumatic injury in which the pulp is destroyed before an inflammatory reaction occurs. An ischemic infarction can develop and may cause a dry gangrenous necrotic pulp. Any noxious stimuli/insult injurious to the pulp as sequelae of inflammation may lead to pulp necrosis. The presence of bacteria, trauma to the pulp, or chemical irritation can cause pulpal inflammation followed by necrosis of the pulp.

Symptoms

The tooth may be completely asymptomatic with a history of previous pain. Many patients report severe pain when the necrotic remnant pulp leach through the apical foramen and elicits an apical periodontal response.

Signs

Greyish/brownish discolouration of the tooth with a dull opaque colour with loss of normal translucency is an indication that the pulp is non-vital. Radiographically, the tooth may be associated with periapical radiolucency, with clinical signs of intra-oral and extra-oral swelling or draining sinus tracts localized with the tooth (Fig. **5**).

Histopathology

Histopathologically, necrotic pulp tissue shows cellular debris and microorganisms, periapical tissue may be normal or with slight evidence of inflammation. Necrosis is of two types, coagulative necrosis, and liquefaction necrosis.

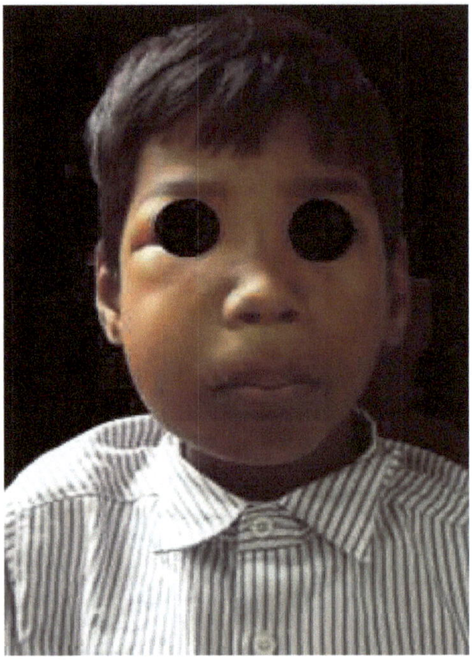

Fig. (5). Extra-oral swelling due to pulp necrosis.

Coagulative Necrosis

The soluble portion of tissue is precipitated into a solid cheesy mass material consisting chiefly of coagulated proteins, fats, and water. Coagulative necrosis is associated with diminishing blood supply to an area.

Liquefaction Necrosis

It occurs when proteolytic enzymes convert the tissue into softened mass, liquid, or amorphous debris. The histopathological appearance of an empty pulp and root canal space is associated with liquefaction necrosis of the dental pulp.

Radiographic Feature

A deep carious lesion extending up to the pulp space is usually appreciated on the radiograph. The presence of apical periodontal space widening, peri radicular, and furcation radiolucency can be seen in long-standing cases. The periapical inflammatory response may also trigger radicular or bone resorption and should be noted in deciduous teeth.

Vitality Test

The tooth does not respond to heat or cold tests. Occasionally, teeth with pulp necrosis may give a false positive response to heat due to the expansion of the gases. In such cases, the pain may be relieved with the application of cold.

Diagnosis

It can only be clinically diagnosed, as no significant findings are present in the tooth. Pain, swelling, mobility, and tenderness to percussion are usually absent with total necrotic condition. Blackish or brownish change in the tooth colour is seen as a result of hemolysis of red blood cells or decomposition of the pulp tissue. Radiographs show a large cavity or restoration or an open approach to the root canal. Sometimes findings are normal except if there is any apical periodontitis. Minimal response to a maximum current of an electric pulp tester occurs when an electric current is conducted through the moisture present in a root canal following liquefaction necrosis to neighbouring vital tissue.

Treatment

The choice of treatment is conventional endodontic therapy. When periradicular lesions and furcation are observed, it is advisable to leave a calcium hydroxide dressing for one or two weeks followed by obturation of the root canals.

Prognosis

The prognosis will be good if proper endodontic therapy is performed, and the tooth is restorable. The tooth should be clinically and radiographically observed at 3-, 6-, and 12-month intervals.

Pulp Degeneration

Pulp degeneration is seldom recognized clinically and is generally present in the teeth of older people. Rarely in young teeth with persistent mild infection or following traumatic injuries.

Symptoms

In the early stages, no definite clinical symptoms are seen but in the later stage there may be tooth discolouration and the pulp does not respond to any stimulation. Pulpal degeneration can be of three types, calcific degeneration, atrophic degeneration, and fibrous degeneration

1. Calcific Degeneration / Dystrophic Calcification

A part of the pulp tissue is replaced by calcified material within the pulp chamber or root canal. It occurs as a response to trauma, caries, periodontal disease, or any other low-grade insult. Calcium salts get attracted to the local alkalinity of the destroyed tissue. Pulp stones range in size from small, microscopic particles to accretions that occupy almost the entire pulp chamber. The mineral phase of pulpal calcifications consists of carbonated hydroxyapatite. It can also be due to excessive deposition of mineralized tissue resembling cementum [9].

Classification of Calcific Degeneration

I. According to the presence of a calcific mass in the pulp chamber or root canal as:
   i. Denticles: Denticles or pulp stones are large, well outlined, more commonly seen in the pulp chamber, laminated, and large enough at times to give an impression of the pulp cavity after removal.
   ii. Diffuse calcifications: They appear as amorphous uniform calcification throughout the pulp chamber and/or root canal space.

II. According to their location:
   a. Free-pulp stones lie freely in the pulp tissue
   b. Embedded-pulp stones are encircled by dentin
   c. Attached-pulp stones are attached to the dentinal walls

III. According to the structure:
   a. True: True denticles or pulp stones are composed of dentin and formed around epithelial cells (remnants of Hertwig's epithelial root sheath).
   b. False: False denticles are formed when a degenerating tissue serves as a nidus for deposition of concentric layers of calcified tissue in a lamellar fashion.

Radiographic Features

The radiograph demonstrates radio-opaque mass-like structures in the pulp chamber or root canal. Partial or complete radiographic obliteration of the pulp chamber may be evident. Calcification of pulp tissue is associated with various degrees of pulp space obliteration (Fig. **6**).

Diagnosis

Yellowish discolouration with dullness and loss of translucency of the crown is a sign of calcific degeneration. Pain threshold to thermal and electric stimuli increases or often the teeth are unresponsive. Palpation and percussion are usually within normal limits.

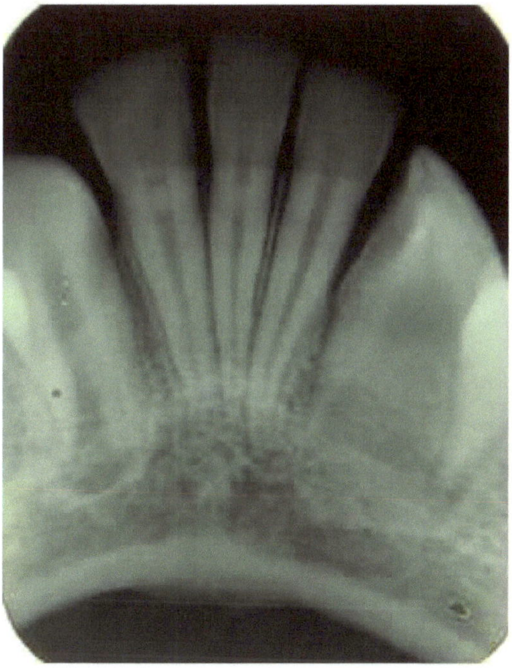

Fig. (6). Calcification of pulp canals.

Treatment

For pulpal degeneration, conventional root canal therapy is the choice of treatment. It usually poses a problem in endodontic treatment due to the presence of pulp stones in pulpal tissues. Use of chelating agents like EDTA is recommended. They can be removed from the pulp chamber using excavators and peeso-reamers. During treatment of calcified canals, it is common to find a total occluded canal space at any level. In the absence of symptoms or evidence of apical pathosis, it is clinically reasonable to the instrument and fills the canal till the level of negotiation. In deciduous teeth, clinical or radiographic evidence of asymptomatic teeth with calcification may be observed until the natural exfoliation of the tooth occurs.

2. Atrophic Degeneration

Atrophy means 'wasting away' or decrease in the size of an organ. It is attributed to faulty nutrition. Usually, it is observed as the teeth grow older, having no clinical diagnostic features. The affected pulp tissue is less sensitive than normal pulp tissue. Histopathologically, an increase in collagen fibres and intercellular fluid is observed. A decrease in the number of cells and only a few stellate cells are seen.

3. Fibrous Degeneration

Fibrous degeneration is characterized by the replacement of cellular elements by fibrous connective tissue that appears as a leathery fibre on removal from a root canal where there are no distinguishing symptoms to aid in clinical diagnosis.

Pulpal degeneration is frequently seen as age-related changes in the dental pulp.

Features of Pulpal Inflammation (Table 1).

Table 1. Features of pulpal inflammation.

-	Potentially Reversible	Probably Irreversible
Pain	Sharp, Momentary: dissipates readily after removal stimulus	Continuous throbbing: Persists for minutes to hours
Stimulus	Requires external stimulus (Cold, heat, sweet)	Spontaneous: dead or injured tissue in chambers or canal. Intermittent: Spontaneous pain of short duration.
History	The recent dental procedure, cervical abrasion	Extensive pulp capping, deep caries.
Electric Pulp test	Premature response	Premature, delayed, or mixed response in advanced stage
Referred pain	Negative	Common
Lying down	Negative	Increases pain
Colour	No change	Discolouration due to tissue necrosis &pulpal haemorrhage.
Radiograph	Restoration, caries, periodontal pocket, cupping of the alveolar crest	Restoration, caries involving enamel, dentin, and encroaching pulp
-	Periapex - Normal	Periapex – widening of PDL

Clinical Characteristics of Pulpal Inflammation (Table 2).

Table 2. Characteristics of pulpal inflammation.

Reversible Pulpitis {Inflammation}	Irreversible Pulpitis {Inflammation}
1. Sensitivity to mild discomfort.	1. Absence or presence of pain
2. Duration of pain is of short or shooting sensation.	2. Patient gives a history of pain
3. Severe pain not present	3. Moderate to severe pain is observed
4. Episodes of discomfort are not frequent	4. Spontaneous pain is present

(Table 2) cont.....

Reversible Pulpitis {Inflammation}	Irreversible Pulpitis {Inflammation}
5. Occasionally hurts to bite unless the tooth is fractured, restoration is displaced, and occlusion is affected.	5. Increasing the frequency of pain, often to the point of being continuous.
6. May also result in irreversible pulpitis if etiology is not eliminated.	6. Lingering pain especially with increasing episodes.
7. After the removal of etiological factors symptoms usually subsided immediately or shortly after that.	7. Some type of analgesia is required by the patient.
8. Aetiologies include exposed dentin, cracked restorations, recently placed restorations, initial carious attack, rapidly advancing caries, and altered occlusion.	8. Heat stimulation often elicits severe lingering pain.
-	9. Might be able to identify specific or multiple stimuli.
-	10. Radiating pain or/is diffuse or localized.
-	11. Trauma to the teeth, extensive restorations, periodontal disease, or extensive recurrent carries is present.
-	12. Changes observed on the radiograph may be absent or include calcifications, resorption, or radiolucencies.

Clinical conditions and their corresponding signs, symptoms, and treatment options (Table 3).

Table 3. Clinical conditions and their corresponding treatment modalities.

Clinical Event	Signs Or Symptoms	Pulpal Status	Treatment Choice
1. Caries without Exposure	No spontaneous symptoms	Healthy	Restore tooth
2. Caries with possible or near exposure	Occasional pain on stimulation	Minimal or reversible pulpitis	Pulpotomy
3. non carious exposure	Asymptomatic	Healthy	Pulpotomy
4. Carious exposure	Minimal history of pain No mobility No radiographic evidence of pathology	Reversible pulpitis	Pulpotomy
5. Carious exposure	Spontaneous pain Swelling Mobility	Irreversible pulpitis	Pulpectomy Intermediate dressing Extraction

(Table 3) cont.....

Clinical Event	Signs Or Symptoms	Pulpal Status	Treatment Choice
6. Carious exposure	Draining sinus Swelling Mobility Radiographic pathology	Necrotic pulp	Pulpectomy Intermediate dressing Extraction
7. Gross caries	Caries through bifurcation Extensive root resorption Tooth non-restorable Extensive periapical pathology	Necrotic pulp	Extraction

Conditions Mimicking Pulpitis

Barodontalgia

Extraoral decompression of the ambient pressure in the plane which causes compensating increase of pressure within the pulp chamber and the root canal is called barodontalgia. Barodontalgia was formerly called aerodontalgia. Such patients may complain of sharp momentary or dull throbbing pain only during decompression or flying at a high altitude. It is usually associated with large carious lesions, fractured amalgam restoration, recurrent caries under restoration, or an incomplete fracture or split the tooth. Mainly, sinusitis can be a contributing factor if maxillary teeth are involved.

Diseases of Periradicular Tissues

Acute Periradicular Disease

a. Acute apical periodontitis –Vital or Non-vital

b. Acute alveolar abscess

c. Phoenix abscess

Chronic Periradicular Disease

a. Chronic alveolar abscess

b. Granuloma

c. Radicular cyst

d. Condensing osteitis

e. External resorption

Periradicular Disease

Acute Alveolar Abscess

A localized collection of pus in the alveolar bone at the root apex of a pulpless tooth can be called an acute alveolar abscess. Sequelae from pulpal pathology through apical foramen into peri-radicular tissues result in an acute alveolar abscess. In primary teeth, the infection spreads into the peri-radicular area through the porous furcation area rather than the apical area usually with diffuse infection. Severe throbbing pain, irritability, sleep depravity, rise in body temperature, malaise, and headache are the main symptoms observed. The affected tooth is painful on chewing with marked mobility and tenderness to percussion. Swelling of soft tissue is observed in association with the involved tooth. A slight widening of the periodontal membrane owing to the fast spread and confinement of infection to the medullary region is seen. Based upon the age and amount of bone loss the treatment of choice may be pulpectomy or extraction.

Chronic Alveolar Abscess

Long-standing low-grade infections with draining sinus are clinical features of the non-vital tooth (Fig. 7). Local lymphadenopathy with furcal radiolucency in primary molars, bone loss, or root resorption is observed radiographically with the associated tooth. Based upon the age and amount of bone loss the treatment of choice may be pulpectomy or extraction.

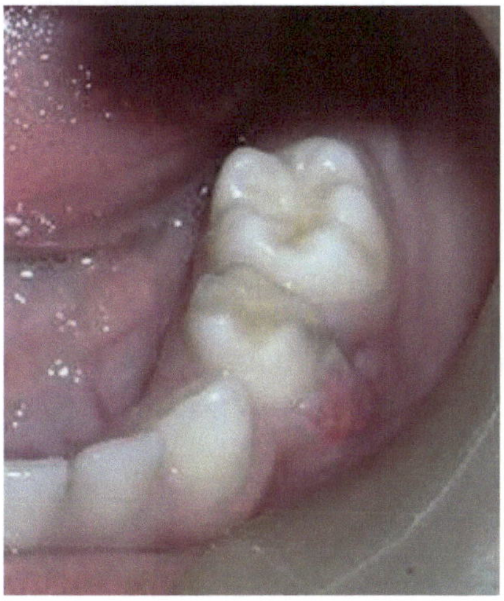

Fig. (7). Chronic Dento-alveolar abscess.

Acute Apical Periodontitis

The first extension of pulpal inflammation into the periradicular tissues is called acute apical periodontitis. Irritants include inflammatory mediators from an irreversibly inflamed pulp or ingress of bacterial toxins from necrotic pulps, chemicals such as irrigants or disinfecting agents, faulty restorations, over instrumentation, and extrusion of obturating materials. The pulp may be inflamed or necrotic.

Moderate to severe spontaneous discomfort along with pain on mastication or occlusal contact are common complaints from patients. In case acute apical periodontitis is an extension of pulpitis, signs, and symptoms will include responsiveness to cold, heat, and electric stimulus. In those cases where acute apical periodontitis is caused by necrosis, teeth do not respond to vitality tests. Excruciating pain is caused by the application of pressure by the fingertip or tapping with the butt end of a mirror handle. Periodontal ligament space widening may be a radiographic feature of acute apical periodontitis. Generally, there is a normal periodontal ligament space and an intact lamina dura [10].

Phoenix Abscess

A phoenix abscess is an acute exacerbation of a chronic periapical lesion. Phoenix abscess can occur immediately following faulty root canal treatment or by untreated chronic apical periodontitis. Phoenix abscess is a painful condition in which the apical portion of a tooth's root becomes inflamed, which may result in swelling and fever. It is an older term, and its use is becoming less common and replaced with descriptive terms like chronic which are suppurative, producing bad taste and halitosis. The treatment for the phoenix abscess is tough as re-root canal therapy is the treatment of choice. In case when re-root canal therapy is not plausible then surgical trephination or extraction of a tooth can be considered.

Condensing Osteitis

[Focal sclerosing osteomyelitis, Focal sclerosing osteitis]

Condensing osteitis is a condition that presents as a localized area of bone sclerosis that forms in response to a low-grade chronic inflammatory stimulus. Clinically, condensing osteitis is occasionally asymptomatic and an area of opaque calcification surrounding the apex of the inflamed tooth is radiographically observed. Treatment requires the elimination of the underlying odontogenic infection, usually by extraction or endodontic therapy. Providing appropriate treatment, there is usually a partial or total resolution of the lesion over time [11].

Prevention of Pulpal Inflammation

To preserve the integrity of the pulp few precautions are to be taken while rendering treatment.

Following are some do's and don'ts:

1. During cavity preparation use of light, intermittent cutting, efficient cooling system, and high rotation speed.

2. Avoid desiccating the dentin and do not over-dry the preparation.

3. Do not apply irritating chemicals to freshly cut dentin.

4. The selection of restorative materials should be carried out carefully taking into consideration the physical and biological properties of the materials.

5. Do not use caustic cavity sterilizing agents.

6. Assuming that all restorative materials will leak, it is mandatory to use a cavity liner or base to seal the exposed dentinal tubules.

7. Do not use excessive force during restoration.

8. Employ polishing procedures that do not subject the pulp to excessive heat.

9. Establish a patient recall system that ensures periodic evaluation of the status of pulp that has undergone injury.

CONCLUSION

Pulpal infections are one of the most common bases of periradicular diseases, as there is an inter-association between pulp and periradicular tissues through numerous foramina of root canals which give rise to inflammatory reactions through the passage of bacterial products and contaminants. It is said that even pulpal infection causes inflammatory changes in the periodontal ligament even before the pulp becomes necrotic. Pain arising from the infected tooth is the most widespread reason why patients seek dental treatment. Pain arises due to diseases involving the pulpal and periradicular tissues, as these tissues are innervated with sufficient blood supply. Also, it is enclosed by surrounding tissues that are incapable of expanding, such as dentin, and has terminal blood flow and a small capillary network at the peri-apical area. These attributes constrain the defensive capacity of the pulp tissue when faced with several other invasions. In addition to the mentioned characteristics, pulp tissue can also be affected by regressive contamination, arising from the secondary canaliculi, periodontal ligament, or the apex during periodontitis, the chapter on diseases of the pulp and peri-radicular tissues concentrates on the classification of pulpal and periradicular diseases and a detailed explanation of them.

CONSENT FOR PUBLICATION

Not applicable.

CONFLICT OF INTEREST

The authors declare no conflict of interest, financial or otherwise.

ACKNOWLEDGEMENT

Declared none.

REFERENCES

[1] Suresh Chandra B, Gopikrishna V. Grossman's Endodontics Practice. 2018; 1-229.

[2] IlanRotstein John I. Ingle. Ingle's Endodontics 7. PMPH USA. Ltd 2017; 1: 1-336.

[3] World Health Organization Application of the international classification of diseases to dentistry and stomatology. 1995.

[4] Abbott PV, Yu C. A clinical classification of the status of the pulp and the root canal system. Aust Dent J 2007; 52(1) (Suppl.): S17-31. [http://dx.doi.org/10.1111/j.1834-7819.2007.tb00522.x] [PMID: 17546859]

[5] Kenneth M, Hargreaves , Louis H Berman. Cohen's Pathways of pulp. 2016; 27-30.

[6] Ali SG, Mulay S. Pulpitis: A review. IOSR J Dent Med Sci 2015; 14(8): 92-7.

[7] Patel N, Vachhani K, Bagda K, Attur K, Desai D, Patel Z. Internal Resorption: An Endodontic Dogma: A Case Report. Int J Adv Res (Indore) 2018; 6(3): 945-50. [http://dx.doi.org/10.21474/IJAR01/6752]

[8] Thomas P, Krishna Pillai R, Pushparajan Ramakrishnan B, Palani J. An insight into internal resorption. ISRN Dent 2014; 2014: 1-7. [http://dx.doi.org/10.1155/2014/759326] [PMID: 24944822]

[9] Goga R, Chandler NP, Oginni AO. Pulp stones: a review. Int Endod J 2008; 41(6): 457-68. [http://dx.doi.org/10.1111/j.1365-2591.2008.01374.x] [PMID: 18422587]

[10] Richard E Walton, Torabinejad Mahmoud. Principles and practice of Endodontics. 2002.

[11] Neville BW, Damm DD, Allen CM, Angela CC. Pulp and Periapical Disease. Colour Atlas of Oral and Maxillofacial Diseases. Elsevier Inc. 2019; pp. 79-92.

CHAPTER 4

Diagnoses of Pulp Pathoses in Children and Investigations

Rajesh Anegundi[1,*], **Dhanashree Sakhare**[2] and **Parag Kasar**[3]

[1] *Pediatric Dentistry, SDM College of Dental Sciences, Dharwad, Karnatakan, India*

[2] *Founder Lavanika Dental Academy, Melbourne, Australia*

[3] *Pediatric Dental Consultant, Deep Clinic Nerul, Navi Mumbai, India*

Abstract: A correct finding of the ailment of the pulp in teeth conceded by caries, dental processes or other forms of injury is vital for arriving at a proper conclusion for the treatment. Essential evidence in this respect is whether the pulp is vital or necrotic. It is similarly important to be able to ascertain whether the pulp is reversibly or irreversibly inflamed, mainly in connection with a carious or traumatic exposure of the tissue. In other words, can the pulp heal and continue in a long□term perception or is it scratched to the extent that it is not curable, and is a root canal treatment required? Diagnostic information is gained from the patient's history of pain or irritation, the experience of trauma or restorative techniques, clinical examinations, results of clinical tests and radiographic assessment of the teeth and the surrounding tissues. A diagnosis is rarely based on a single finding, but rather on a set of reflections. The clinical condition may be so complex that a proper diagnosis and treatment outcome requires a diagnostic process comprising several steps

Keywords: Clinical, History, Pathosis, Pulp, Radiograph.

INTRODUCTION

The chief complaint is generally the first information to be obtained. It is expressed in the patient's own words describing the condition that prompted him or her to seek treatment. The chief complaint is recorded in non-technical language. The children are sometimes able to tell and describe the condition but there are times when the chief complaint has to be obtained from the parent or an accompanying person when the child is very young and unable to describe the complaint or in a medically and physically challenged child.

* **Corresponding author Rajesh Anegundi:** Pediatric Dentistry, SDM College of Dental Sciences, Dharwad, Karnataka, India; E-mail: rajroopa2@yahoo.co.in

Correct treatment begins with a correct diagnosis. Arriving at an accurate diagnosis requires knowledge, skills, and art; the knowledge of identifying the diseases from their signs and symptoms, skills to apply proper test procedures, the art of synthesizing impressions, facts, and experience into understanding. To arrive at an accurate diagnosis of pulp status, histological evaluation is practically impossible therefore clinicians should co-relate history, examination, and diagnostic tests together.

Misdiagnosis implies the inability to derive the correct diagnosis with resultant incorrect treatment and mistrust between the patient and dentist. To avoid misdiagnosis and to rule out orofacial pain of non-pulpal or peri-radicular origin, a step-by-step systematic approach to diagnosis and treatment planning must be followed.

Symptoms and signs of pulpal diseases are snippets of information that allow the clinician to paint an entire picture of the pulpal condition. Symptoms refer to the information that the patient or their relatives can relay and explain to the health worker while signs are elicited by the operating dental surgeon to help in diagnosing the disease.

HISTORY AND RECORD

To avoid irrelevant information and to prevent errors of omission and clinical tests, the clinician must practice a fixed routine for examination protocol. Thus, the criteria for an accurate clinical diagnosis are that the clinician should include a good case history, a thorough clinical examination, relevant investigations, or diagnostic tests.

Demographic Data

The demographic data includes the name, age, and gender of the patient. Education level, socioeconomic status, address, contact number, religion, birth date, and registration details like case paper number should also be included. In the case of children, additional details like the nickname, name of the school, friends and teachers should also be recorded to help in initiating conversations with the child and make the child more comfortable. Whenever possible, the child's hobbies, favorite cartoons, TV shows, likes and interests should also be recorded to maintain a fluent conversation during the child's visits.

Medical History

Detailed comprehensive medical history is an absolute necessity before the commencement of any dental treatment. Any present or previous medical history the clinician can determine, whether medical consultation or premedication, is required before diagnostic examination or clinical treatment is undertaken. The dentist should be aware of the maledictions that the patient is following to avoid any adverse drug reaction and to understand the patient's susceptibility and reaction to infection and bleeding. This will help in understating the patient's susceptibility and reactions to infection and bleeding.

Dental History

Understating the patient's attitudes toward oral health, care and treatment can be assessed by recording the dental history. Dental history reveals past dental experience and clues to the patient's psychological makeup as well as explains subtle clinical findings.

Clinical Diagnostic Examination

In the diagnosis of pulpal pathology, the clinical diagnostic method includes a subjective and objective examination. Subjective symptoms are those explained by the patient himself or herself.

Pain [1]

One of the first main complaints from the patient is pain and it must be recorded carefully as it plays an important role in diagnosing pulpal or peri radicular pathology. Intensity, spontaneity, and persistent nature of pain are strongly indicative of pulpal and/or peri radicular pathosis. The pain of high intensity is usually intermittent, whereas low-intensity pain is often continuous and protracted. Spontaneous pain occurs without an eliciting stimulus. It awakens the patient or begins without stimulus; it is spontaneously combined with intense pain usually indicating severe pulpal and/or peri radicular pathosis. Persistent type of pain is of a lingering type that continues evenly and increases in intensity after the stimulus is removed. Pain can be of non-dental origin, periodontal origin, or dental origin.

Non-dental pain is of systemic conditions like trigeminal neuralgia, acoustic neuroma, herpes zoster, diabetic odontalgia and myocardial infarction, which present infrequently in the dental office. However, the pain of atypical facial neuralgia is most frequently referred by physicians to dentists for consultation and creates a diagnostic problem when deep fillings are present. Periodontal pain is usually due to periodontal disease. There can be a rather large amount of bone loss without any pain as pus can usually drain out of a periodontal pocket so press ure does not build up. If periodontal inflammation progresses deeper down into the bone, pus may not be able to drain, leading to the development of pain.

Dental Pain

The clinician should ask the patient the following kinds of pain that the patient is having.

a. The kind/type of pain,
b. Location of the pain,
c. Duration of the pain,
d. What causes the pain?
e. What alleviates the pain?
f. Whether the pain is referred to another site or not

The patient explains the pulpal pain generally in one of two ways. The sharp, piercing and lancinating pain is due to the excitation of the A-delta nerve fibres (myelinated principal sensory fibres) in the pulp. This pain may reflect on a reversible or acute state of pulpitis. The dull, boring, and gnawing pain is due to excitation and a slower rate of transmission of the unmyelinated C nerve fibres. This type of pain is usually associated with an irreversible and often chronic state of pulpitis. Determining the category of pain is an important tool in diagnosing pulpal diseases.

Duration of Pain

The duration of pain is another feature that helps in finding out the pulpal condition. Duration of pain needs to be recorded at the time since the onset of symptoms and the duration of pain in relation to the stimulus. Pulpal pain may last only if an irritant is present or at other times pain may last for minutes to hours.

Localization of Pain

The ability to localize the pain is important. Pain is localized when the patient can point to a specific tooth or site with assurance and speed and reproducibility when asked to do so.

Referred Pain

Referred pain implies that the pain is referred to other areas and even beyond the mouth. Most commonly it is manifested in other teeth within the same or the opposing quadrant. Patients may report that their dental pain is exacerbated by lying down or bending over. This occurs because of the increase in blood pressure to the head, which increases the pressure on the confined nerves located in the enclosed pulp chamber.

Swelling

Swelling may be present intraorally restricted to the infected tooth or extra orally as cellulitis caused by the inflammatory exudates associated with a pulpally affected tooth. Locations like buccal fascial planes, and the submandibular region are commonly involved due to mandibular teeth. In the maxillary arch, swelling can spread in the buccal or periorbital space.

Examination

The clinical procedures performed to examine the status of the pulp and peri-radicular tissues are as follows:

1. Visual and tactile inspection
2. Percussion
3. Palpation
4. Mobility and depressibility
5. Periodontal examination
6. Anesthesia test
7. Occlusal pressure test
8. Gutta-percha point tracing
9. Transillumination
10. Staining
11. Radiographs
12. Vitality tests
13. Sensibility tests

The other Methods are

1. Xeroradiography
2. ComputerizedTomography
3. Magnetic resonance imaging.
4. Radiovisiography
5. Computerized expert system
6. Digital subtraction radiography
7. Dual-wavelength spectrophotometry.
8. Ultrasound.
9. Infrared Thermographicimaging.
10. Tuned aperture computed tomography
11. Dental operating microscope
12. Xenonradioisotope
13. Photoplethysmography

Visual and Tactile Inspection

The visual and tactile examination is a common procedure routinely done. A thorough visual and tactile examination depends on checking the colour, contour and consistency.

In the case of soft tissues any deviation from the healthy *i.e.*, pink colour is readily recognized when inflammation is present. A change in contour occurs when there's swelling. Similarly, an alteration inconsistency from normal, healthy firm tissue to that of a soft, fluctuant, or spongy tissue indicates a pathologic condition. The dental hard tissues should be visually examined after thoroughly cleaning any food debris and drying the tooth. Teeth that are discoloured, opaque and less lifelike in appearance should be carefully evaluated. Discolouration of teeth indicates the pulp may already be inflamed, degenerated or necrotic. Not all discoloured teeth will require endodontic treatment as staining may be caused by old amalgam restorations, root canal filling materials and medicaments or systemic medication, such as tetracycline staining. Many discolourations however are the result of disease commonly associated with necrotic and gangrenous pulp, internal or external resorption, and carious exposure.

Crown contours should be examined for cracks, fractures, wear facets and restorations. Consistency of the hard tissue relates to the presence of caries and internal or external resorption. The technique of visual and tactile examination is straightforward. It can be done with one's fingers, eyes, an explorer, and a periodontal probe. The patient's teeth and periodontium should be examined in good light under dry conditions. A sinus tract (fistula) might escape detection if it is covered by saliva or an interproximal cavity may escape notice if it is filled with food debris.

The visual examination should include the soft tissue adjacent to the involved tooth, for detection of swelling. The periodontal probe should be used routinely to determine the periodontal status of the suspected tooth and adjacent teeth. Sinus tracts opening into the gingival crevice or deep infrabony pockets may go overlooked because of failure to use the periodontal probe. The crown of the tooth should be carefully evaluated, to determine whether it can be restored properly after any previous restorations.

Palpation

Palpation refers to the firm pressure that is applied on the mucosa overlying the apex by a fingertip to examine tissue consistency and pain response. A positive response to palpation indicates periradicular inflammation. The pain is primarily due to the extension of inflammation of the coronal pulp tissue that is engaging the mesencephalic Ruffini nerve fibres. These are located at the periapical-third of the root. Pain or tenderness on palpation is important for arriving at a diagnosis and for proper treatment planning.

Percussion

The percussion test helps the clinician to determine the condition of the periodontal tissues surrounding a tooth. In percussion, the crown of a tooth is gently tapped with the end of a blunt instrument to ascertain whether the tooth is tender or not. A painful response to percussion denotes inflammation of the periodontal membrane. Observing the child's response by watching the eye reflexes are indicative of perceived pain. The painful response differs when an adjacent tooth is percussed. Although percussion may be a simple method of testing, it may be misleading if used alone. In performing the test, several teeth are percussed in a random order to eliminate bias on the part of the patient (Fig. **1**). Pain following percussion is usually an indication of inflammation of the periodontal ligament that may arise due to inflammatory exudate or bacterial exotoxins leaching from the apical foramen, presence of abscess or trauma to the periodontal ligament.

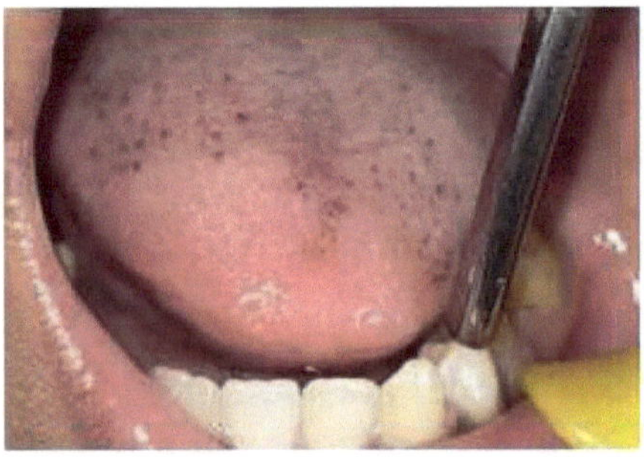

Fig. (1). Tenderness is checked in the vertical and horizontal direction by firmly tapping the tooth with a blunt instrument.

Mobility-Depressibility Testing

The mobility test is performed to evaluate the integrity of the attachment apparatus surrounding the tooth. The test consists of moving a tooth laterally in its socket by using the handles of two instruments. The objective of this test is to determine whether the tooth is firm or loosely attached to its alveolus. The amount of movement is indicative of the condition of the periodontium, the greater the movement poorer the periodontal status. Similarly, the test for depressibility involves the movement of a tooth vertically in its socket. This test may be performed with an instrument. The presence of depressibility indicates that the possibilities for retaining the tooth are questionable. Mobilometers are electronic devices that aid in determining tooth mobility. The apparatus essentially consists of two electrodes or prongs which hold the facial and lingual surface of the teeth. The degree of mobility tested is then reflected as a numerical reading either on the instrument itself or an attached computer screen. Mobility in a primary tooth may result from physiological or pathological causes. Fig. (**2**) Radiographic evaluation of the remaining root of a primary tooth, the crown position, and the amount of root formation of the underlying permanent successor will determine whether the mobility is physiological or pathological.

Periodontal Examination

A dental examination is incomplete without careful evaluation of the periodontal support. The periodontal probe should be an integral part of all endodontic tray setups. Using a periodontal probe, the clinician examines the gingival sulcus and records the depths of all pockets. Multirooted teeth are carefully probed to determine whether there's any furcation involvement. A lateral canal exposed to the oral cavity by periodontal disease may become the portal of entry for toxins that cause pulpal degeneration. To distinguish lesions of periodontal origin from those of pulpal origin, thermal and electric pulp tests, along with periodontal examination are essential.

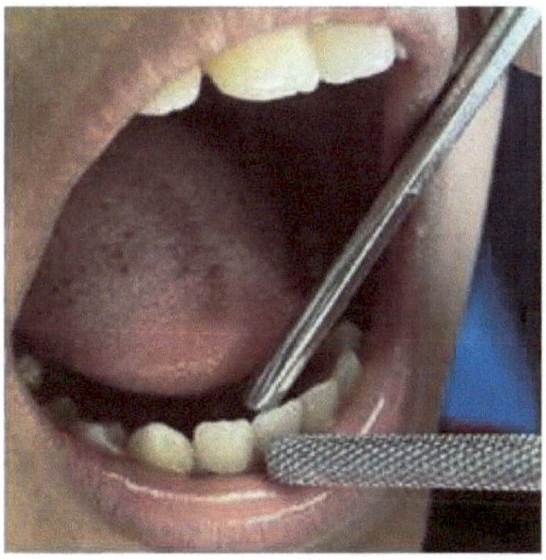

Fig. (2). Mobility should be checked with two blunt instruments.

Palpation, percussion, mobility, depressibility and probing, test the integrity of the tooth-supporting structures and are not diagnostic when the disease is confined within the pulp cavity.

Anesthetic Testing

An anaesthetic test is performed when there is a diffuse strong pain of vague origin at the time of the test when all other tests have failed. The objective of anaesthetic testing is anaesthetizing a single tooth at a time until the pain disappears and is localized to a specific tooth. An anaesthetic test is performed by infiltration or intra-ligament injection and injecting the foremost most posterior tooth within the area suspected of being the cause for pain. If pain persists, when the tooth has been fully anaesthetized, the next tooth mesial to it is anaesthetized and it is continued until the pain disappears. If the source of the pain cannot be determined if it is in maxillary or mandibular teeth, then an inferior alveolar nerve block should be given. Cessation of pain naturally indicates involvement of a mandibular tooth and localization of the specific tooth is done by the intraligament injection when the anaesthetic has spent itself. This test may be a last resort and has a plus over the test cavity during which iatrogenic damage is possible.

Occlusal Pressure or Biting Test

A clinical test that simulates the chief complaint is the occlusal pressure test or biting test. Orangewood stick, Burlew rubber disc, and Wet cotton rolls are used to perform an occlusal pressure test. An interesting clinical observation in patients with tooth infractions or cracked tooth syndrome is that the pain is often experienced when biting force is released rather than during the downward chewing motion [2].

Gutta-Percha PointTracing

It involves the placement of a gutta-percha point through the sinus or fistulous tract followed by a radiograph. This will help in localizing the endodontic lesion to the specific tooth. This test also aids in the differential diagnosis between a periodontal and an endodontic lesion.

Transillumination & Magnification Test

Fiberoptic lighting and chair side magnification tests are good enough in searching the cracks, fractures, unfound canals, proximal lesions, and obstructions in the root canal [3], (Fig. **3**). Loss of translucency, light colour changes and cracks may not be apparent in poor light, in such cases, a transilluminator may aid in detecting enamel or crown cracks (Fig. **4**).

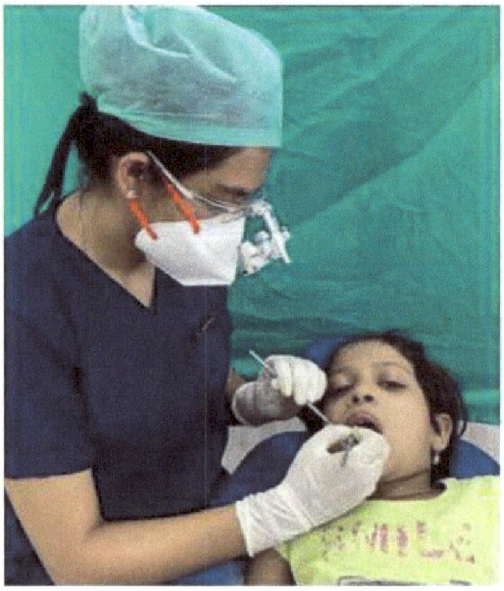

Fig. (3). Magnification with loupes.

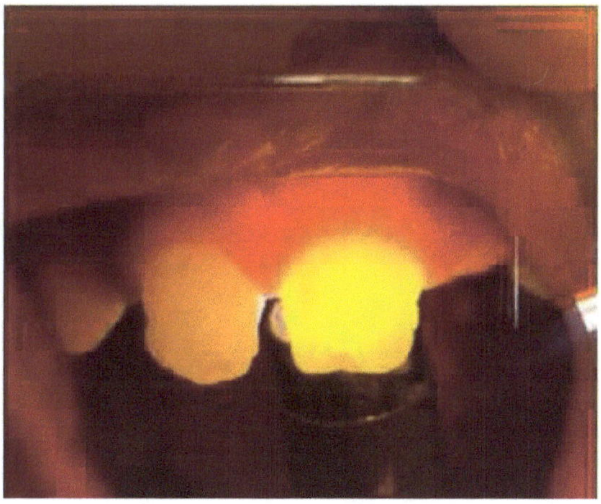

Fig. (4). Transillumination.

Staining Test

A staining test is used for the identification of a cracked tooth. We remove the filling from the suspected tooth and place 2% iodine dye or disclosing tablet or any staining dye in the cavity preparation. The fracture lines can be identified with food colouring placed on the dried occlusal surface.

Radiographs

After the clinical examination, radiographs of good quality are essential in making a diagnosis. Visual examination of the oral structures that would otherwise be unseen by the naked eye. Recent pre-operative radiographs are prerequisites for pulp therapy in primary and young permanent teeth. Besides providing information on the child's dental development, they may demonstrate pathological entities, which contraindicate some forms of pulp therapy or indicate failed treatment. The radiograph is a two-dimensional image of a three-dimensional object and sometimes misinterpretation is a constant risk. To utilize radiographs properly, the clinician must have the knowledge and skill necessary to interpret them correctly. A thorough understanding of the underlying normal or abnormal pathosis and the changes that can occur due to ageing, trauma, disease, and healing is required.

Radiographs can contain information on:

1. The extent of dental caries

2. The number shape, course, width, and length of the root canals.

3. Calcification changes in pulp chambers and root canals.

4. Incompletely formed roots with immature apices

5. Signs of internal and external root resorption

6. Widening of the periodontal ligament space and thickening of lamina dura.

7. Bone resorption.

8. Radiolucencies in periapical areas.

9. Previous Pulpal treatment.

10. Trauma.

11. Root fractures.

12. Displacement of teeth.

12. Pulp vitality and sensibility test Vitality tests.

There is a lot of uncertainty regarding the use of terminology vitality test. Vitality means that blood supply is present within the tissues. Hence only a test that measures or assesses pulp blood flow can be called a vitality test. Vitality tests are also sometimes called blood flow determination.

1. Pulse oximetry

2. Laser doppler flowmetry.

Sensibility Tests

The tests which assess the pulpal nerve fibre's response to a stimulus are called sensibility tests. Sensibility tests are used to determine whether a pulp is likely to be responsive or not [4]. Commonly used tests are:

1. Thermal tests

2. Electric pulp test

3. Test cavity

The pulp vitality and sensibility tests have a little value in primary teeth as they might indicate pulp vitality. The response does not identify the degree of pathoses present. The patient may give a response that they feel is correct rather than an accurate one. In permanent teeth, these tests can be performed and comparisons can be made with normal teeth.

Cold Test

The cold test works on the principle of hydrodynamic theory [5]. It causes contraction of dentinal fluid within the dentinal tubules, which can cause rapid outward movement of fluid within the tubules. This movement of dentinal fluid leads to hydrodynamic forces that act on nerve fibres and is responsible for sharp sensation in the pulp. To perform the cold testing, the teeth must remain isolated and dry. 15 seconds interval application of cold is preferred to get a good response from the patient. The cold test is more effective on anterior teeth than on multi-rooted posterior teeth. A false-negative response is often expected when cold is applied to teeth with constricted canals due to calcific metamorphosis. A false-positive response may result if cold water contacts gingival tissue or is transferred to adjacent teeth with vital pulps multi-rooted teeth [4].

The most common techniques for cold test

1. Stream of cold air test

2. Regular ice

3. Carbon dioxide (dry ice)

4. Compressed gases

5. Dichloro-difluoromethane [DDM]

6. Ethyl chloride

Stream of Cold Air Test

A stream of cold air from a 3-way syringe is directed against the crown of a previously dried tooth and also at the gingival margin. It is not very specific as the air stream cannot be directed towards individual teeth separately.

Sticks of Ice

After the tooth is isolated with cotton rolls and dried, an ice stick is applied to the facial surface of the tooth. This stimulus applied over a vital pulp usually results in sharp, brief pain regardless of pulp status (normal or reversible or irreversible pulpitis). However, an intense and prolonged response usually indicates irreversible pulpitis. In contrast, necrotic pulps don't respond.

Carbon Dioxide Test [6, 7]

Carbon dioxide snow in the form of dry ice has been used for the application of cold to teeth. (Fig. **5**). The use of dry ice is more effective and reliable even in immature teeth it produces lower intrapulpal temperatures than other methods. This test is even reliable in immature teeth.

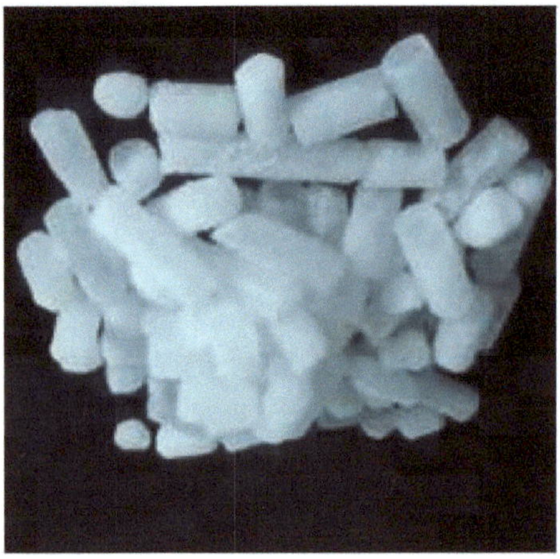

Fig. (5). Dry ice.

Ethyl Chloride Spray Test

In this test, ethyl chloride is sprayed copiously on a cotton pellet and held against the middle 3rd of the facial surface. A positive response indicates pulp vitality in a tooth whose pulp is normal or abnormal. This ethyl chloride evaporates rapidly by absorbing heat and cooling the tooth surface. Ethyl chloride is effective even on teeth covered with cast metal crowns (Fig. **6**).

Thermal Testing

One of the most common symptoms associated with a symptomatic inflamed pulp is pain induced by hot or cold stimulation [2]. The thermal test can be performed using different techniques. The different thermal test is heat test and cold test. Response to cold indicates a vital pulp, regardless of whether that pulp is normal or inflamed [4]. An abnormal response to heat usually indicates the presence of a pulpal disorder indicating the need for endodontic treatment. Long thermal test results should be correlated with other clinical examinations. Thermal tests are usually not conducted on primary teeth because of their unreliability to respond. In children, it is difficult to assess pulp status by heat or cold due to fear and anxiety which can give false readings. Secondly, the heat might damage the pulp, since pulp horns are highly placed in deciduous teeth and if the kid is uncooperative the heat might cause injury to the soft tissue. In heat test, initially, A-fibrcs are stimulated leading to sharp localized pain and with continuous stimulation, C fibres are activated causing a dull radiating pain. Heat test duration should be limited to not more than 5 seconds as damage to the pulp tissues can be expected.

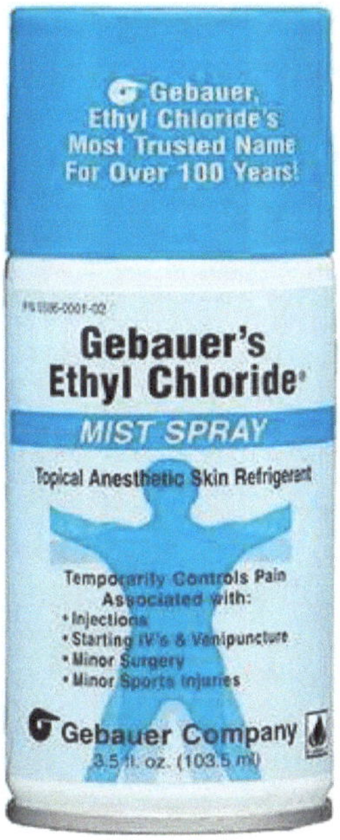

Fig. (6). Ethyl chloride spray.

The Technique of Performing Thermal Tests

The heat test is often performed using different techniques that deliver different degrees of temperature. The preferred temperature for performing a heat test is 65.5°C/150° F. various modes of application of heat have been listed:

1. Hot burnisher or flame heated instrument.

2. Hot Gutta-percha stick.

3. Hot water bath

4. Hot airblast

5. Polishing of crown with dry rubber cups.

6. Touch-n-Heat test.

Before testing, the patient should be told what tests are going to be performed and the reason. Additionally, the patient should be explained what is to be expected. The tests should be first performed on teeth that are to be used as controls *i.e.*, corresponding or the opposite side of the same arch. By doing so, the patient gets an idea of how the tests will feel. The clinician should also inform the patient how to respond when a sensation is experienced, for example, the patient should be instructed to raise a hand as soon as any sensation is felt. When heat or cold tests are performed on an interior tooth the medium should be placed on the middle of the third of the labial surface and posterior teeth should be on the occlusal third of the buccal surface. However, placing the stimulus on exposed dentin should be avoided because an accelerated or exaggerated response can be expected. Also, the stimulus should not be applied against restorations unless the enamel surface is unavailable. Nonmetallic restorations are poor conductors so tests give a delayed response or no response and the same way metallic restorations are good conductors. The teeth in the quadrant must first be isolated and then dried with 2x2 inch gauze and a saliva ejector placed. When a response occurs, the heat should be removed immediately. Care should be taken to avoid using excessive heat or prolonged application of heat to the tooth.

Responses to Thermal Tests

The patient's responses to heat and cold testing are identical because the neural fibres in the pulp transmit only the sensation of pain according to the hydrodynamic theory which is proposed by Brannstrom [6].

Electric Pulp Testing

The electric pulp test is more accurate than some of the other tests used to determine pulp vitality. Historically the electric pulp tester has been used in dentistry since asearlyas1867and has evolved over the years into the present digital electronic

pulp tester. It is a valuable tool for diagnosis because not only does it help the clinician in determining pulp vitality but also aids in thermal and periodontal tests in differentiating radiographic signs of pulpal, periodontal, or non-odontogenic causes. The electric pulp tester is designed to stimulate a response by electrical excitation of the neural elements within the pulp. A positive response is an indication of vitality and helps in determining the status of the pulp. No response to the electrical stimulus can be an indication of pulp necrosis indicating the need for clinical procedures like pulpectomy or root canal treatment. In children, the response from the electric pulp test is not reliable since the complete development of the plexus of Raschkow does not occur until the final stages of root development [8]. For children with a history of trauma where root formation is not complete, an electric pulp test may not show any response as the pulp may be in a state of shock (Fig. 7).

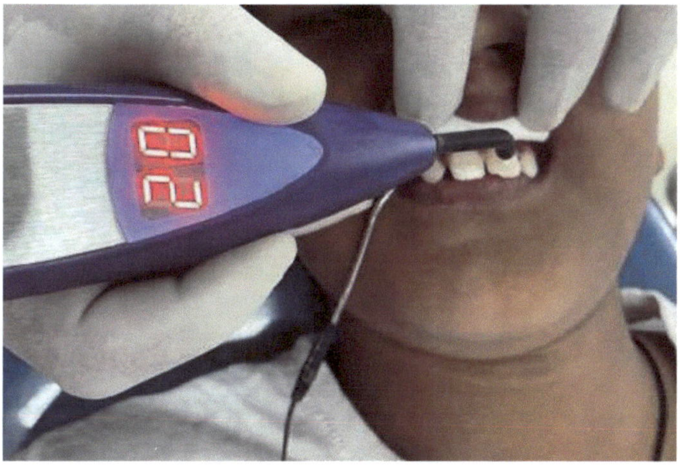

Fig. (7). Electric pulp tester.

Technique

Describe the test to the patient in a way that will reduce anxiety and will eliminate a biased response. To eliminate a biased decision, an electric pulp tester should first be performed on a normal healthy tooth adjacent or contralateral. This aids in determining the patients' threshold level. It is very important to clean, dry, and isolate the teeth. Clean the surface of the tooth and isolate it with a cotton roll, saliva ejector and thoroughly dry with the air syringe. A small amount of conductive gel is placed on the electrode. An electrical circuit is established by using a lip clip or having the patient touch the metal handle. The electrode is placed on the facial or lingual surface, and the level of current is gradually increased until it surpasses the perception threshold. The sensation may be tingling, stinging, full or hot or pain. Patients should be instructed to raise a hand as soon as they begin to feel slight tingling or sensation. Record the result according to the numeric scale on the pulp tester. Each tooth should be tested 2 or 3 times and the reading averaged.

Factors Affecting the Level of Response

Enamel thickness: Thicker the enamel, the more delayed the response. Thin anterior teeth respond faster and broad posterior teeth show slower response because of the greater thickness of enamel and dentin.

Probe placement on the tooth: Placing the probe on the occlusal third of posterior teeth and the incisal third of anterior teeth may help in limiting false stimulation of gingival tissue. Others include dentin calcification, restoration, and presence of enamel defects and the patient's level of anxiety.

Advantages of Electric Pulp Tester

1. The intensity of the stimulus is comfortable for the patients.

2. The digital display of many electric pulp testers provides instant, easy and reliable information.

3. In some electric pulp testers, a red indicator light flashes on and off when a maximum stimulus is reached.

4. Gives a quantitative reading which can be compared with the reading of the control tooth and during the follow-up visits.

Disadvantages of Electric Pulp Tester

1. It cannot be used on patients having cardiac pacemakers because of potential interference with the pacemaker.

2. Some electric pulp testers are very expensive.

3. Electric pulp tester is not useful on recently erupted teeth with immature apex.

4. Recently traumatized teeth cannot be tested.

5. No indication is given regarding the state of vascular supply which would give a more reliable measure of the vitality of the pulp.

6. Readings from posterior teeth with partial vital pulps may be misleading because in multi-rooted teeth one canal may have vital pulp tissue and other canals necrotic tissue.

7. Electrical testers do not measure the degree of health or disease of a pulp.

Limitations of Pulp Testing

False reading from the electric pulp tester could be misleading and this could be a false-positive response or a false-negative response. The false-positive response means the pulp is necrotic but the patient nevertheless the patient signals that he experiences sensation. The false-negative response means the pulp is vital but the patient appears unresponsive to electric pulp tests.

False-positive Results

Non-vital teeth sometimes give a false-positive response. Anxious young patients give premature responses as anticipation of unpleasant sensations. In multi-rooted teeth, necrotic breakdown in one root canal can conduct electric signals and mislead pulpal response. Contact with the larger metal restoration like bridge, acrylic, ceramic, or class II restoration and gingival allow the current to reach the attachment apparatus. Liquefaction necrosis may conduct current to the attachment apparatus and the patient may slowly raise his hand near the highest range. Failure to isolate and dry the teeth properly before attempting to test also gives a false-positive result.

False-negative Result

The false-negative results may be due to inadequate contact between electrode and enamel. The dental trauma, calcification, partial necrosis, incomplete root development, patients with high pain threshold, and psychotic disorder may cause false-negative results. Patient heavily pre-medicated with analgesics, narcotics, alcohol, or tranquillizers can also result in the same. Non-working batteries or forgetting to turn on the pulp tester may also show a false-negative response.

Types of Pulp Testers

Two types of electric pulp tester are available.

I. 1) Current is varied

2) Voltage is varied

II. 1) Monopolar

2) Bipolar

Commercially Available Testers are
Analytic technology pulp tester Digilog pulp tester Greenwood pulp tester Pelton crane pulp tester Parkell pulp tester (battery operated)

Test Cavity

This method allows one to determine pulp vitality. This method is performed when other diagnostic methods have not yielded satisfactory results and as a last.

The test cavity is made by drilling through the enamel-dentin junction of an un-anaesthetized tooth. The drilling should be done at a slow speed using a small round bur and without a water coolant. Sensitivity or quick sharp pain felt by the patient is an indication of pulp vitality and no endodontic treatment is indicated. Sedative cement is then placed in the cavity, and the search for the source of pain continues. If no pain is felt, cavity preparation may be continued until the pulp chamber is reached. If the pulp is completely necrotic, endodontic treatment can be continued painlessly in many cases without anaesthesia [2].

Other Methods of Pulp Diagnosis Radiovisiography [9]

Radiovisiography digitizes ionizing radiation and provides an instantaneous image on a monitor thereby reducing radiation exposure by 80% and the need for harmful chemicals for processing of the films. Advantages of

Radiovisiography include the elimination of X-ray film, significant reduction in exposure time and instantaneous image display.

Xeroradiograph

Xeroradiograph is another new dental radiographic technique where an x-ray is exposed with a conventional x-ray machine. The advantages of this include less radiation than conventional, x-rays, and can be delivered as a dry or laminated permanent copy. Compared to conventional xeroradiography shows images of sharper clarity and finer detail [9].

Pulse Oximetry Test Pulse Oximetry

Direct measurement of pulp circulation is the only real measure of pulp vitality. Pulse oximetry tests are based on the passage of light through a tooth and have been considered as a possible means of detecting pulp vitality with greater objectivity requiring no subjective response from the patient. The pulse oximeter is a non-invasive oxygen saturation monitor that provides continuous pulse rate readings. The liquid crystal display gives oxygen saturation, pulse rate and plethysmographic waveform readings. Pulse oximetry uses red light and infrared wavelength to transilluminate a tissue bed and detect absorbance peaks due to pulsative circulation. This information is used to calculate the pulse rate and oxygen saturation. These characteristics infer that the pulse oximeter is also capable of evaluating the blood vasculature status within a tooth and therefore pulp vitality. The tooth to be tested is sandwiched between a photoelectric detector and red and infrared light-emitting diodes. This method is superior to other vitality tests since it does not rely upon sensory nerve response.

Dual-wavelength Spectrophotometry

Dual-wavelength spectrophotometry is a method that detects the presence or absence of oxygenated blood at 760 and 850 nm in pulsatile circulation; it is a non-invasive, inexpensive method and does not rely on subjective patient response and results in objective observations. The limitation is that it detects only the presence of haemoglobin not the circulation of blood [10].

Photoplethysmography

Photoplethysmography is another noninvasive diagnostic tool to detect vascularity within the dental pulp. This method is advantageous due to less signal contamination derived from periodontal blood flow and also less signal noise.

Laser Doppler Flowmetry [11]

The drawbacks of electric pulp testing lead to the development of newer methods. A method that determines and registers the blood flow rather than the neural response was preferred. Laser doppler flowmetry was thus introduced first in 1972 to determine blood flow in the retina of rabbits by Ross and Benedek as a non-invasive method to measure blood flow. The crux of the laser doppler flowmetry is based on the detection of movement of blood cells in the pulpal blood vessels giving a true picture regarding pulp vitality. The advantages of laser doppler flowmetry are non-invasive, easy to apply, providing a continuous record, demonstrating the establishment of the vitality of teeth and the detected output signal can be fed onto an analogue printer. The disadvantages are the inability to calibrate the readings in absolute units and output may not be linearly related to blood flow.

Computerized Tomography (CT)

Computed tomography was introduced in the mid-1970s. Computed tomographic systems are also referred to as computed axial tomography scanners (CAT). Observation of structures that are difficult to visualize with conventional x-rays can be visualized with computerized tomography and thus providing a 3-dimensional image of roots, root canals and teeth. Computerized tomography is expensive requires a larger dose of radiation and time.

One cannot depend solely on the diagnostic tests to arrive at a diagnosis. The clinician's knowledge, skill and art combined with these diagnostic tests will help one to make the right diagnosis and treatment plan.

CONCLUSION

Dental pulp tests are investigations that offer valuable diagnostic and treatment planning information to the dental clinician. If pathosis is present, pulp testing joint with information taken from the history, examination, and other investigations such as radiographs leads to the diagnosis of the underlying disease which can usually be reached easily. Dental pulp testing is a beneficial and essential diagnostic aid in Pediatric Dentistry. Pulp sensibility tests include thermal and electric tests, which extrapolate pulp health from the sensory response. Whilst pulp sensibility tests are the most used in clinical practice, they are not without limitations and shortcomings. Pulp vitality tests attempt to examine the presence of pulp blood flow, as this is perceived as a better measure of true health than sensibility. Laser Doppler flowmetry and pulse oximetry are examples of vitality tests. Whilst the prospect is encouraging, there are still many practical issues that need to be addressed before vitality tests can replace sensibility tests as the standard clinical pulp diagnostic test. In this chapter, the stress is laid on careful interpretation and close monitoring as false results can lead to misdiagnosis which can then lead to incorrect, inappropriate, or unnecessary treatment.

CONSENT FOR PUBLICATION

Not applicable.

CONFLICT OF INTEREST

The authors declare no conflict of interest, financial or otherwise.

ACKNOWLEDGEMENT

Declared none.

REFERENCES

[1] Suresh Chandra B, Gopikrishna V. Grossman's Endodontics Practice. 13th ed. Wolters Kluwer 2018; pp. 1-229.

[2] Ingle JI, Bakland LK. Endodontic Diagnostic procedures.Endodontics. 5th ed. Hamilton, London: BC Decker Inc 2003; pp. 203-58.

[3] Robeson TM, Heymann HO, Swift EJ. Sturdevant's Art and Science of Operative Dentistry. India: Elsevier Science Health Science Div 2006; p. 1040.

[4] Cohen S, Hargreaves KM. Pathways of pulp. In: Louis St, Mosby , Eds. Elsevier's publication 2006.

[5] Brannstrom M. The hydrodynamics of the dental tubule and pulp fluid: its significance in relation to dentinal sensitivity. In: Proceedings of the Annual Meeting of the American Institute of Oral Biology.

[6] Pantera EA Jr, Anderson RW, Pantera CT. Reliability of electric pulp testing after pulpal testing with dichlorodifluoromethane. J Endod 1993; 19(6): 312-4. [http://dx.doi.org/10.1016/S0099-2399(06)80463-2] [PMID: 8228753]

[7] Ehrmann EH. Pulp testers and pulp testing with particular reference to the use of dry ice. Aust Dent J 1977; 22(4): 272-9. [http://dx.doi.org/10.1111/j.1834-7819.1977.tb04511.x] [PMID: 277144]

[8] R G, Gopakumar M. Diagnostic Aids in Pediatric Dentistry. Int J Clin Pediatr Dent 2011; 4(1): 1-7. [http://dx.doi.org/10.5005/jp-journals-10005-1073] [PMID: 27616851]

[9] Van der Stelt PF. Better Imaging: the advantages of digital radiography. J Am Dent Assoc 2021; 7S-13S.

[10] Ingle IJ, Bakland LK, Baumgartner JC. Endodontics. 6th ed. Hamilton, London: BC Decker Inc 2008; p. 1555.

[11] Olgart L, Gazelius B, Lindh-Strömberg U. Laser Doppler flowmetry in assessing vitality in luxated permanent teeth. Int Endod J 1988; 21(5): 300-6. [http://dx.doi.org/10.1111/j.1365-2591.1988.tb01139.x] [PMID: 3074062]

CHAPTER 5

Pediatric Endodontics

I. K. Pandit[1,*], **Vitrat Galhotra**[2] and **Parag D. Kasar**[3]

[1] *DAV Dental College, Yamuna Nagar, Haryana 135001, India*

[2] *AIIMS Raipur, Chhattisgarh 492099, India*

[3] *Department of Pediatric Dentistry, Terna Dental College, Navi Mumbai, Maharashtra 400706, India*

Abstract: Pediatric endodontics is an integral part of dental practice that aims to preserve fully-functional primary teeth in the dental arch. Despite advances in the prevention of dental caries in pediatric dentistry, the occurrence of pulpal-involved primary teeth and their premature loss continue to be a common problem. The benefits of preserving primary teeth are of utmost importance. Primary teeth aid in mastication, phonation, and guidance of permanent tooth bud, harmonized temporal and spatial development of permanent teeth and prevent the detrimental psychological effects due to tooth loss. Despite the emphasis, prevention in primary teeth remains much talked about and rarely practiced. Restoration of a child's dentition to a healthy, functional status is often complicated by the severity of dental caries, particularly in the primary dentition, which often falls prey to the ravages of decay. Moreover, primary dentition is often regarded as transient and hence, undeserving of much time or effort. The intervention is only sorted when the child experiences pain due to the decay. Unfortunately, the delay incurred due to dental caries renders the tooth non-restorable.

Keywords: Pediatric Endodontics, Root Canal Treatment, Pulpectomy, Pulpotomy, Technique.

INTRODUCTION

Primary teeth should be preserved until their normal exfoliation time to maintain arch length and function to provide proper guidance for the eruption of permanent teeth, enhance aesthetics and mastication, prevent aberrant tongue habits, aid in speech, and prevent the psychological effects associated with the tooth. Paediatric dentistry is a unique speciality that deals with the total oral health care of children. Anciently, Pediatric dentistry has evolved from an extraction-oriented practice, where primary teeth with inflamed pulps were mostly extracted and did not focus on preserving the pulp, to a speciality based on emphasizing the prevention of oral

* **Corresponding author I. K. Pandit:** DAV Dental College, Yamuna Nagar, Haryana 135001, India; E-mail: drpandit3080@gmail.com

Satyawan Damle, Ritesh Kalaskar & Dhanashree Sakhare (Eds.)

and dental diseases where extraction of teeth with symptomatic pulpits becomes obsolete [1]. The aim of pulp therapy in the primary dentition is to retain the primary tooth as a fully functional part of the dentition, problems related to the loss of teeth. Clinically, the choice of pulp therapy is based on interpretation despite the assessment difficulties and imprecision of pulp tests related to the primary dentition.

The choice of treatment modalities in primary teeth is generally based on the severity of the symptoms clinically and/or radiographically. When indicated, pulp capping or pulpotomy of the deciduous tooth is relatively an easy procedure with generally good clinical results. Pulpectomy on the other hand is a heavier treatment for the child and is more complicated due to anatomical complexities that are not found in the permanent tooth.

A review of the anatomy of primary teeth readily explains the frequent need for pulp therapy to maintain the integrity and health of oral tissues (Fig. **1**).

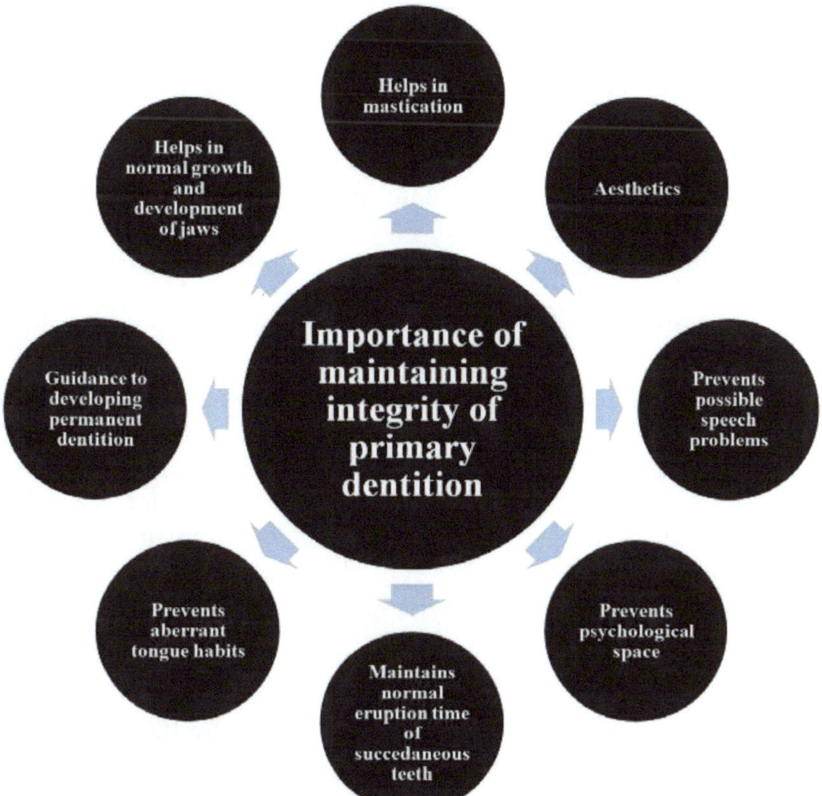

Fig. (1). Importance of Primary Teeth.

Ideally, Finn [1] and Ash [2] described basic differences between primary and permanent teeth that can be summarized as follows:

The enamel of primary teeth is thinner than on permanent teeth. Also, the thickness of the dentin between the pulp chambers and the enamel in primary teeth is comparably less than that of permanent teeth. The pulp horn in primary teeth is closer to the dentin-enamel junction, and dental caries can progress into the dentin more rapidly, leaving the tooth more susceptible to infection. Thus, pulp exposures caused by caries occur more frequently in deciduous teeth. If the infection spreads to the alveolar bone, then there are chances that the succedaneous teeth may also be affected.

Historical Perspective

At the beginning of the twentieth century, it became obvious that microorganisms were the reason for pulp inflammation, and more attention was drawn to disinfecting agents that, although effective, were very cytotoxic. The first method of pulp capping was described by ***Phillip Pfaff***, a dentist at the court of the Prussian King **Friedrich II in Berlin** in **1756** who used gold foils [3]. Various agents for direct pulp capping had been recommended ever since. The first scientific clinical study to correlate the different pulp capping materials was conducted by ***Dätwyler*** in **1921**, where zinc oxide-eugenol showed the best results. ***Hermann*** (1920) introduced calcium hydroxide as a root canal filling material [3]. Between 1928 and 1930, ***Hermann*** studied the action of calcium hydroxide on vital pulp tissue and prove that it was a biocompatible material [3].

There has been a paradigm shift in the approach regarding reversibly inflamed pulp from an **"aggressive"** approach involving total excavation of the carious dentin increasing the danger of exposing the pulp, towards a more **"conservative"** approach in which dental caries may be left in the pulpal wall to prevent pulpal exposure. This approach is being slowly spread among dental professionals and may become the treatment of choice for deep caries in modern paediatric dental practice. If minimally invasive dentistry is reluctantly accepted by the professional community, teeth with reversible pulp inflammation, that could otherwise be conservatively treated, will become pulpally infected.

The Primary Pulp

1. The dental pulp is considered a specialized connective tissue of mesenchymal origin surrounded by tubular dentin walls occupying the pulp chamber and the root canal. The specific cells present in dental pulp known as Odontoblasts are responsible for the synthesis and deposition of the collagen-rich dentin organic matrix which will be further mineralised to the pulp tissue. So, the dentin and

pulp remain associated during the development & throughout life and are commonly referred to as the pulp-dentin complex. The pulp-dentin complex is surrounded by enamel, (crown) and root as well as cementum, periodontal ligament, and bone [3].

Accordingly, the functions of the dental pulp are as follows (Fig. **2**):

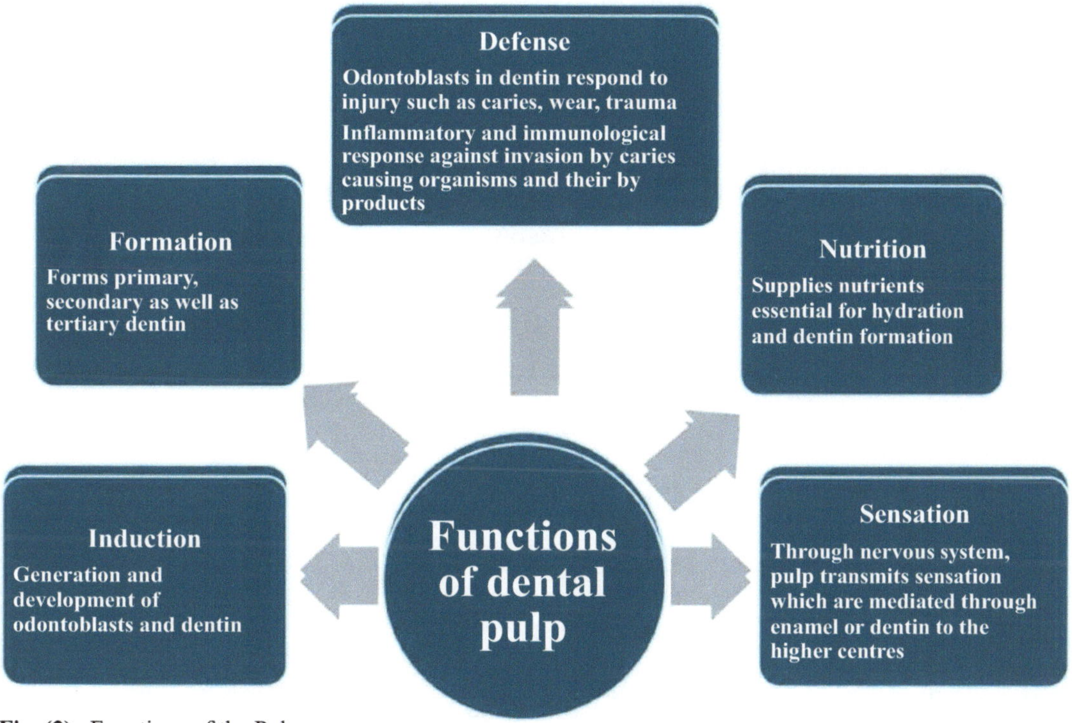

Fig. (2). Functions of the Pulp.

Factors Affecting the Pulp -Dentin Complex Response to Stimuli in Primary Teeth:

Although the life span of primary teeth is shorter and their dentin is thinner as compared to that of permanent teeth, the pulp-dentin complex response to dental caries in human primary teeth is like that of permanent teeth, including a reduction in the number of the odontoblasts and an increase in the number of inflammatory cells. These are found under very deep lesions and are less in more distant regions, being almost absent in the radicular apical pulp. The primary dentition is frequently subjected to noxious stimuli such as trauma or caries with associated pulpal inflammation [4]. The same factors affect both the pulp-dentin responses in primary as well as permanent teeth.

Based on the Remaining Dentin Thickness, Three Situations can be taken into Consideration:

Initial carious lesion (or) shallow cavity preparations [Remaining Dentin Thickness (RDT) > 500 μm]: A localized reactionary dentin may be formed facing the restoration site, and intratubular mineralization (dentin sclerosis) occurs, resulting in a significant decrease in the dentin permeability and pulp protection [5].

1. Carious lesion progression implies a deep cavity preparation [Remaining Dentin Thickness (RDT) < 500 μm]: These lesions may lead to partial death of odontoblast. Depending on the pulp inflammatory intensity, progenitor/stem cells can migrate to the injury site and differentiate to give rise to a new generation of odontoblast-like cells. These cells are responsible for the deposition of a specific type of tertiary dentin termed reparative dentin [6].

2. During a subsequent restorative process, deep cavity preparations with RDTs (Remaining Dentin Thickness) between 250 and 400μm lead to poor tertiary dentin repair activity. This results from impaired odontoblast dentin secretory activity due to cellular injury [7].

Diagnosis

Then encountering deep carious lesions affecting the primary dentition, limitations exist regarding the confirmation of the vitality status of the pulp. Percussion and palpations tests, operative diagnosis combined with bitewing radiograph and selected periapical radiographs are complementary information that must be obtained. Figs. (**3** - **5**) illustrate the pulpal diagnosis tree for deep carious lesions in immature permanent teeth, treatment options and problems encountered in paediatric endodontics.

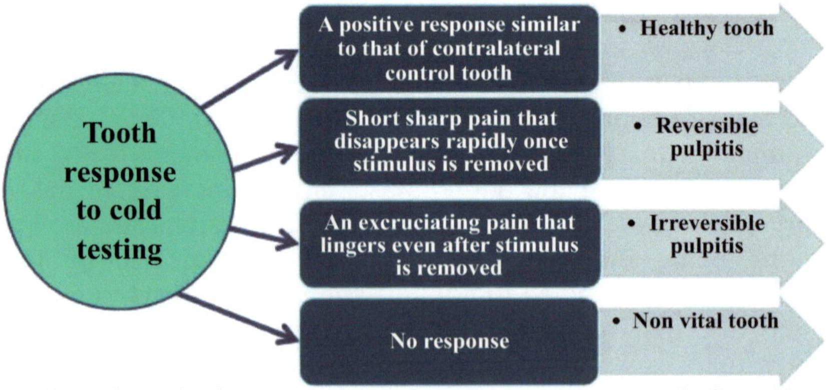

Fig. (3). Pulpal diagnosis tree for deep carious lesions in immature permanent teeth after cold application.

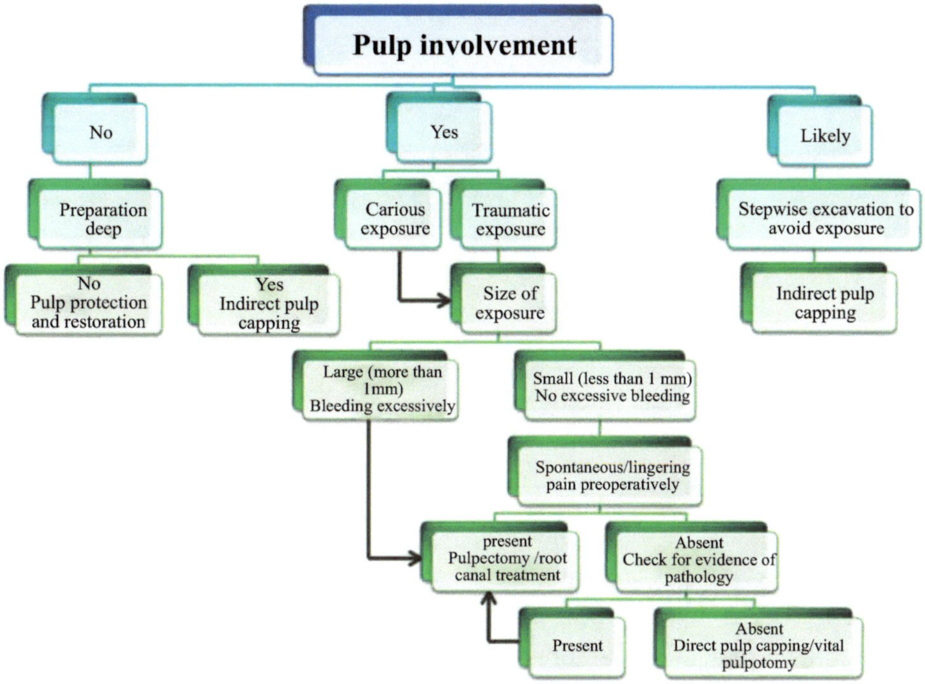

Fig. (4). Procedure (process) for the management of deep caries.

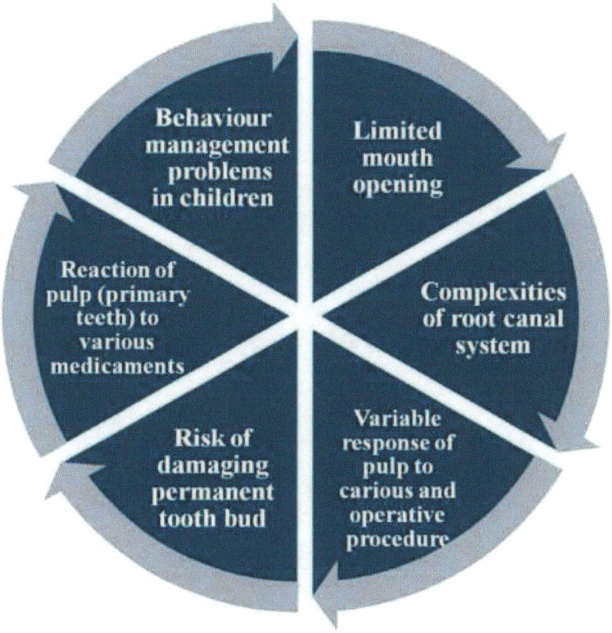

Fig. (5). Problems Encountered in Pediatric Endodontics.

Vital Pulp Therapy for Primary Teeth (Fig. 6)

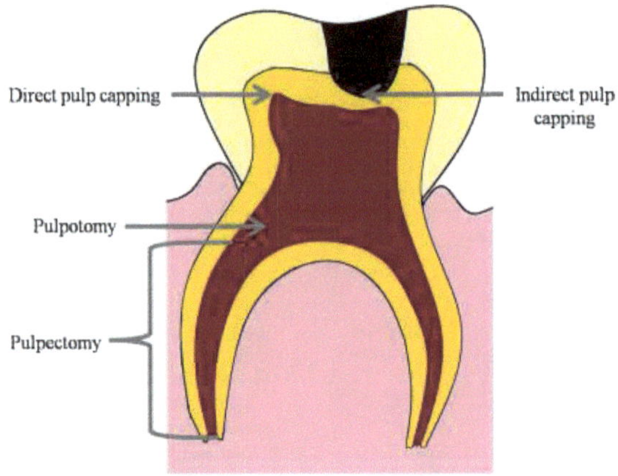

Fig. (6). Criteria for case selection.

INDIRECT PULP CAPPING

- It is defined as a procedure wherein the deepest layer of the remaining affected carious dentin is covered with a layer of biocompatible material to prevent pulpal exposure and further trauma to the pulp [8].
- **McDonald** defined it as a procedure in which only the gross caries is removed from the lesion and the cavity is sealed for a time with a bio-compatible material [9].
- **Materials Used for Pulp Capping: (Fig. 7).**

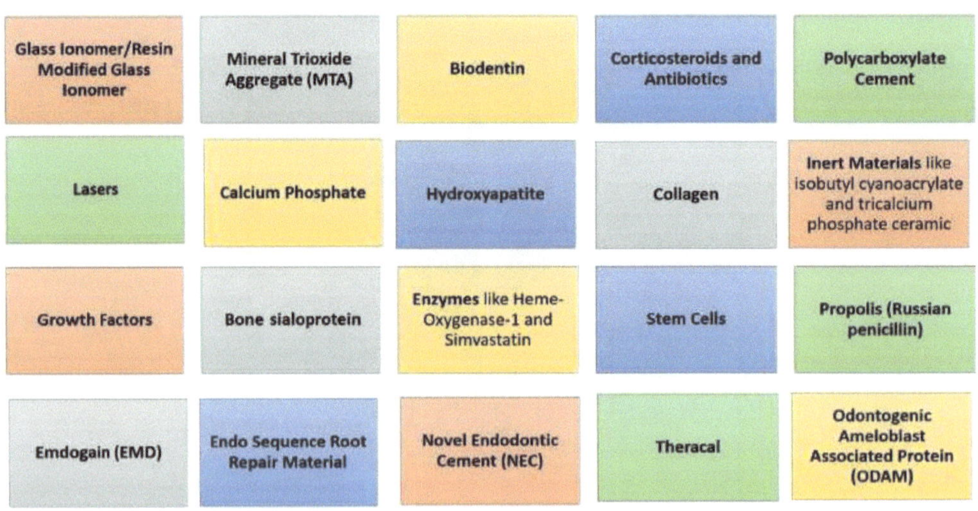

Fig. (7). Materials used for pulp capping.

- Calcium hydroxide
- Mineral Trioxide Aggregate (MTA)
- Resin-modified glass ionomer
- Biodentine

Indicators and Contraindications (Table 1)

Table 1. Indications and contra indications.

Indications	Contraindications
Teeth with deep caries, which are free from pulpitis.	Teeth with deep caries and symptoms of pulpitis.
No history of spontaneous toothache.	History of spontaneous pain.
No tenderness to percussion.	Tenderness to percussion.
No abnormal mobility.	Abnormal mobility.
No radiographic evidence pathologic resorption.	Radiographic evidence of interradicular bone loss or root resorption.

- Primary tooth with deep caries that exhibits no signs of pulpitis or with reversible pulpitis when the removal of deepest carious dentin leads to pulp exposure [10].

- **Objectives [11]:**

1) The involved dentin should be sealed from the oral environment by the restorative material.

2) There should be no evident post-treatment signs or symptoms such as sensitivity, pain or swelling.

3) There should be no radiographic evidence of pathologic external or internal root resorption or other pathologic changes.

4) There should be no harm to the succedaneous developing tooth.

Procedure (Fig. 8a).

Single Appointment Procedure

1. Use local anaesthesia and isolation with a rubber dam.
2. Establish cavity outline with high-speed air turbine handpiece.
3. Remove all caries using a caries detector dye that is infected dentin must be removed.

4. Stop the excavation as soon as the firm resistance of sound dentin is felt.
5. If there is a probability of exposure while removing further caries, then a conservative approach is chosen by placing a hard calcium hydroxide base and temporizing the tooth (Fig. **8b**).
6. Cavity flushed with saline and dried with cotton pellet.
7. Site is covered with calcium hydroxide [Ca $(OH)_2$].
8. Remainder cavity is filled with reinforced Zinc Oxide Eugenol (ZOE) Cement.
9. Final restoration is done followed by placement of crown.

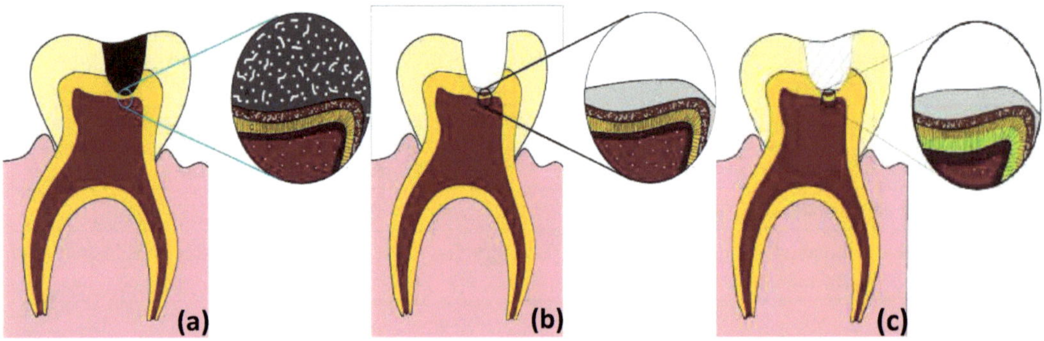

Fig. (8). Procedure of Indirect Pulp Capping. **(a)** Caries approaching pulp: Necrotic zone, soft leathery dentin, affected dentin; **(b)** Zone of leathery dentin left to avoid pulp exposure and is covered with calcium hydroxide (L) liner followed by interim restoration; **(c)** 6-8 weeks after showing reparative dentin (R) formation.

2nd Appointment Procedure (6-8 weeks later) (Fig. 8c)

1. Between the two appointments the tooth should be asymptomatic and temporary restoration should be intact.
2. Reparative dentin bridge (Fig. **8c**) is formed (clinical and radiographical confirmation), and a permanent restoration followed by full-coverage restoration is chosen.
3. But if there is some amount of caries remaining in re-entry, carefully removal of caries, now somewhat sclerotic may reveal sound dentin without pulp exposure.
4. Previous remaining carious dentin will have become dried out, flaky and easily removed.
5. The area around the potential exposure will appear whitish and may be soft, which is pre-dentin.
6. The cavity preparation is washed and dried gently.
7. Cover the entire floor with Ca $(OH)_2$.
8. Reinforced ZOE cement or GIC is filled in the cavity.
9. Final restoration like stainless steel crown is then placed.

- **Stepwise Excavation**
  1. Deep caries excavation should be done in two visits.
  2. First excavation is intended to remove the superficial necrotic, infected, and affected dentin by completely excavating the periphery of the lesion. This excavation does not excavate caries near the pulp to avoid a pulpal exposure.
  3. A retentive temporary restorative material is placed leaving soft, moist, discoloured dentin on the pulpal floor. The remaining dentin is then covered with calcium hydroxide and glass ionomer restoration.
  4. Stepwise excavation is intended to allow remineralisation of the affected dentin and the formation of more tertiary dentin.
  5. After, 8-12 weeks, the carious lesion is re-entered in by removing the temporary restoration and a final complete excavation is done leaving the central yellowish or greyish hard dentin in the floor of the pulp.
  6. A final restoration is then placed to seal the pulp from any microleakage.

DIRECT PULP CAPPING

- **Kopel (1992)** defined it as the placement of a medicament or non-medicated material on a pulp that has been exposed in course of excavating the last portions of deep dentinal caries or because of trauma [12].
- **Materials Used for Pulp Capping:**
  - Calcium hydroxide
  - Mineral Trioxide Aggregate (MTA)
- **Indications:**
  - This procedure is indicated in primary teeth with a normal pulp following a minimal pulp exposure of 1mm or less when there is a favourable condition [13].
- **Objectives:**
  1. The vitality of the tooth should be maintained.
  2. There should be no evident post-treatment signs or symptoms such as sensitivity, pain or swelling.
  3. There should be no radiographic evidence of pathologic external or internal root resorption or other pathologic changes.
  4. It should result in Pulp healing and reparative dentin formation.

- **Procedure (Fig. 9a to 9h Clinical and Histological Stages in DPC)**

  1. Rubber Dam Provides only Means of Working in a Sterile Environment, so it must be used.
  2. Once the exposure is encountered (Fig. **9b**), further manipulation of pulp is

avoided.

3. Cavity should be irrigated with saline, chloramine T or distilled water.
4. Haemorrhage is arrested with light pressure from sterile cotton pellets
5. Place the pulp capping material (Fig. **9c**), on the exposed pulp with the application of minimal pressure to avoid forcing the material into the pulp chamber.
6. Place temporary restoration.
7. Final restoration is done after determining the success of pulp capping which is done by determining the dentinal bridge (Fig. **9d**).
8. Maintain the pulp vitality, lack of pain and minimal inflammatory response.

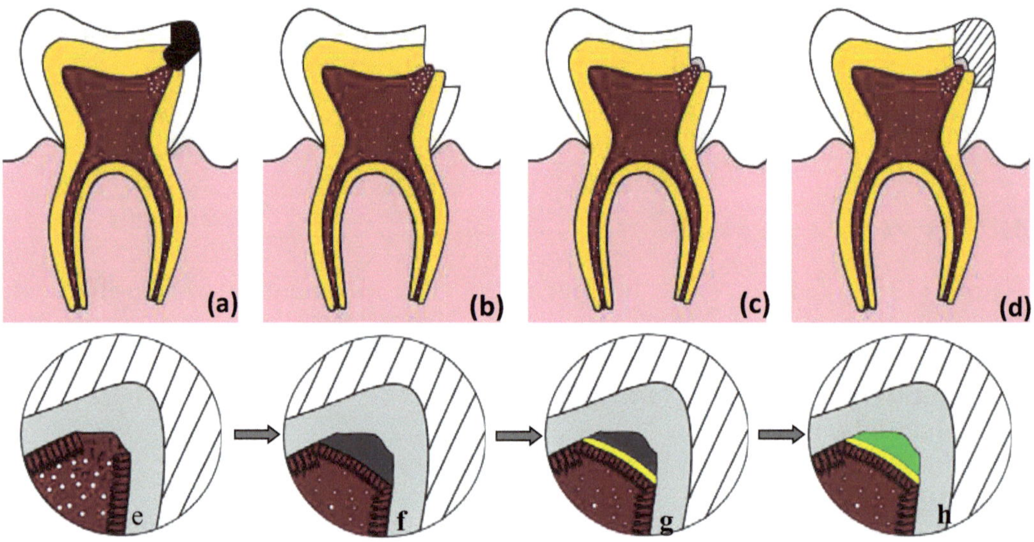

Fig. (9). Procedure of Direct Pulp Capping. **(a)** Caries involving pulp with no clinical symptoms or radiographic pathology; **(b)** Accidental carious exposure with no signs of irreversible pulpitis; **(c)** Application of calcium hydroxide liner; **(d)** Final restoration; **(e)** Disruption of odontoblastic layer and formation of zone of necrosis; **(f)** Differentiation of neoodontoblasts adjacent to zone of necrosis; **(g)** Initial deposition of tertiary dentin; **(h)** Deposition of reparative dentin and calcification in zone of necrosis.

PULPOTOMY

- **Finn (1995)** defined pulpotomy as the complete removal of the coronal portion of the dental pulp, followed by the placement of a suitable dressing or medicament that will promote healing and preserve the vitality of the tooth [9].
- **American Academy of Paediatric Dentistry (1998)** defined pulpotomy as the amputation of the affected, infected coronal portion of the dental pulp preserving the vitality and function of the remaining part of the radicular **pulp** [14].
- **Indications:**
  1. Indicated when a caries removal results in pulp exposure in a primary tooth with reversible pulpitis after traumatic pulp exposure.

2. When there are no radiographic signs of infection or pathologic resorption.
3. When the remaining radicular portion of pulp must be judged to be vital without suppuration, purulence, necrosis, or excessive haemorrhage that cannot be controlled by cotton pellet after several minutes after the amputation of coronal **pulp** [15].

- **Objectives:**
  1. Remaining radicular portion of the pulp must remain asymptomatic without any adverse clinical signs or symptoms such as sensitivity, pain or swelling [15].
  2. No postoperative radiographic signs of pathologic external root resorption. Internal root resorption may be stable and self-limiting.
  3. No harm to the succedaneous tooth.

Procedure (Figs. 10 & 11)

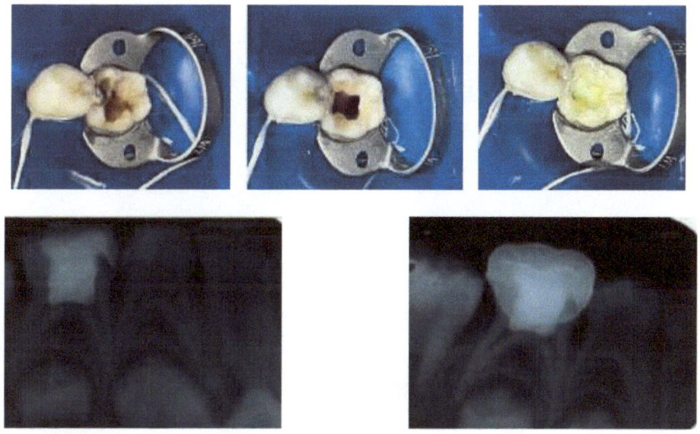

Fig. (10). a: Deep carious lesion. **b:** Access opening and amputation of pulp. **c:** MTA placement. **d:** Post-Operative IOPA. **e:** Post-Operative IOPA with SS crown

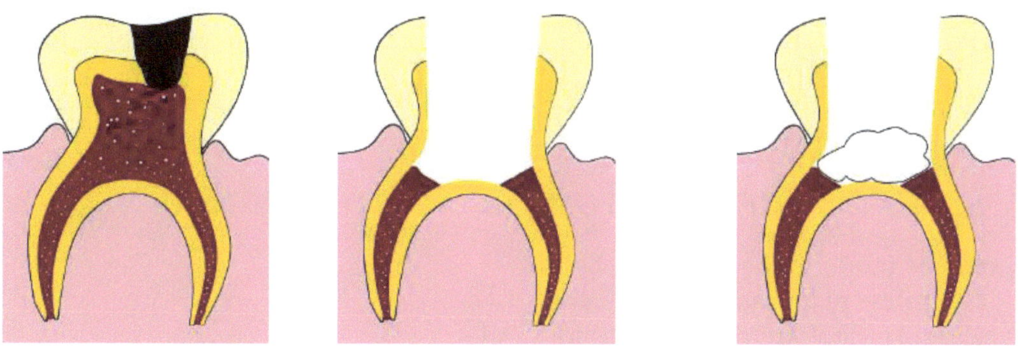

(a) (b) (c)

(Fig. 11) contd.....

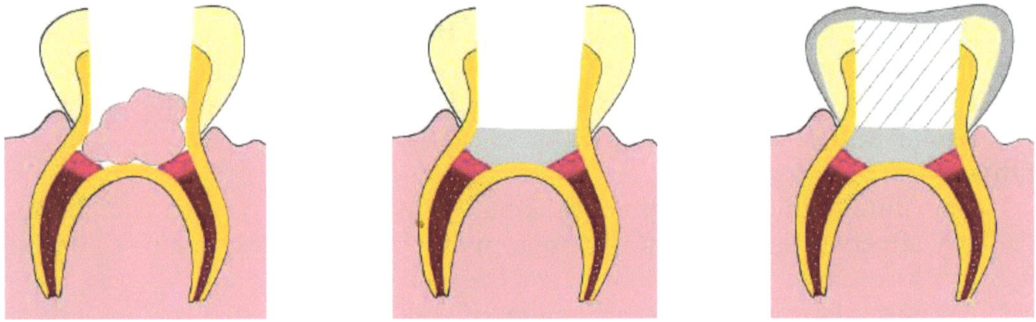

(d) (e) (f)

Fig. (11). **(a)** Carious tooth with reversible pulpitis; **(b)** Caries excavation followed by coronal amputation of pulp; **(c)** Bleeding arrested with sterile cotton pellet. **(d)** Placement of a medicament-soaked cotton pellet; **(e)** Pulp stumps covered with thick ZnOE paste; **(f)** Pulpotomies tooth with permanent restoration and ss crown.

1. The primary tooth to receive the pulpotomy should be selected based on the clinical and radiographic indications (Fig. **10a** & **11a**).
2. Anaesthesia should be given, and isolation should be done preferably using a rubber dam to avoid pulp chamber contamination with salivary microorganisms (Fig. **10a**).
3. **Caries removal should be done** before entering the pulp chamber (Fig. **10b**)
4. After caries removal is completed, a #330 carbide bur under copious irrigation is used to expose the pulp chamber (Fig. **11b**).
5. Coronal pulp is removed with a slow speed bur and haemostasis are achieved by the application of a cotton pellet for not more than 5mins (Fig. **10b**, Fig. **11c**).
6. Once haemostasis is obtained, medicament such as glutaraldehyde, and MTA is placed on the pulp stump and allowed to remain in contact for a stipulated time (Fig. **10c**, Fig. **11d**).
7. The pulp stumps are covered with a thick paste of zinc oxide eugenol cement (Fig. **10d**, Fig. **11e**)
8. The tooth is restored with a semi-permanent restoration like stainless steel crown. (Fig. **10e**, Fig. **11f**).

CLASSIFICATION OF PULPOTOMY (RANLY) (TABLE 2):

A. Extent of pulp tissue removal
   a. Complete pulpotomy
   b. Partial pulpotomy (Cvek's pulpotomy)
B. Medicament used
   a. Formocresol pulpotomy
   b. Glutaraldehyde pulpotomy

c. Calcium Hydroxide pulpotomy
d. Ferric sulphate pulpotomy
e. MTA pulpotomy

C. Method of pulp tissue removal
a. Surgical pulpotomy – pulp removed by sharp spoon excavator
b. Electrosurgical pulpotomy – pulp removed by electrocautery
c. Laser pulpotomy – pulp remover by Laser's

- Some of the important studies for each method is illustrated in the following table obtained from Ranly, 1994 (Table **3**).

Table 2. Classification of pulpotomy by Ranly.

Types	Other Name	Features	Examples
Vital Pulpotomy			
Devitalisation	Mummification, cauterization, fixation.	It is intended to mummify the vital tissue	Single sitting: • Formocresol • Electrosurgery • Laser Two stages: • Gysi Triopaste • Easlick's formaldehyde • Paraform devitalising paste
Preservation	Minimal devitalisation, noninductive	This implies maintaining the maximum vital tissues, with no induction of reparative dentin	• ZnO Eugenol • Glutaraldehyde • Ferric sulphate
Regeneration	Inductive, reparative	This has the formation of the dentin bridge	• $Ca(OH)_2$ • Bone morphogenic protein • Mineral trioxide aggregate • Enriched collagen • Freeze-dried bone • Osteogenic protein
Nonvital Pulpotomy			
Mortal pulpotomy	-	It is done in compromised cases	• Beechwood cresol • Formocresol

Table 3. Review of studies regarding different pulpotomy procedures.

Timeline	Devitalizing	Preserving	Regenerating
1930	Multiple Visits with Formocresol [Sweet CA]	-	-

(Table 3) cont.....

Timeline	Devitalizing	Preserving	Regenerating
1938	-	-	Ca $(OH)_2$ Pulpotomy for Primary Teeth. (Teuscher and Zander1938)
1962	2 Visit FC Pulpotomy [Doyle WA *et al*]	-	-
1965	5 min FC Pulpotomy (Spedding *et al.*1965)	-	-
1970	Dilution of FC (Straffon& Han 1970)	-	-
1971	-	ZOE evaluated (Magnusson 1971) Ledermix introduced humans (Hansen *et al* 1971)	-
1975	Dilution of FC; (Morawa 1975)	Glutaraldehyde proposed pulp therapy (s-Gravenmade)	-
1978	-	Glutaraldehyde proposed pulpotomy (Ranly&Lazzari)	-
1980	-	GA proposed (Kopel)	-
1981	Dilution of Formocresol [Garcia-Godoy]	-	-
1984	-	-	Enriched collagen [Fuks] Hard setting CaOH [Heilig]
1985	Laser [Shoji]	-	-
1988	-	-	Freeze-dried bone [Fadavi *et al*]
1989	-	-	Demineralized Dentin [Nakashima]
1991	-	Ferric Sulphate [Fei]	Bone Morphogenetic protein [Nakashima]
1993	Electrosurgical Pulpotomy [Mack]	-	Osteogenic Protein [Rutherford]
1996	Argon laser [Wilkerson]	-	MTA animal [Ford]
2001	-	-	MTA Human [Eidelman]
2002	-	Sodium Hypochlorite animal [Hafez]	-
2006	-	Sodium Hypochlorite human [Vargas KG]	-

FORMOCRESOL PULPOTOMY (FIG. 12)

Formocresol has been extensively used in the past for pulpotomy procedures in primary teeth. Buckley formocresol is prepared by mixing 19% formaldehyde, 35% tricresol, and 15% glycerine in water. A 1:5 dilution of this mixture is used as a medicament in deciduous pulpotomy. It works on the principle of fixation or mummification of the remaining radicular pulp. It was first introduced by Sweet (1930) for multi-visit pulpotomy. Doyen (1962) recommended the two-visit formocresol pulpotomy. A single application of five minutes was recommended by Redid (1966), while presently the universally accepted method is a one-minute application of formocresol after haemostasis. The reduction in application time has been recommended as formaldehyde which is a component of formocresol is a known carcinogen. By limiting the time of application, the diffusion and leakage of the medicament through the apical foramen are reduced. The amount of medicament used is further reduced by blotting the excess medicament on a dry gauze prior to placement in the pulp chamber.

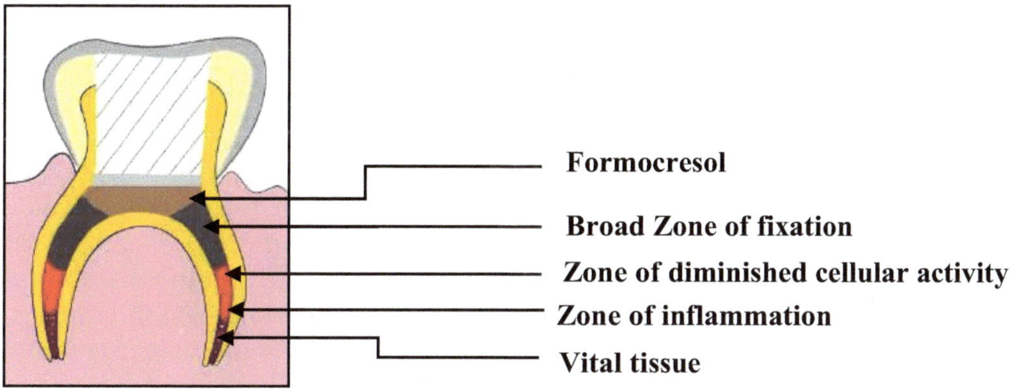

Fig. (12). The zones have been described as: Broad acidophilic zone of fixation; Zone of diminished cellular activity; Zone of inflammation; Zone of vital pulp.

After the application of formocresol distinct zones have been identified in the remaining pulp as described by Massler and Mansukhani (1959).

GLUTARALDEHYDE PULPOTOMY (FIG. 13)

Due to the mutagenic properties of formocresol, Gravenmade (1973) recommended the use of glutaraldehyde for pulpotomy. It has better fixation properties due to the presence of two aldehyde rings in its molecular structure. This also limits the diffusion of the medicament within the pulp and beyond the apical foramen. Atkinson has described the following zones of the pulp after glutaraldehyde application.

i. Zone of fixation
ii. Zone of pro-inflammatory fibroblasts
iii. Zone of vital pulp

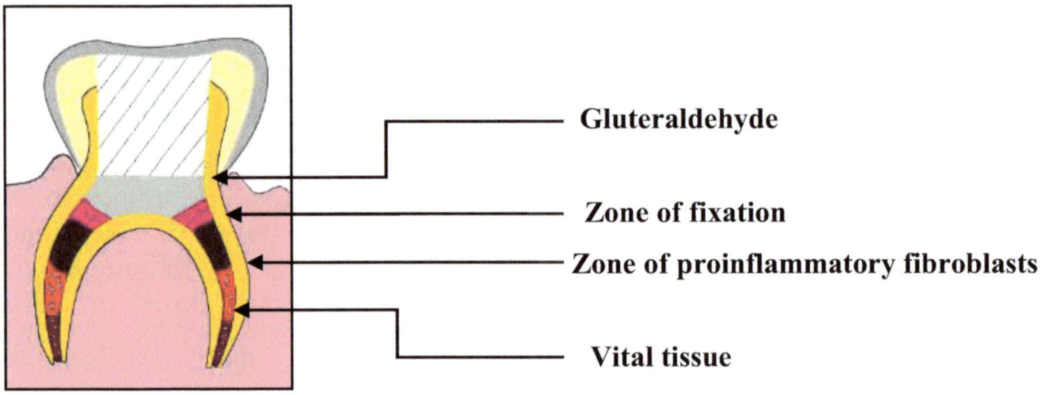

Fig. (13). Zones in radicular pulp after glutaraldehyde pulpotomy.

CALCIUM HYDROXIDE PULPOTOMY

Calcium hydroxide pulpotomy was first recommended by Teusher and Zander (1938). When used in young permanent teeth it helps in the apexogenesis of immature root apices. In deciduous teeth, the use of calcium hydroxide has been reported with signs of post-operative internal resorption. Though these resorptive changes have been attributed to improper case selection and the presence of inflammation of the radicular pulp. When used with appropriate case selection, calcium hydroxide has a good clinical success rate.

Due to its high alkaline pH, it helps in the reduction of microorganisms and promotes calcific barrier formation

FERRIC SULPHATE PULPOTOMY

Complete control of haemorrhage from the pulp amputation site is an important requisite for the successful outcome of pulpotomy. Ferric sulphate does not cause fixation of the dental pulp. As it is a heavy metal salt, it causes agglutination proteins in the peripheral capillaries and helps in the formation of a blood clot. The precipitated mettalo protein complexes clog the blood vessels and act as a barrier to the irritants of the zinc oxide eugenol base thereby promoting healing in the remaining radicular pulp.

MINERAL TRIOXIDE AGGREGATE (MTA)

Whilc many new materials have been tried for pulpotomy MTA is a suitable alternative to calcium hydroxide. MTA introduced by M. Torabinejad is a non-resorbable hard-setting cement available as an amorphous powder and has an exceedingly long setting time. It shows a high alkaline pH like calcium hydroxide but as it is not affected by leaching it provides a better sealing ability. Earlier MTA was available as grey MTA which causes staining of the crown of the tooth after pulpotomy procedures. The newer forms of MTA have shown limited discolouration.

PULPECTOMY (FIGS. 14 - 17)

- **Finn** defines pulpectomy as the removal of all pulpal tissue from the coronal and radicular portion of the tooth.
- **Mathewson (1995)** defined it as the complete removal of the necrotic pulp from the root canals of primary teeth and filling them with an inert resorbable material to maintain the tooth in the dental arch.

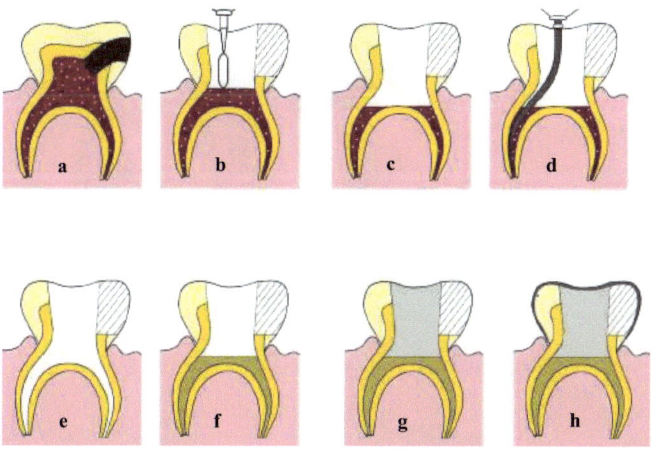

Fig. (14). Pulpectomy. **a**. Carious tooth, **b**. access opening, **c**. coronal pulp amputation, **d**. cleaning and shaping of radicular space. **e**. Complete cleaning and shaping, **f**. Obturation, **g**. final restoration, **h**. Semi-permanent restoration with ss crown.

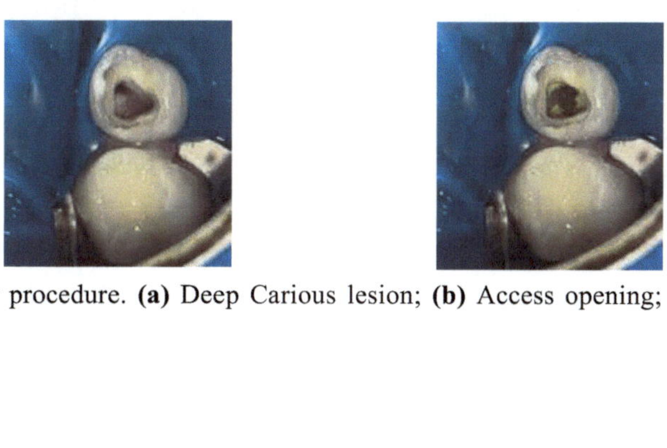

Fig. (15). Pulpectomy procedure. **(a)** Deep Carious lesion; **(b)** Access opening; **(c)** Preparation of root canals; **(d)** Obturation.

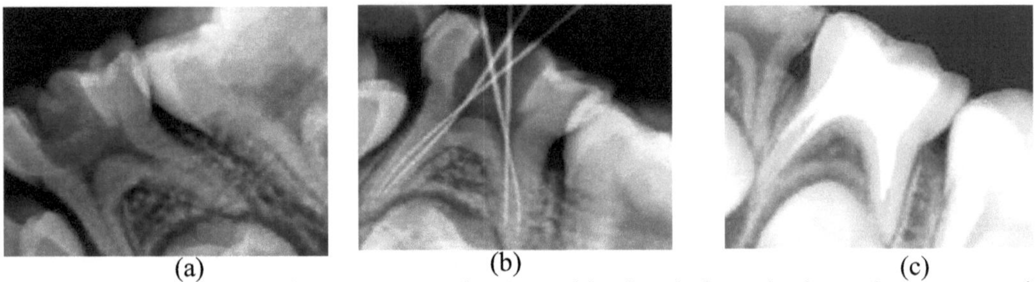

Fig. (16). Pulpectomy procedure. **a.** preoperative, **b.** working length determination and **c.** post-operative IOPA images.

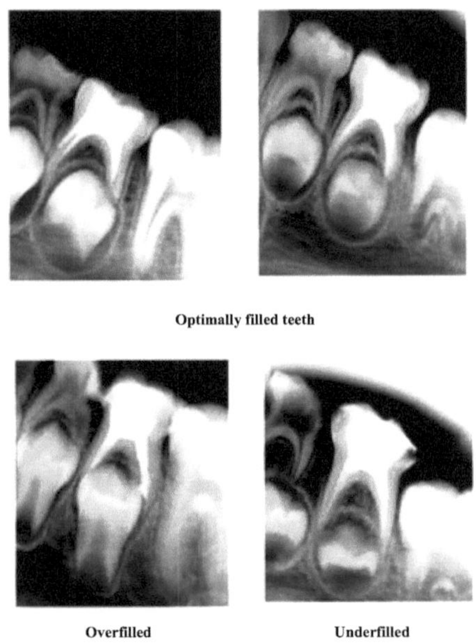

Fig. (17). IOPA images showing optimally filled, overfilled and underfilled root canals after pulpectomy procedure.

INDICATIONS

1. Performed when radicular pulp exhibits clinical signs of irreversible pulpitis or pulp necrosis while the roots show minimal or no resorption [16].
2. The tooth should be clinically restorable

- **Contraindications**
  1. Non-restorable crowns
  2. Perforation to the pulpal floor
  3. Serious reduction in bone support and/or extreme tooth mobility
  4. Radiographic indication of extensive internal or external root resorption
  5. Periapical radiolucency involving the follicle of the permanent tooth

6. Underlying dentigerous or follicular cysts
7. Medically compromised children.

- **Access And Debridement**

1. Inflamed or necrotic pulp is removed, and access preparation is refined to view all canals orifices (Figs. **14a, b, c, 15b**).

2. Primary molar roots are usually curved and flared to allow for the development of the succedaneous tooth.

3. Endodontic files are selected and adjusted to stop 1-2 mm short of the radiographic apex, with the preliminary working length estimated with a preoperative radiograph (Fig. **14d**, **16b**).

4. Pre-bending of the instrument should be done to avoid perforation on the inner and outer portions of the root.

5. Mechanical removal of the remnants from the canal is performed using a series of 21mm long K-type files. Avoid unnecessary shaping of the canal since that can damage the tooth and lead to perforation in the furcation or lateral walls (Fig. **15c**).

- **Irrigation**

1. Disinfecting with irrigating solutions is an important step in assuring optimal bacterial decontamination of the canals (Fig. **14e**).

2. Canals are irrigated with 0.2% – 2% chlorhexidine solution or with 1% - 5% sodium hypochlorite. [According to AAPD guidelines]

- **Filling The Canals/(Obturation)**

1. Instruments required to fill the canals depend mainly on the type of material used.

2. Thick pastes such as ZOE should be used with root canal pluggers

3. Thinner pastes like Calcium hydroxide & iodoform-based materials are inserted with a lentulo spiral mounted on a slow handpiece or with the tips provided by the manufacturer (Fig. **14f**, **15d**, **16c**).

MATERIALS (TABLE 4)

Table 4. Different obturating materials.

Root filling material	Components	Usage	Difficulties	Antibacterial activity
Zinc oxide eugenol	-	Without setting accelerators may be pushed into the root canals using a suitable root canal plugger	Tends to resorb at a slower rate than the roots of the primary teeth [17]	Strong antibacterial Effectiveness
Calcium hydroxide with iodoform	Vitapex (New Dental Chemical ProductsCo. Ltd., Tokyo, Japan)/ Diapex: 30%calcium hydroxide,40.4% iodoform, and22.4% silicone oil.	Introduced into the root canal using disposable tips or a lentulo spiral mounted on a slow-speed handpiece	Aqueous vehicles cause depletion of paste from root canals before the time of physiological tooth replacement A viscous vehicle promotes lower solubility of the paste. Oily vehicles have the lowest solubility and diffusion of calcium hydroxide pastes [18].	showed no antibacterial activity against most pure cultures.
Calcium hydroxide	Sealapex Calcicur	Introduced into the root canal using a lentulo spiral. Also available in Auto-mix syringes or application cannula	Showed minimal antibacterial activity against most pure cultures. Overfilling and voids	-
Iodoform based	Metapex (Meta Biomed Co. Ltd. Cheongju City, Korea): calcium hydroxide with iodoform Kri-paste (PharmachemieAG, Switzerland): iodoform (80.8%), camphor, parachlorophenol, menthol.	A sterile syringe with disposable plastic needles injects the paste into the canal	-	-

(Table 4) cont.....

Root filling material	Components	Usage	Difficulties	Antibacterial activity
Zinc oxide and iodoform	Maisto's paste zinc oxide and iodoform, with para-chlorophenol camphor, lanolin, and thymol Endoflas (Sanlor&cfa. S. en C.S. from Columbia South America): tri-iodmethane and iodine dibutyl orthocresol (40.6%), zinc oxide (56.5%), calcium hydroxide (1.07%), and barium sulphate (1.63%) with a liquid consisting of eugenol and paramonochlorophenol	introduced into the root canal using a spiral lentulo mounted on a slow-speed handpiece	-	-

CONCLUSION

The benefit of preserving primary teeth is of utmost importance. Primary teeth aid in mastication, phonation, the guidance of permanent tooth bud, harmonized temporal and spatial development of permanent teeth and prevents the detrimental psychological effects due to tooth loss. Despite the repeated emphasis, prevention in primary teeth remains a much talked about and rarely practised treatment modality and the therapeutic approach mainly remains curative. Restoration of a child's dentition to a healthy, functional status is often complicated by the severity of dental caries, particularly in the primary dentition which often falls prey to the ravages of decay. Moreover, the primary dentition is often regarded as transient and hence, undeserving of much time or effort. The intervention is only sorted when the child experiences pain due to tooth decay. Unfortunately, the delay incurred prior to seeking treatment for dental caries renders the tooth nonamenable to conventional restorative procedures. Maintaining the integrity and health of the primary dentition is the main objective of pulp treatment.

CONSENT FOR PUBLICATION

Not applicable.

CONFLICT OF INTEREST

The authors declare no conflict of interest, financial or otherwise.

ACKNOWLEDGEMENT

Declared none.

REFERENCES

[1] Finn SB. The children's dentist, his practice, and his community. In: Finn SB, editor. Clinical Pedodontics. 4th ed. Clinical Pedodontics, Philadelphia: WB Saunders 1973.

[2] Ash M. Wheeler's dental anatomy, physiology, and occlusion. Philadelphia: WB Saunders 1992.

[3] Fuks A, Peretz B. Pediatric endodontics: Past and present perspectives and future directions. In Pediatric Endodontics: Current Concepts in Pulp Therapy for Primary and Young Permanent Teeth. Springer International Publishing, 2016; 1-5.
[http://dx.doi.org/10.1007/978-3-319-27553-6_1]

[4] Yu CY, Abbott PV. Responses of the pulp, periradicular and soft tissues following trauma to the permanent teeth. Aust Dent J 2016; 61(1) (Suppl. 1): 39-58.
[http://dx.doi.org/10.1111/adj.12397] [PMID: 26923447]

[5] Berbari R, Khairallah A, Kazan HF, Ezzedine M, Bandon D, Sfeir E. Measurement reliability of the remaining dentin thickness below deep carious lesions in primary molars. Int J Clin Pediatr Dent 2018; 11(1): 23-8.
[http://dx.doi.org/10.5005/jp-journals-10005-1478] [PMID: 29805230]

[6] Fuks AB, Peretz B. Pediatric Endodontics: Current Concepts in Pulp Therapy for Primary and Young Permanent Teeth. Springer International Publishing, 2016; 1-5.

[7] Gateva N. Pulp Therapy for the Young Permanent Dentition – clinical features and diagnostic. PHD 2016.

[8] Markose A. Vital Pulp Therapy. Int J Curr Res 2018; 10(08): 72961-4.

[9] Nallanchakrava S, Virginia M, Niharika P, Khan HS. An update on materials used for vital pulp therapy in primary teeth: A review international journal of advances in pediatric dentistry 2019; 4(1): 1-8.

[10] Coll JA, Seale NS, Vargas K, Marghalani AA, Shamali S, Graham L. Primary tooth vital pulp therapy. Systematic review and meta-analysis. Pediatr Dent 2017; 39(1): 16-27.E15-E110.

[11] Pulp therapy for primary and immature permanent teeth. Pediatr Dent 2017; 39(6): 325-33.

[12] Kashyap N. A Review of Direct Pulp Capping: New Treatment Approaches and Modalities. EC Dental Science 2020; 19(2): 1-11.

[13] Garrocho-Rangel A, Esparza-Villalpando V, Pozos-Guillen A. Outcomes of direct pulp capping in vital primary teeth with cariously and non□cariously exposed pulp: A systematic review. Int J Paediatr Dent 2020; 30(5): 536-46.
[http://dx.doi.org/10.1111/ipd.12633] [PMID: 32078201]

[14] Devi Praja V, Muttath A, Duraisamy V, Selvarajan N, Suresh Kumar V, John JB. A clinical and radiographic comparison of platelet-rich fibrin and lyophilized platelet-derived preparation as pulpotomy agent in primary molars. J Pharm Bioallied Sci 2020; 12(5) (Suppl. 1): 155.
[http://dx.doi.org/10.4103/jpbs.JPBS_48_20] [PMID: 33149448]

[15] Fuks A, Kupietzky A, Guelmann M. Pulp therapy for the primary dentition. In: Nowak AJ, Christensen JR, Mabry TR, Townsend JA, Wells MH, Eds. Pediatric Dentistry- Infancy through Adolescence 6th ed. 2019; 329-51.

[16] Coll JA, Vargas K, Marghalani AA, *et al.* A systematic review and meta-analysis of nonvital pulp therapy for primary teeth. Pediatr Dent 2020; 42(4): 256-461.

[17] Rajsheker S, Mallineni SK, Nuvvula S. Obturating Materials Used for Pulpectomy in Primary Teeth- A Review. Journal of Dental and Craniofacial Research 2018; 3(1): 3.
[http://dx.doi.org/10.21767/2576-392X.100019]

[18] Venkatesh N S. Smriti Jha, Parin V Bhanushali, Ayisha Moureen Comparative assessment of diffusion of calcium and hydroxyl ions from calcium hydroxide formulations used for obturation in primary teeth international journal of scientific study, february 2017; 4(11).

CHAPTER 6

Management of Young Permanent Teeth (Apexogenesis, Apexification and Regenerative Endodontics)

Varinder Goyal[1,*], Dhanashree Sakhare[2] and Vidya Iyer[3]

[1] *Department of Pediatric and Preventive Dentistry, Guru Nanak Dev Dental College & Research, Institute Bhatinda-Patiala Road, Sunam, Punjab, India*

[2] *Founder, Lavanika Dental Academy, Melbourne, Australia*

[3] *Department of Pediatric and Preventive Dentistry, CSI College of Dental Sciences & Research, Madurai, India*

Abstract: Traumatic injuries suffered by the anterior teeth mostly occur before completion of the root formation which may have consequences like inflammation or necrosis of the pulp. The most sensitive part of a young permanent tooth to trauma is the Hertwig's epithelial root sheath (HERS). However, root formation can still continue to occur if there is a disruption of vascularity and cellularity in the apical region, even in the presence of pulpal inflammation and necrosis of the traumatized teeth. Hence, every effort should be made to maintain the viability of HERS as it acts as a source of undifferentiated cells which could give rise to the formation of the hard tissue and it also protects the tooth against the ingrowth of the cells of periodontal ligament into the root canal, which might result in intracanal bone formation and cessation of root development. In cases where complete destruction of Hertwig's epithelial root sheath occurs, the development of a normal root comes to a halt but, this does not mean that there is an end to the deposition of hard tissue in the region of the root apex. Although, once the sheath has been destroyed, there can be no further differentiation of odontoblasts but, the hard tissue can still be formed by cementoblasts which are present in the apical region or by fibroblasts of the dental follicle and periodontal ligament cells that undergo differentiation after the injury. This chapter is specifically oriented towards discussion of the viable methodology and treatment modalities of vital, nonvital immature young permanent teeth.

Keywords: Apexification, Apexogenesis, $Ca(OH)_2$, Immature teeth, Pulp, Vital/Non-vital teeth.

* **Corresponding author Varinder Goyal:** Department of Pediatric and Preventive Dentistry, Guru Nanak Dev Dental College & Research, Institute Bhatinda-Patiala Road, Sunam, Punjab, India; E-mail: virinderg@gmail.com

Satyawan Damle, Ritesh Kalaskar & Dhanashree Sakhare (Eds.)

INTRODUCTION

The formation of dentin is among one of the main functions of the dental pulp. Whenever the pulp undergoes a pathological change before the complete development of the root, its growth gets disrupted. In cases like caries or an exposure where a pulp is reversibly inflamed, the treatment of choice is to maintain pulp vitality by pulp capping or pulpotomy. However, if the pulp irreversibly inflamed or necrotic, apexification is the treatment of choice. The traditional apexification procedure consisted of multiple and long-term application of calcium hydroxide for creation of an apical barrier which would aid in the obturation of the root canal. Currently, the apexification procedure involves the use of mineral trioxide aggregate (MTA) for the formation of an apical barrier against which a three-dimensional obturation can be done. In addition to this, the novel procedures like pulp regeneration have received an immense attention as an option for such teeth.

Major Causes of Pulpal Diseases

1. Microbiota

2. Iatrogenic injury caused by trauma

3. Dental procedure generating thermal stimulation

4. Chemical agents

The pulp tissue can be affected by dental traumatic injuries and restorative procedures. The thermal irritation can occur during tooth preparation or finishing procedures, dry cutting, using dull burs, deep periodontal curettage, orthodontic movement. Also, the heat generated from the polymerization shrinkage of resin materials or lasers and air abrasion devices can cause an injury to the associated tooth pulp. The chemical irritants of the pulp include cavity cleansers such as alcohol, chloroform, hydrogen peroxide, sterilizing and desensitizing substances as well as some of the substances present in various restorative materials and cavity liners.

Pathogenesis

1. Pulpal inflammation is a complex process that involves a wide variety of neuronal and vascular interactions and reactions.

2. The unique responses of the pulpal tissue against the irritants and associated physiological feedback mechanisms can further lead to its injury.

3. Damage to the subjacent cells of the sub-odontoblastic zone and cells deeper to it causes irreversible pulpitis and eventually complete pulpal necrosis.

4. As the necrotic pulp space is relatively inaccessible to the immune response, it becomes a reservoir of the infective process.

5. Interaction of these irritants with the host tissue results in the release of non-specific mediators and immune reaction in the periapical tissues.

Factor Affecting Treatment

1. Status of the pulp and stage of root development

2. Number of visits required

3. Risk of fracture of the root

4. Extent of pulpal damage

5. Restorability of tooth

6. Patient preferences

7. Finances

Types of Open Apices

1. Blunderbuss: Derived from the Dutch word "Donderbus" which means "thunder gun" referring to an 18th century weapon with a short and wide barrel. These are the flaring root canal walls where the apex is funnel-shaped and wider than the coronal aspect of canal (Fig. **1**).

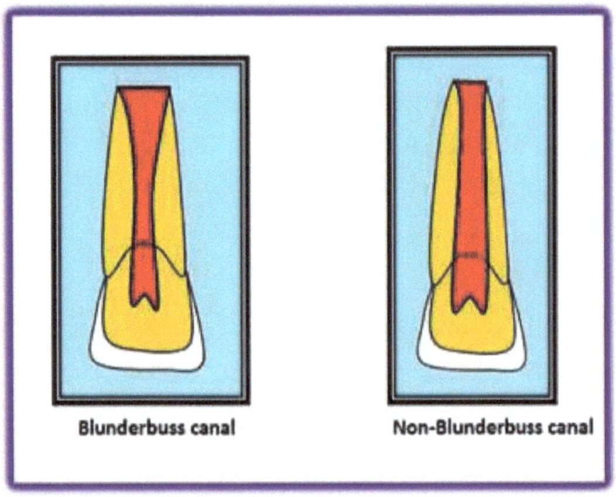

Fig. (1). Types of open apices.

2. Non blunderbuss: These consist of parallel/almost parallel root canal walls.

Treatment of Teeth with Vital Pulp and Open Apices (Apexogenesis)

Apexogenesis is a procedure that addresses the shortcomings associated with capping of an inflamed dental pulp with an incomplete root development. The main goal of apexogenesis is to preserve the vital pulp tissue so that continued root development with apical closure may occur.

Rationale

- When a pulp exposure occurs in an immature tooth, it can be repaired unaided just by protecting the tooth from further injury or an insult or else bioactive materials can be used to achieve the desired outcome [1].
- The idea is to preserve as much vital pulp tissue as possible, as it promotes continued vital functions of the pulp and root development.
- Healing and repair of a tooth with an exposed pulp with a predictable long-term pulp tissue preservation, in both primary and permanent teeth are possible with a variety of methods.
- Treatment of immature teeth has changed dramatically in recent years as new concepts and materials have been developed.
- Therapeutic apexogenesis on vital pulp therapy is the treatment of choice for traumatized or carious teeth with vital pulp and open apices. These approaches include a simple protective lining in direct pulp treatment in deep cavities and direct pulp capping or pulpotomy in case of pulp exposure

Material

1) Calcium Hydroxide

- Calcium hydroxide-based materials have been the gold standard for direct pulp capping for decades.
- Mechanism of action: They cause disinfection and coagulation necrosis at the junction of necrotic and vital tissues, with mild irritation to the pulp which leads to the formation of a hard tissue barrier [2].
- Hard setting calcium hydroxide pastes are less caustic than pure calcium hydroxide. However, they do not prevent bacterial leakage.
- There is a tendency of calcium hydroxide-based materials to get dissolved ultimately, leading to the formation of tunnel defects which may act as potential pathways for microleakage.
- Long term success rate of calcium hydroxide pastes ranges from 13% to 96%. This variability might be attributed to the inability of this material to biologically activate odontoblasts or accelerate reparative dentine formation.

- Repair responses like calcium hydroxide have been reported for several other materials proposed as capping agents for vital pulp therapy. Figs. (**2**, **3** and **4**).

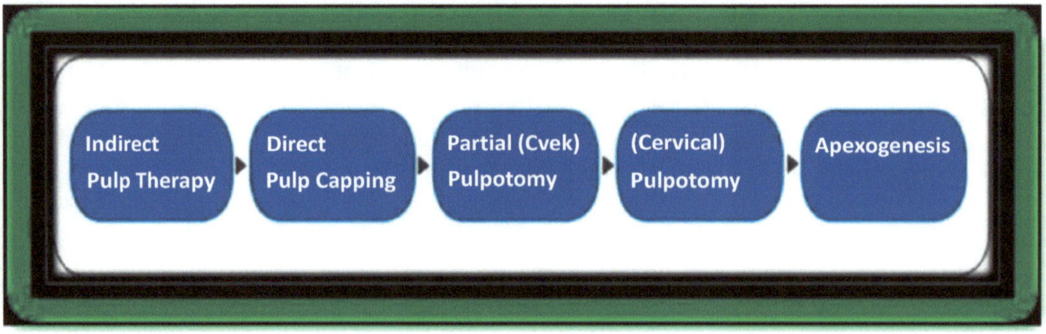

Fig. (2). Apexogenesis method.

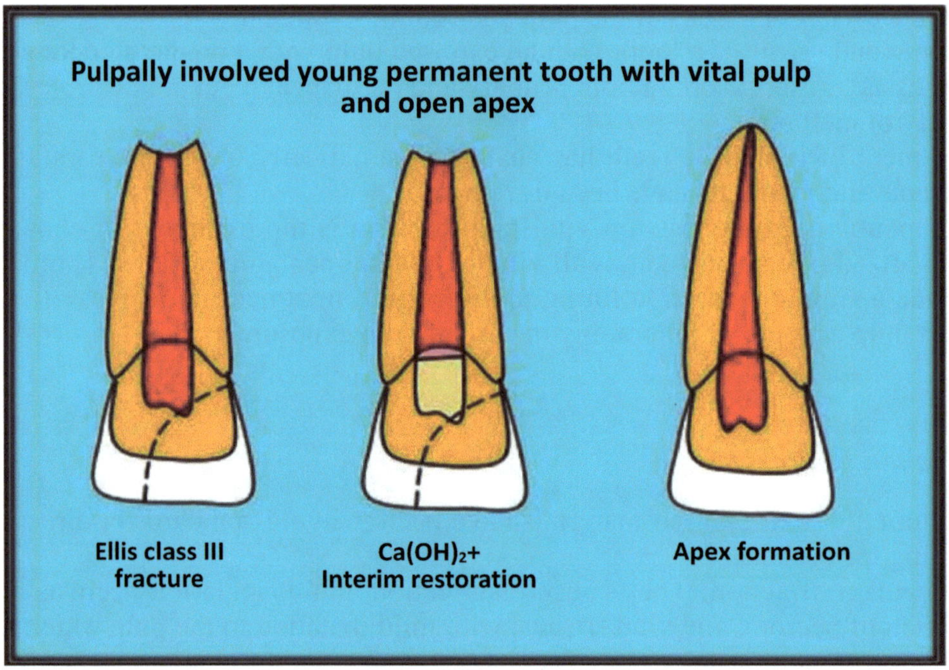

Fig. (3). Apexogenesis procedure.

2) Mineral Trioxide Aggregate (MTA)

- It is an alternative to calcium hydroxide based capping material and was developed by Torabinejad and co-workers at Loma Linda University in 1990s and has received much attention since then.
- It is biocompatible, seals well, has antibacterial properties and sets in the presence of moisture.

- Almost 30 years of clinical and experimental success has been reported for various applications of MTA in dentistry. The first commercially available product was ProRoot MTA. The Grey (GMTA) and White MTA(WMTA) form an essential part of today's armamentarium for capping of pulp and pulpotomy procedures in primary teeth.
- Despite having features similar to those of Ca $(OH)_2$, MTA causes less inflammation, less hyperemia, less pulpal necrosis, and a thicker dentinal bridge formation. With these features, MTA appears to be an alternative gold standard substitute to calcium hydroxide in case of vital procedures. Also, it eliminates some of the disadvantages associated with calcium hydroxide such as slower pulp healing, material stability, resorption, and subsequently inadequate long-term sealing ability [3].

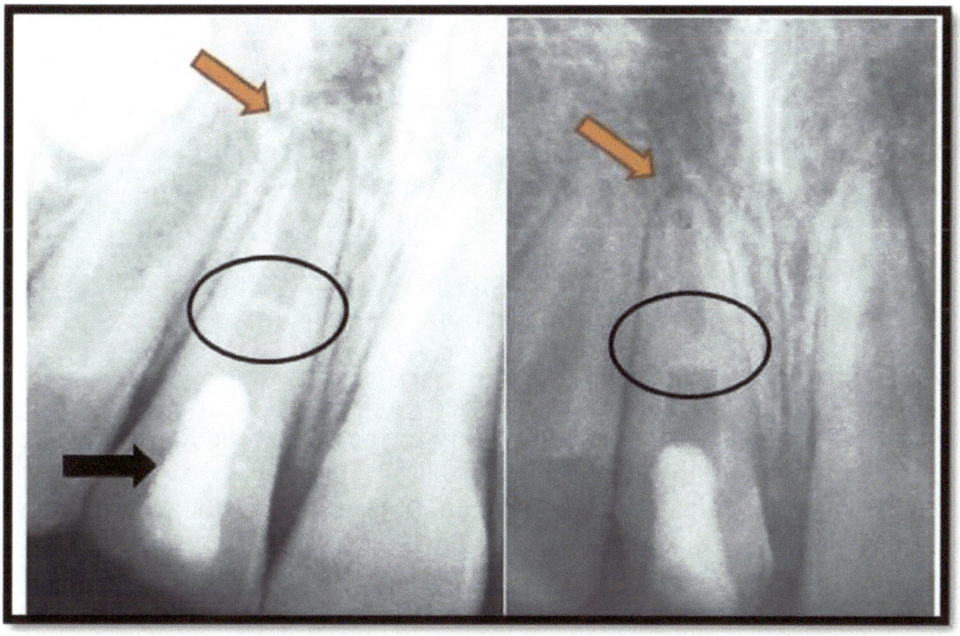

Fig. (4). Apexogenesis *via* pulpotomy.

Other Materials

3) A Variety of Biological Molecules

4) Growth Factors

5) Enamel and dentin matrix proteins.

- **Extracellular matrix molecules** are secreted by dentin-forming cells during tooth development and can play a key role in reparative dentin formation.

- **Bone Morphogenetic Protein**, also known as **Osteogenic protein**, has proved to be a promising material, promoting odontogenic differentiation in large direct pulp exposures in permanent teeth when used as a pulp capping agent.
- **Enamel matrix derivative (EMD)** may potentially play a role in the process of calcification of dental pulp tissue in a process mimicking normal odontogenesis.
- Over the last decade, many **Self-etch systems** have become popular. The histological response of total-etched and non-etched compomer restored cavity preparations that have shown biological compatibility with pulp tissues like that of calcium hydroxide mediated hard tissue repair. Histological comparisons of calcium hydroxide and resin pulp capping in a recent report by **Murray *et al.*** tend to support resin adhesives as an alternative to calcium hydroxide. However, calcium hydroxide apparently stimulates far more odontoblast like cells.

Apexification

It is a technique of inducing the root end closure in an immature nonvital permanent tooth/teeth by removing the coronal and radicular tissue and placing a suitable biocompatible material. Once an apical closure of the tooth/teeth is obtained, root canal therapy needs to be completed [4].

Goal: To obtain an apical barrier to prevent the passage of toxins and microorganisms into periapical tissues from root canal.

Rationale

- In the pulpless tooth, with an incompletely formed apex, the thin fragile dentinal walls made it difficult to achieve an apical seal.
- When a portion of the root removed to obtain a seal, the crown root ratio remains poor.
- Since this situation is usually present in the pediatric patient, a less traumatic approach is always desirable.
- These problems are overcome by stimulating the formation of a hard tissue barrier to allow for optimum filling of the canal and reinforcing the weakened root against fracture both during and after apexification.

Objective

- It should induce root closure at the apices of immature roots and should be evidenced by regular radiographic assessment.
- Post-treatment clinical signs or symptoms such as prolonged sensitivity, pain or swelling should not be present.

- There should be no evidence of abnormal canal calcification or internal and external root resorption lateral root pathosis or breakdown of peri-radicular supporting tissues during or following therapy.

Indications

- Permanent teeth with incompletely formed roots that become non vital after a traumatic injury or after carious exposure.
- Certain anatomic aberrations like dens invaginatus.
- Teeth with radiographic signs of rarifying osteitis where healing of the bone will be observed gradually after apexification.

Method for Apical Closure

Conditions like trauma or caries can trigger the loss of pulpal vitality as well as directly affect the development of root in an immature permanent tooth, resulting in short root with very thin walls, predisposing it to a greater risk of fracture. Fig. (5).

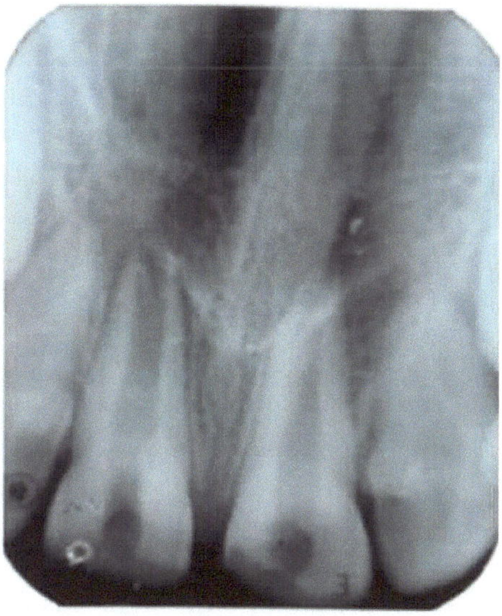

Fig. (5). Immature tooth with open apex.

The desired treatment to be carried out in such a situation is the elimination of the pulpal tissue followed by disinfection of the root canal system through different irrigants. The most commonly used among them being sodium hypochlorite (NaOCl) and Ethylenediaminetetraacetic acid (EDTA).

This procedure may involve a single or multiple appointments for placement of the calcium hydroxide inside the root canal to eliminate infection and stimulate the calcification process to achieve the desired apical closure. After several appointments, the walls of the root canal of the tooth should radiographically show more thickness and a rounded apex, which allows the root canal to be sealed with conventional techniques using gutta-percha and a sealant. Ca $(OH)_2$ can alter the mechanical properties of dentin and make these teeth more susceptible to root fracture. However, the traditional use of Ca $(OH)_2$ is being gradually replaced by mineral trioxide aggregate (MTA) as a one-step technique. The MTA can be placed as an apical plug to produce the disinfection and root end closure. It can even be used as a material for filling of canals [5].

Technique

1. Local anesthesia of the tooth
2. Placement of the Rubber dam.
3. Coronal access is gained and should be wide enough to include the pulp horns to prevent future contamination and disclosure.
4. The length of the canal is estimated using radiographs.
5. Exceptionally light filing (because of the thin dentinal walls) is performed with copious irrigation using 0.5% to 2.5% sodium hypochlorite or 0.2% chlorhexidine solution followed by sterile saline solution.
6. The canal is dried with paper points and then a calcium hydroxide dressing in consistency of a paste is applied with the help of lentulospirals, specially designed syringes or other systems followed by condensation with endodontic pluggers. If rotary instruments are used, care should be taken to prevent instrument breakage.
7. A cotton pledget is placed over the calcium hydroxide and the seal is completed with a layer of reinforced zinc oxide-eugenol cement.
8. The tooth is monitored clinically and radiographically at 3 months intervals.
9. When a calcified barrier is visible in the radiograph, the tooth is reopened and biomechanically cleaned by sodium hypochlorite irrigation. **The different materials for apexification** are given in Fig. (**6**).
10. The apical area should be examined using a file to the predetermined working length to detect the completeness of the apical barrier formation.
11. If the barrier is incomplete and the patient feels the touch of the file, the apexification procedure is re-established until a complete barrier is formed. When a hard tissue barrier is indicated on radiographs and can be probed with an instrument, routine endodontic procedures may be completed (Fig. 7).

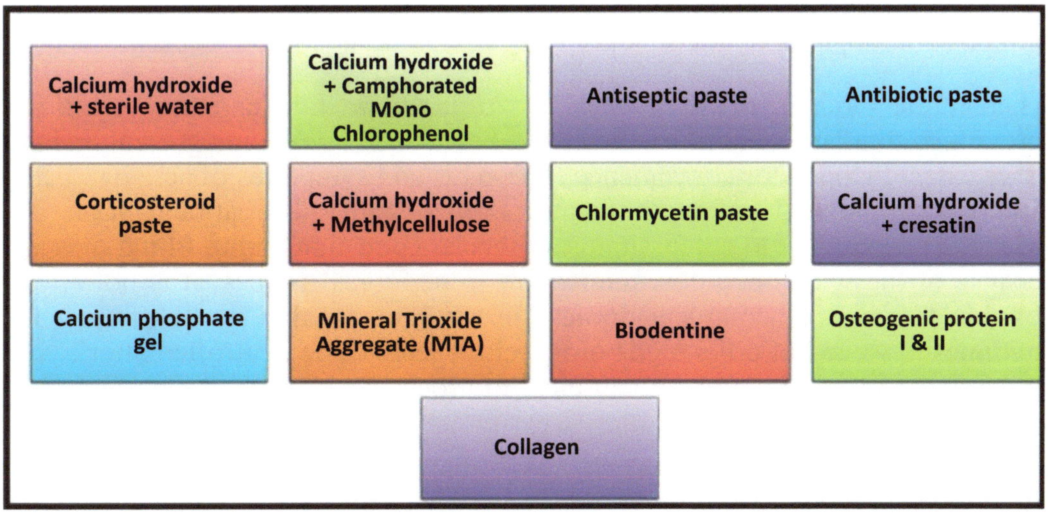

Fig. (6). Materials used for apexification.

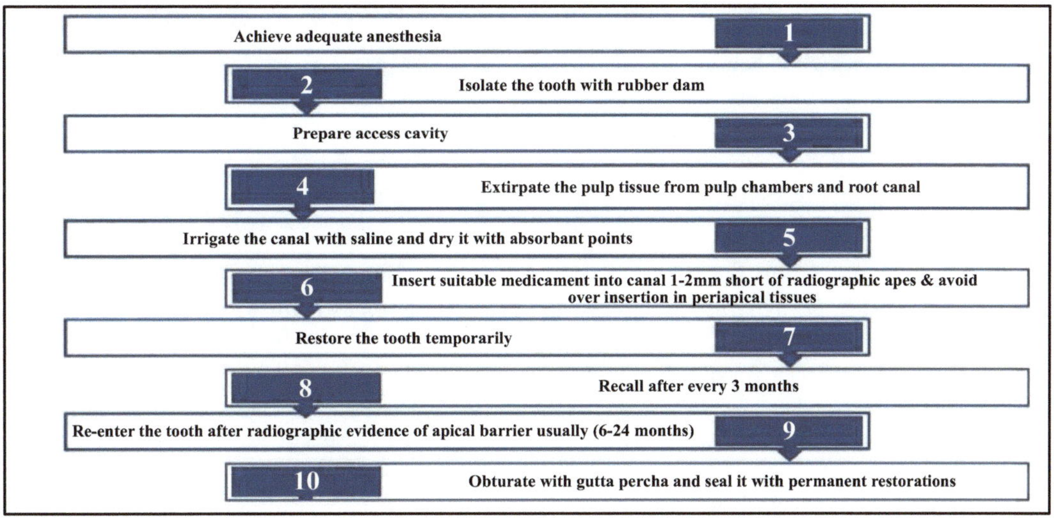

Fig. (7). Exhibiting apexification procedure.

Frankline Weine (1984) recommended that the apexification procedure must be completed in two appointments. After instrumentation, irrigation and drying of the canal during the first appointment, he advised using a sterile, dry cotton pellet in the pulp chamber for 1 to 2 weeks. The placement of a calcium hydroxide dressing in the canal is optional at the first appointment. During the second appointment, the debridement procedures are repeated before filling the canal with a thick paste of Calcium Hydroxide and CMCP or Calcium Hydroxide in a methylcellulose paste.

Whether the tooth is filled in one or two appointments (or more) should be determined to a large extent by the clinical signs and symptoms present and to a lesser extent by operator convenience. The signs and symptoms of active infection should be eliminated before the canal is filled with the treatment paste. The absence of tenderness to percussion is a especial good sign before filling the canal because of the wide-open communication to periapical tissues, it is not always possible to maintain complete dryness in the root canal (Fig. **8**). If the canal continues to weep but other signs of infection seem to be controlled after two or three appointments, the dentist can elect to proceed with the calcium hydroxide paste treatment.

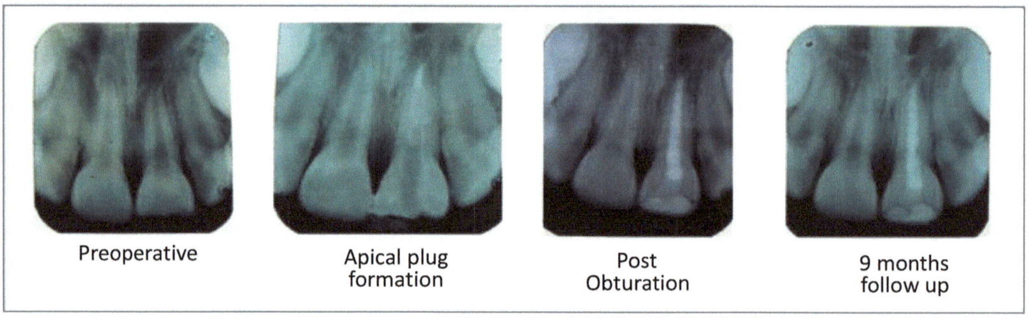

Fig. (8). Radiographic representation of One Step Apexification procedure.

Apexification has been found to be a predictable procedure, and an apical barrier has been found to be formed in 74% to 100% of cases (Table **1**, Figs. **9** and **10**).

Table 1. Difference between apexification and apexogenesis.

Apexogenesis	Apexification
Increases radicular length	Leads to apical barrier formation thus no increases in radicular length
Sufficient crown-root ratio	In-sufficient crown-root ratio
Can bear masticatory forces	Cannot bear sufficient masticatory forces
Continued root development decreases the fracture risk against lateral condensation	Leaves thin dentinal walls, increases the fracture risk, against lateral condensation

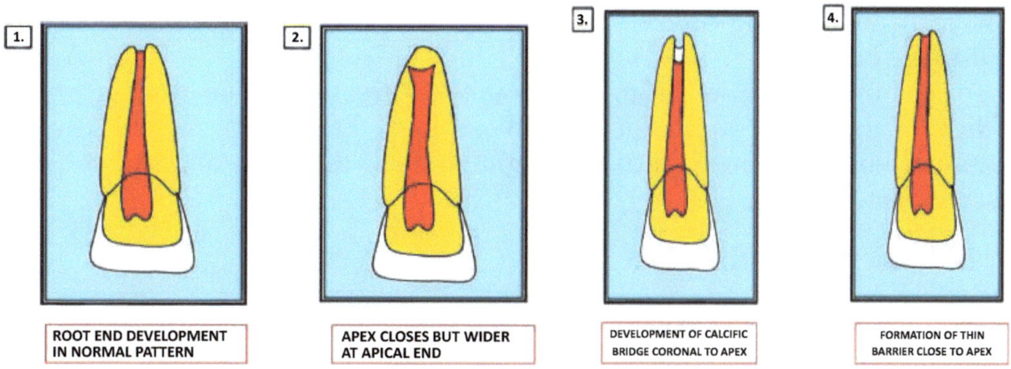

Fig. (9). Types of root apex closures which can occur after apexification.

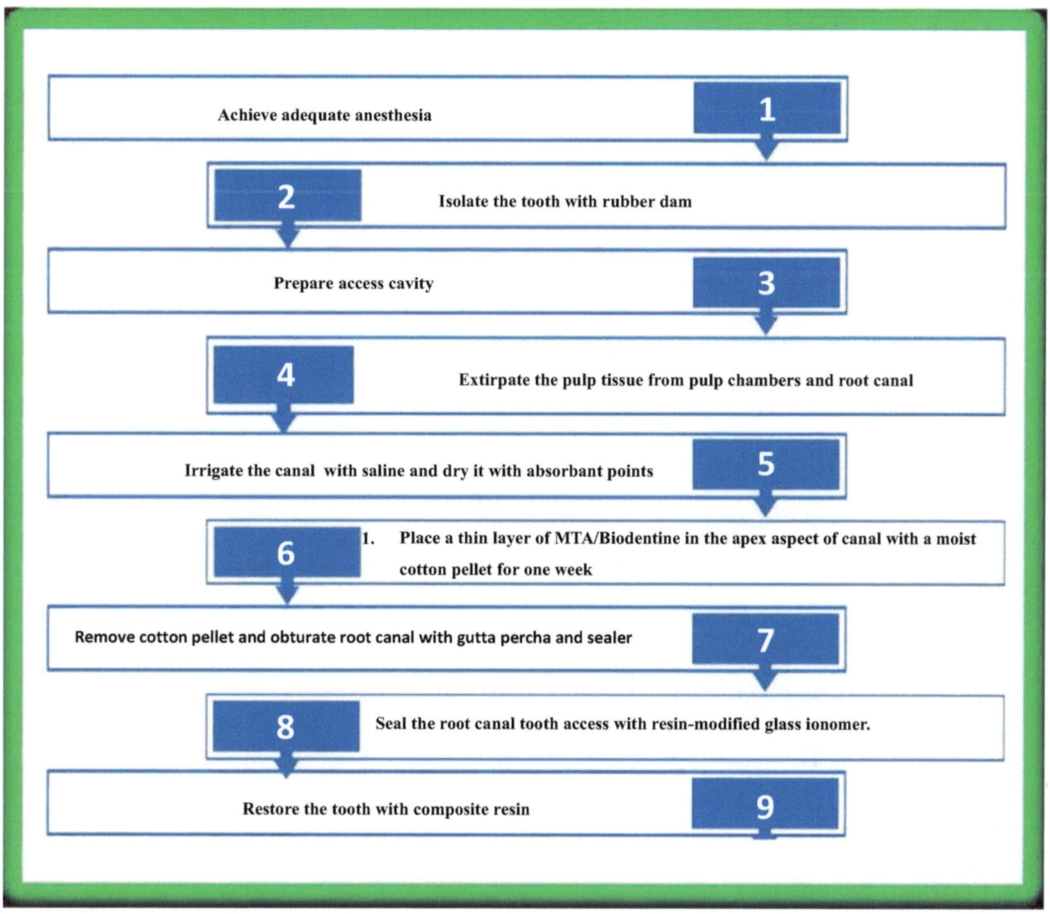

Fig. (10). One step apexification procedure.

- The patient is required to present for treatment multiple times. Thus, compliance is needed due to long duration period required for creation of a physiologic hard-tissue barrier.
- The tooth may fracture during the course of treatment due to thin cervical portion of the tooth. In addition to this, a study has indicated that long-term treatment with calcium hydroxide might weaken the roots and make it more susceptible to fracture [10].

Apical Barrier Method (MTA)

Recently, it has been suggested that the process of apexification will be replaced by using MTA as a sealing material. MTA was introduced to function as an apical barrier, reducing the time needed for completion of the treatment and for restoration of the tooth. The treatment may be completed in just a few visits.

Technique

1. After completion of the biomechanical cleaning of the root canal, MTA can be placed at the apical portion of the immature root and will act as an apical plug after setting, MTA cannot be removed from within the canal and retreatment, if necessary, can only be done by apical surgery. Therefore, complete debridement and disinfection of the root canal and of the dentin walls mandatory. To improve disinfection of the canals, Torabinejad suggested using an intracanal medication with calcium hydroxide for 1 week [6, 7].

2. Remove the calcium hydroxide from the root canal with irrigation and dry the canal with paper points.

3. The MTA powder is mixed with saline or sterile water according to the manufacturer's instructions. The material is then placed at the apical area using prefitted carriers or endodontic pluggers. MTA should be positioned exactly at the foramen, because the material must be in direct contact with periapical tissues. However, enthusiastic overfilling should be avoided (Fig. **11**).

4. The thickness of an apical plug must be 3 to 4 mm. After completion, the extension of the apical plug is checked radiographically [8].

5. If the apical plug is not satisfactory, the MTA is removed using the saline irrigation, and the filling procedure is repeated.

6. When the radiographic appearance looks ideal, a moist paper point or cotton pellet is placed in direct contact with the MTA, and the access cavity is closed with a temporary seal and allowed to set for 3-4 hours [9].

7. After the material is set, the same day or at the next visit, the root canal filling can be completed, and the tooth is restored with a composite resin.

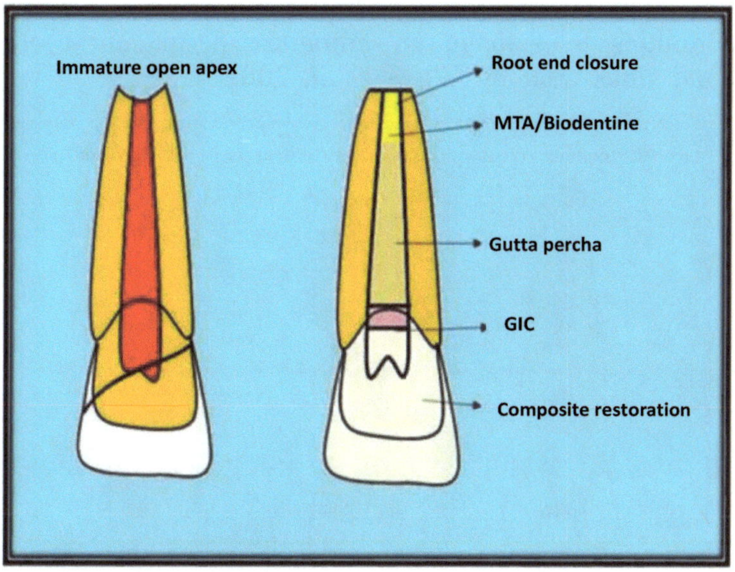

Fig. (11). Diagrammatic representation.

The MTA Apical Seal has Several Advantages

- Less patient compliance is required.
- Dentin will not lose its physical properties.
- The material allows for earlier restoration of the tooth, thus minimizing the likelihood of root fracture as compared to that of calcium hydroxide (Fig. **12**).

Regenerative Endodontics

Regenerative endodontics is an exciting and developing field that has emerged for the treatment of immature teeth with infected root canals. It has been described as a "paradigm shift" in the management of the infected teeth which can result in the continued root maturation and apical closure of same.

Immature permanent teeth with necrotic pulp/apical periodontitis are traditionally treated with apexification procedures using calcium hydroxide to induce apical hard tissue barrier formation or apical MTA plugs before root canal filling . The calcium hydroxide apexification procedure usually takes multiple treatment visits over an extended period [10]. The prolonged exposure to calcium hydroxide dressing could increase the risk of fracture of the root. An MTA plug is able to shorten the time of treatment. The treatment outcome of calcium hydroxide apexification and apical MTA plug appears to be compatible. However, an apexification procedure has no potential to restore the vitality of damaged tissue in the canal space and promote root maturation (thickening of the root canal walls and/or apical closure) of immature permanent teeth with necrotic pulp. In the year 2001, a new treatment option termed as 'revascularization' was introduced in the field of endodontics to manage an immature permanent tooth with apical periodontitis and sinus tract by Waya *et al.* 2001.

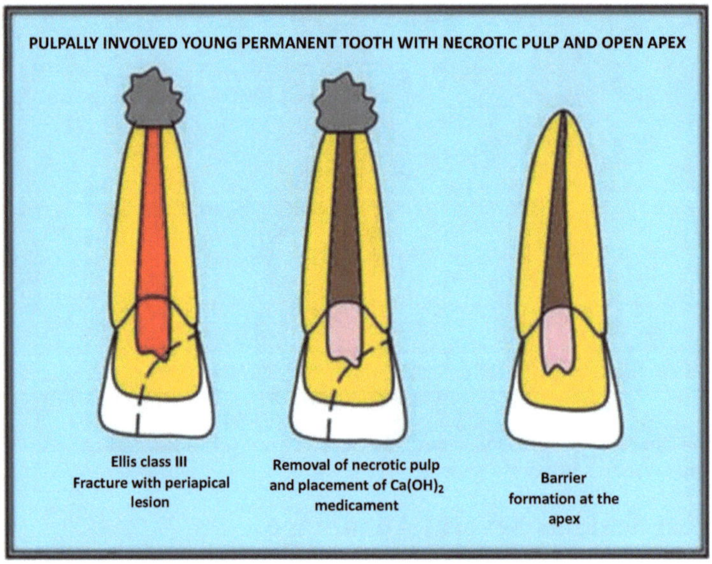

Fig. (12). Successful apical bridging Of one stage procedure has been formed.

Regenerative Endodontic Procedures

Several researchers recently published clinical as well as research work that offer a biologically based alternative to conventional endodontic treatment of these complex clinical cases. In general, these studies have evolved from the trauma literature, where the following precepts have been established:

1. Revascularization occurs most predictably in teeth with open apices.
2. Instrumentation and irrigation with NaOCl are not sufficient to reliably create the conditions necessary for revascularization of the infected necrotic tooth.
3. Placement of $Ca(OH)_2$ in root canal systems prevents revascularization coronal to the location of the $Ca(OH)_2$.
4. The use of the "3 mix-MP" triple antibiotic paste, consisting of ciprofloxacin, metronidazole, and minocycline, is effective for disinfection of the infected necrotic tooth, setting the conditions for subsequent revascularization.

History

It should be appreciated that research on the regeneration of a pulp- dentin complex has a long history. Revascularization of the pulp space in a necrotic, infected tooth with apical periodontitis was attempted by Nygaard-Ostby and Hjortdal in the 1960s but was primarily unsuccessful. However, the materials and instruments available 40 -50 years ago were probably not appropriate to create an environment like the avulsed tooth, *i.e.*, a canal that is free of bacteria, containing a scaffold for new tissue to grow and to be largely resistant to further bacterial penetration. With currently available technologies it could be possible to effectively disinfect an infected pulp, artificially place a scaffold, and then effectively seal the access cavity to res ensuing infection.

There are Some Important Points that can be Taken from the Studies Done so Far

- **First,** although structurally weak, it is important to realize that the immature permanent tooth in general has a very wide apical opening that likely is conducive to tissue ingrowth.
- **Second**, these patients are young (8-13 years old) and studies suggest that younger ages have greater healing capacity or stem cell regenerative capabilities.
- **Third,** none of the cases used instrumentation of the root canal walls, where the researchers used NaOCl as an irrigant.
- **Fourth**, both $Ca(OH)_2$ paste, and combinations of multiple antibiotics have been used in these patients. The outcome differences between these two medicaments reveal an important aspect of regenerative techniques, because many of the reported cases with $Ca(OH)_2$ display intra-canal calcifications which impede the continued thickening of the dentinal walls of these immature teeth. In addition to this, other investigators have suggested that the use of $Ca(OH)_2$ might kill any remaining pulpal cells, including stem or progenitor cells known to be present in dental pulp tissue. On possibly to disrupt the apical papilla and its resident stem cells, which is critical for continued root development.
- **Fifth**, the formation of a blood clot might serve as a protein scaffold, permitting - dimensional ingrowth of tissue.
- **Sixth,** nearly all these studies report continued thickening of the dentinal walls and subsequent apical closure.

The Procedure can be Explained as Follows

- Recently, several clinical studies demonstrated that despite the formation of periapical abscesses with extensive periarticular bone resorption as the result of root canal infection in immature teeth, conservative treatment may allow root development to reach maturation.

- The interest generated from this clinical observation appears to be underscored by the discovery of some of the dental stem cells which may shed light on the understanding of the repair of the pulpodentin complex, healing within the root canal space and the continued maturation of roots after endodontic treatment of the immature permanent teeth [11, 12].
- **Rationale**
  - Certain important types of cells and tissues must have survived after an insult, thereby allowing the root to undergo maturation, for example, the HERS (Hertwig's epithelial root sheath) and SCAP (Stem cells from the apical papilla). SCAP have been proposed to be the cell source of root odontoblasts.
    A. Case selection -

Currently there is no evidence-based guideline that can be established to help clinicians to determine which condition of cases that can be treated with this conservative approach. As mentioned, the presence of radiolucency in the periradicular region can no longer be used as a determining factor, nor is the vitality test. Since there is a lack of clinical studies on the success rate of treating immature teeth with periradicular bone resorption, clinicians may consider always choosing the conservative approach first. Apexification is only undertaken when the attempt is failed. It is also said if one happens to see soft tissue while observing under a microscope one should carry out the conservative treatment.

Disinfection Protocol

The management of these immature teeth can be initiated:

- Minimal or no instrumentation.
- Irrigation with 2.5-5.25% NaOCI, 3% hydrogen peroxide.
- Intra-canal medication with antimicrobial agents consisting of equal parts of ciprofloxacin in a paste form at the concentration of 20mg/ml.

This gentle treatment regimen is just an attempt to conserve whatever viable tissues may have remained in the canal system that harbour stem cells, SCAP in the apical papilla and DPSCs in the pulp.

A clinical protocol to treat immature teeth after a thorough irrigation is summarized as follows:

ROOT CANAL REVASCULARISATION *VIA* BLOOD CLOTTING
POSTNATAL STEM CELL THERAPY
PULP IMPLANTATION
SCAFFOLD IMPLANTATION
INJECTABLE SCAFFOLD DELIVERY
3-D CELL PRINTING
GENE DELIVERY

- The antimicrobial paste is to be introduced into the canal carefully to a depth slightly deficient of the remaining vital tissue with a lentulo spiral and the accessed cavity sealed with 2mm thick inner layer and 2 mm-thick durable cement such as glass ionomer outer layer [13]
- After 2 weeks, the patient should return for evaluation. If the tooth is asymptomatic and lacks clinical signs of pathology, the canal will be re-accessed to visually examine the condition under a microscope [14]. If there is no observable virulent exudate, the canal system will be irrigated with NaOCl and chlorhexidine followed by sterile normal saline and then cement which is to be placed over it [14].
- The accessed cavity will then be sealed with glass ionomer or resin-modified glass ionomer cement and the tooth should be followed up periodically to observe the maturation of the root [15].

Blood Clot Formation in Canal Space (Figs. 13 and 14)

- Some investigators induce hemorrhage by an endodontic explorer penetrating slightly into the remaining pulp tissue or periapical tissue allowing the blood clot to form in the canal and stopped at a level 3 mm below CEJ [16, 17].
- MTA then placed over the blood clot.
- The blood clot is considered as a scaffold and source of growth factors to facilitate the regeneration and repair of tissues into the canal.

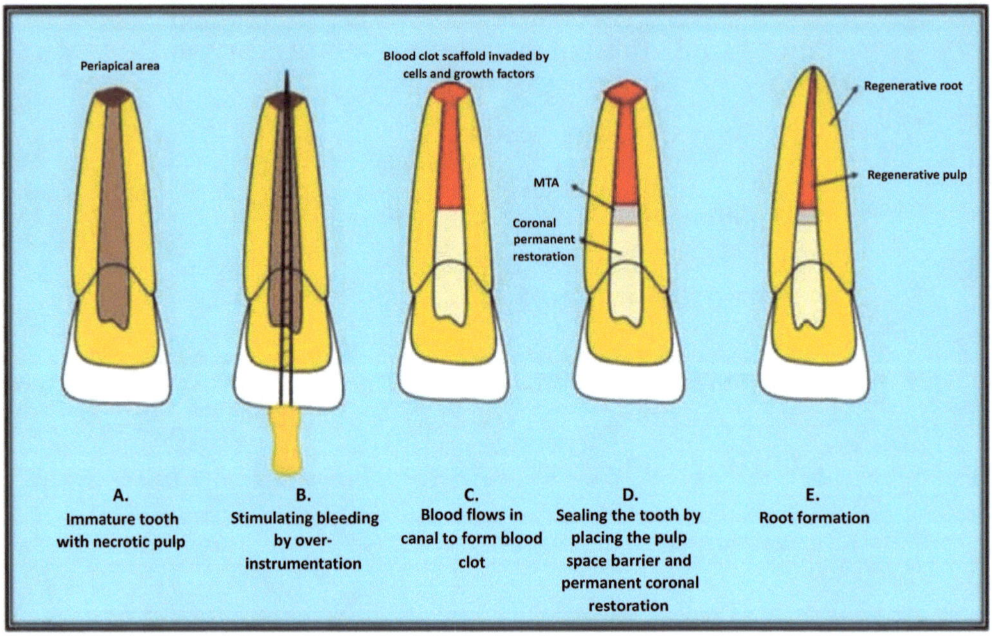

Fig. (13). Revascularization procedure.

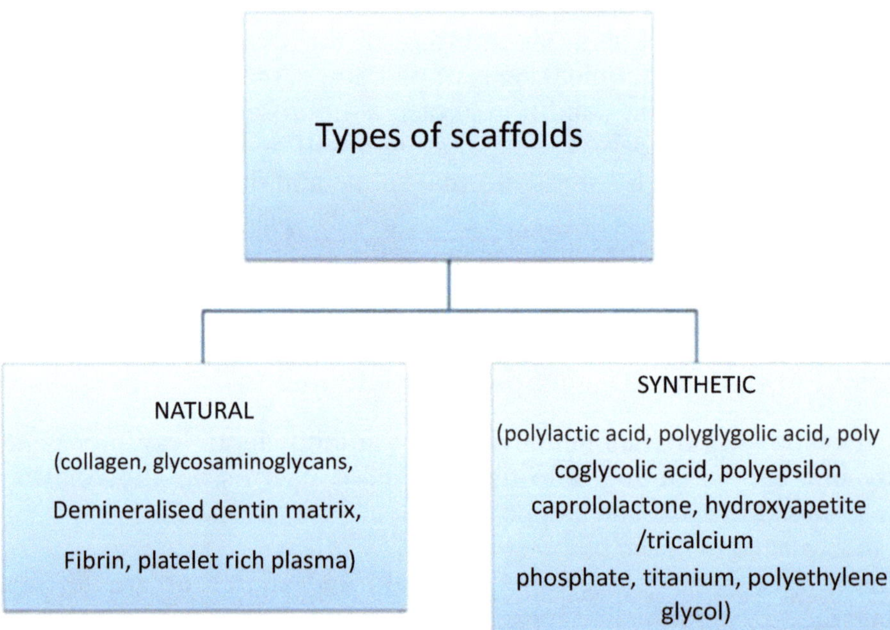

Fig. (14). Types of scafold.

Outcome

- Given a condition that is free of infection, many tissues are programmed and capable of self-regeneration to repair the damaged portion. The literature is replete with the finding that if disinfection can be performed effectively, pulp tissue can heal, and a new dentin bridge will form.
- Whether the thickened root is formed by pulp tissue from the remaining vital pulp and dental papilla at the apical region, or that is formed by PDL tissue that has grown into the root canal from the apical foramen and deposited the cementum onto the inner surface of the root dentin, is not clear.
- The dental papilla at the apex contains stem cells (SCAP) that have been recently described to be more robust stem cells than DPSCs. The SCAP may survive the infection to allow maturation while the survived DPSCs in the remaining vital pulp, rebuild the lost pulp tissue in the canal and may give rise to replacement odontoblasts to substitute for the damaged primary odontoblasts.

3Mix-MP

- Antibiotics (3Mix)
  - Ciprofloxacin 200mg
  - Metronidazole 500mg
  - Minocycline 100mg
- **Carrier (MP)**
  - Macrogol ointment
  - Propylene glycol

Protocol for preparation

Antibiotics (3Mix)

- Be sure to not cross-contaminate.
- Remove sugar coating from tablets with surgical blade, crush individually in separate mortars
- Open capsules, crush in individually in separate mortars
- Grind each antibiotic to a fine powder
- Combine equal amounts of antibiotics (1:1:1) on mixing pad

Carrier (MP)

- Equal amounts of macrogol ointment and propylene glycol (1:1)
- Using clean spatula, mix on pad
- Result should be opaque

- **Separate out small portions of 3Mix and incorporate into MP using the following:**
  - 1:5 MP:3Mix) → creamy consistency
  - 1:7 (standard mix) → smears easily but does not crumble
  - If result is flaky or crumbly, then too much 3Mix has been incorporated

- ***Storage***

- Antibiotics must be kept separately in moisture-tight porcelain containers
- Macrogol ointment and propylene glycol must be stored separately
- Discard if the mixture is transparent (evidence of moisture contamination)

Bioroot Engineering

- Dental implants have recently gained momentum as a preferred option for replacing missing teeth instead of bridges or removable dentures [18].
- However, although dental implants have had great improvements over the past decades, the fundamental pitfall is the lack of a natural structural relationship with the alveolar bone (*i.e.*, the absence of PDL). In fact, it requires a direct integration with bone onto its surface as the prerequisite for success. The lack of natural contours and its structural interaction with the alveolar bone make dental implants a temporary option until a better alternative is available.
- The other approach is to use SCAP and PDLSCs to form a bio root. Using a minipig model, autologous SCAP and PDLSCs were loaded onto HA/TCP and gelfoam scaffolds respectively and implanted into sockets of the lower jaw. A post channel was precreated to leave space for post insertion. Three months later, the bio root was exposed, and a porcelain crown was inserted. This approach is relatively a quick way of creating a root onto which an artificial crown can be installed [19].
- The bio root is different from the natural root and the root structure is developed by SCAP in a random manner. Nevertheless, the bio root is encircled with periodontal ligament tissue and appears to have a natural relationship with the surrounding bone. What remains to be improved is the mechanical strength of the bio root, which are approximately two-thirds of a natural root (Fig. **15**).

Materials for Regeneration

- An even more daring goal would be to regain the tooth substance that was lost prior to the pulpal exposure.
- Stem cells, morphogenic or growth factors, and the scaffold of an extracellular matrix are key elements involved in the regeneration of a function dentin-pulp complex.

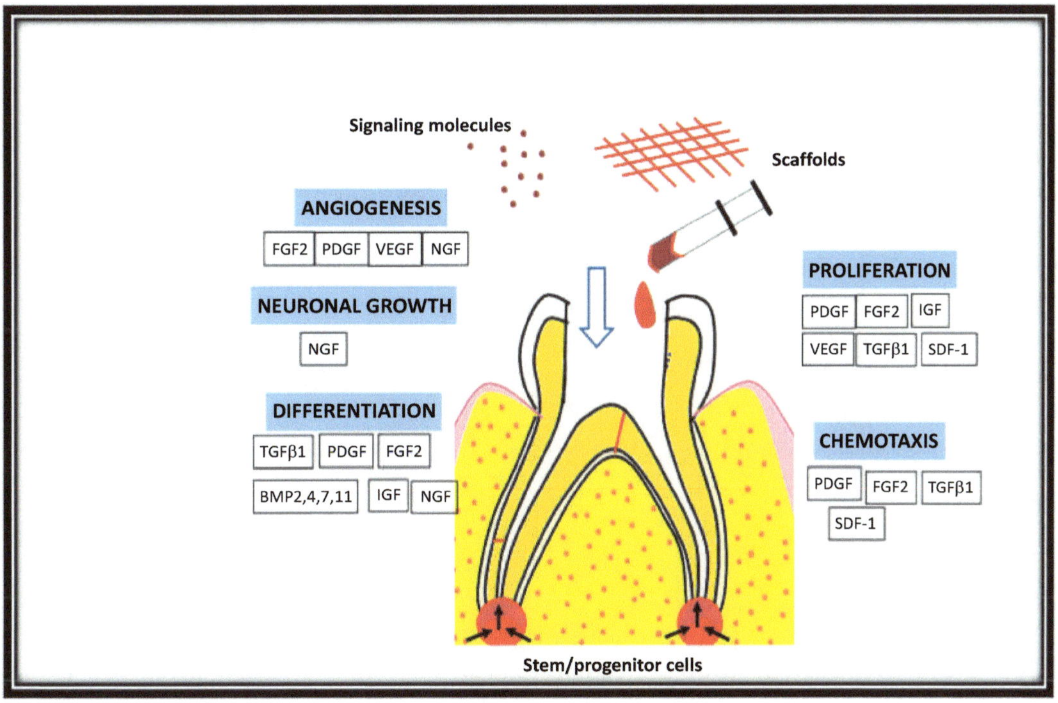

Fig. (15). The recruited stem/progenitor cells proliferate around injury and differentiate into a specific cell phenotype to replace the damaged cells. The replacement cells are stimulated to produce extracellular matrix that is essential for tissue to function biologically.

Mechanism of Action

- An environment free from wound infection and that the materials, after the initial exposure to the pulp, become relatively innocuous. Initiation of reparative dentin formation might not be attributed to any specific dentinogenic effect, but it appears that the stimulation of the wound healing process is affected by infection control.
- Bridge formation beneath a pulp capping material could be due to the properties of the capping materials such as sealing ability, alkalinity, and biocompatibility.
- The process of MTA - induced reparative dentinogenesis might primarily involve a "non-specific" wound healing mechanism of the exposed pulp, inducing cytological and functional changes within the pulpal cells, which result in the formation of fibronectin and reparative dentin at the surface of the mechanically exposed dental pulp. The application of MTA might provide a healing environment for the regeneration of pulp and dentin by osteoblastic-cementoblastic differentiation of human periodontal ligament cells but the exact mechanisms of its action as a pulp capping agent in humans are not completely understood.

- MTA does not contain calcium hydroxide; however, it contains calcium hydroxide, which forms calcium hydroxide with tissue fluids, producing a substance like hydroxyapatite adjacent to body fluids. An increase of the pH value to approximately 12.5 results in the release of calcium ions during the first few hours, this results in a mechanism like that of calcium hydroxide whereby a hard tissue bridge is formed following the development of inflammation and a narrow zone of tissue necrosis in subjacent pulp.
- In cell culture studies, the bioactivity, biocompatibility, and antibacterial properties of MTA may be caused in part by providing a mild calcium stimulus to cells in proximity of the material. These properties may contribute to the healing or regeneration of PDL tissue, which serves as a promising scaffold.
- EMD has been shown to increase the level of mineralization markers by stimulating the expression of osteo protegrin.

Prognosis

Although controversies exist regarding clinical outcomes, risk factors, primary *versus* permanent teeth and optimal treatments, numerous pulps that have been extirpated in the past could now be saved through the conservative approach of direct pulp capping with high success rates ranging from 93-98% after MTA pulp capping of cariously exposed permanent teeth.

The success rate is markedly different for mechanical exposure and carious exposure; the repair of mechanical exposure produces a 92% success rate compared with mere 33% for the carious exposures. Most of the failures in these reports remain asymptomatic; the pulp tends to become necrotic slowly. Clinical success is judged by the absence of clinical and radiographic signs of pathosis and the verification of continued dentin deposition both radiographically and clinically. Hard tissue barriers sometimes can be seen at the treated exposure site as early as six weeks after treatment.

SUMMARY

1. The two main concerns regarding direct pulp capping are canal obliteration and internal resorption. These calcific changes of the pulp tissue might signal a biological breakdown in tissue function.
2. Although direct pulp capping of mature teeth has less than a 50% chance of success. It is universally accepted that vital pulp therapy is the treatment of choice for immature teeth with incompletely developed apices.
3. In a recent systematic review on complete or ultraconservative removal of decayed tissue, partial removal of caries should be done rather than complete removal to reduce the risk of carious exposure. This step enables continued physiological dentin deposition and complete root development throughout the

length of the root, providing greater strength and more resistance to future vertical root fractures.

4. A successful outcome of patient treatment using the new direct pulp capping materials and techniques is less expensive and requires less treatment time.

CONCLUSION

The dental pulp is an ectomesenchymally derived connective tissue with certain unique properties such as being encased in hard tissues, which limits its collateral circulation. The pulp provides a matrix for binding of its cells and provides support allowing communication between the cells. In addition to immune cells, the dental pulp contains odontoblasts, which are specialized cells capable of producing dentin. In the absence of a vital pulp, dentin deposition is arrested. When an immature tooth is affected by caries or trauma, the pulp requires proper management according to the degree of inflammation and its vitality. Maintenance of pulp vitality will allow continued root development along the entire root length. If the pulp is irreversibly inflamed or necrotic, root-end closure procedures are required when the apex is not fully formed.

CONSENT FOR PUBLICATION

Not applicable.

CONFLICT OF INTEREST

The authors declare no conflict of interest, financial or otherwise.

ACKNOWLEDGEMENT

Declared none.

REFERENCES

[1] Song JS. Pulp treatment for immature permanent teeth. J Kor Den Assoc 2019; 57(8): 464-73.

[2] Shah D, Lynd T, Ho D, *et al.* Pulp-dentin tissue healing response: A discussion of current biomedical approaches. J Clin Med 2020; 9(2): 434.
[http://dx.doi.org/10.3390/jcm9020434] [PMID: 32033375]

[3] Mathew J, Syriac G, Nair M, Rahul J. Conventional multivisit calcium hydroxide apexification with rare apexogenesis like outcome and novel single visit mta apexification followed by root reinforcement with fiber post: Two case reports. Saudi J Oral Dent Res 2017; 2(2): 43-8.

[4] Vidal K, Martin G, Lozano O, Salas M, Trigueros J, Aguilar G. Apical closure in apexification: A review and case report of apexification treatment of an immature permanent tooth with biodentine. J Endod 2016; 42(5): 730-4.
[http://dx.doi.org/10.1016/j.joen.2016.02.007] [PMID: 26994597]

[5] Guerrero F, Mendoza A, Ribas D, Aspiazu K. Apexification: A systematic review. J Conserv Dent 2018; 21(5): 462-5.

[http://dx.doi.org/10.4103/JCD.JCD_96_18] [PMID: 30294103]

[6] Muhamad AH, Azzaldeen A, Hanali AS. Mineral trioxide aggregate (MTA) in apexification. Endodontology 2013; 25(2): 97-101.
[http://dx.doi.org/10.4103/0970-7212.352338]

[7] Ramnani K, Shetty R, Shetty S. Evaluation of outcomes of recent materials used for single visit apexification. J Adv Med Den Sci Res 2018; 6(6): 76-80.

[8] Ahlawat B, Kumar A, Chaudhary N, Laxmy V, Bhardwaj V. Apexification with rapid MTA plug technique. Indian J Sci Res 2015; 153-7.

[9] Lin JC, Lu JX, Zeng Q, Zhao W, Li WQ, Ling JQ. Comparison of mineral trioxide aggregate and calcium hydroxide for apexification of immature permanent teeth: A systematic review and meta-analysis. J Formos Med Assoc 2016; 115(7): 523-30.
[http://dx.doi.org/10.1016/j.jfma.2016.01.010] [PMID: 26911724]

[10] Majeed HA, Sherazi UR, Munir B. Comparison of effectiveness of mineral trioxide aggregate and calcium hydroxide in apexification procedure. Pak Oral Dent J 2018; 38(2)

[11] Thakur S, Thakur S, Parthi A, Bakshi S, Kridutt V. Management of an open apex with mineral trioxide aggregate apexification: A case report. International Journal of Preventive and Clinical Dental Research 2020; 7(2): 36.
[http://dx.doi.org/10.4103/INPC.INPC_6_20]

[12] Galler KM. Clinical procedures for revitalization: current knowledge and considerations. International endodontic journal 2016; 49(10): 926-36.
[http://dx.doi.org/10.1111/iej.12606]

[13] Kim SG, Kahler B, Lin LM. Current developments in regenerative endodontics. Current Oral Health Reports 2016; 3(4): 293-301.
[http://dx.doi.org/10.1007/s40496-016-0109-8]

[14] Boufdil H, Mtalsi M, El Arabi S, Bousfiha B. Apexification with Calcium Hydroxide *vs.* Revascularization. Case Rep Dent 2020; 2020: 1-6.
[http://dx.doi.org/10.1155/2020/9861609] [PMID: 32550029]

[15] Aly MM, Taha SEED, El Sayed MA, Youssef R, Omar HM. Clinical and radiographic evaluation of Biodentine and Mineral Trioxide Aggregate in revascularization of non-vital immature permanent anterior teeth (randomized clinical study). Int J Paediatr Dent 2019; 29(4): 464-73.
[http://dx.doi.org/10.1111/ipd.12474] [PMID: 30702789]

[16] Staffoli S, Plotino G, Nunez Torrijos B, *et al.* Regenerative endodontic procedures using contemporary endodontic materials. Materials (Basel) 2019; 12(6): 908.
[http://dx.doi.org/10.3390/ma12060908] [PMID: 30893790]

[17] Chisini LA, Grazioli G, Francia A, Martin ASS, Demarco FF, Conde MCM. Revascularization *versus* apical barrier technique with mineral trioxide aggregate plug: A systematic review. G Ital Endod 2018; 32(1): 9-16. [Anamaria Matichescu].
[http://dx.doi.org/10.1016/j.gien.2018.03.006]

[18] Matichescu A, Ardelean LC, Rusu LC, *et al.* Advanced Biomaterials and Techniques for Oral Tissue Engineering and Regeneration-A Review. Materials (Basel) 2020; 13(22): 5303.

[19] Arangannal P, Jeevarathan J, Amudha S , Aarthi J, Vijayakumar M. 'Bioroot' –A Nascent Paradigm In Tooth Regeneration. Eur J Mol Clin Med 2020; 7(2): 6474-81.

CHAPTER 7

Endodontic Instruments and Irrigants

M.H. Raghunath Reddy[1] and **H. Sharath Chandra**[1,*]

[1] *SJM Dental College and Hospital, Chitradurga, Karnataka, India*

Abstract: Pulpectomy is the treatment of choice for pulpally involved deciduous teeth, which potentially eliminates inflamed or necrotic pulp, bacteria, and toxins, relieving pain and promoting periradicular healing by cleaning and shaping the root canals. Over the years, cleaning and shaping of the root canals are done by manual endodontic instruments like files and reamers which are still considered to be the gold standard. With the advent and advances in Nickel Titanium rotary files, rotary endodontic instruments have been widely used for cleaning and shaping the root canals in Pediatric Dentistry. Of rotary files is less time-consuming thereby reducing stress to both the child and the dentist, giving consistent and predictable results even in narrow and curved root canals due to superelasticity and shape memory of nickel-titanium alloy

Keywords: Nickel-Titanium files, Paediatric rotary files, Pulpectomy, Rotary endodontics.

INTRODUCTION

Paediatric dentistry has emerged as a highly specialised branch in which endodontic procedures of deciduous teeth are the major treatment. An endodontic procedure of deciduous teeth preserves function, and esthetics and ensures normal eruption and it is preferred over extraction. It offers quite a few challenges in paediatric patients ranging from limited cooperation of the child to complex root canal morphology. Prerequisite for successful endodontic treatment includes removal of infected or inflamed pulp, toxins and bacteria from the root canals which results in effective infection control thereby relieving pain and permitting healing of periradicular tissue.

The primary objective of cleaning and shaping root canals is to remove soft and hard tissue, giving access for irrigating solutions to the apical part of the canal, creating space for the delivery of medicaments and obturating material along with retaining the integrity of radicular structures [1]. Endodontic instrumentation over

* **Corresponding author H. Sharath Chandra:** SJM Dental College and Hospital, Chitradurga, Karnataka, India; E-mail: sharathchandrah2012@gmail.com

Satyawan Damle, Ritesh Kalaskar & Dhanashree Sakhare (Eds.)

the years was done by stainless steel files manually, as they have excellent tactile control with sharp and long-lasting cutting surfaces. With limited flexibility of the hand files, accessing narrow constricted canals is difficult and manual preparation of curved canals is laborious resulting in inconsistent preparation of the canals (Fig. **1**) [2].

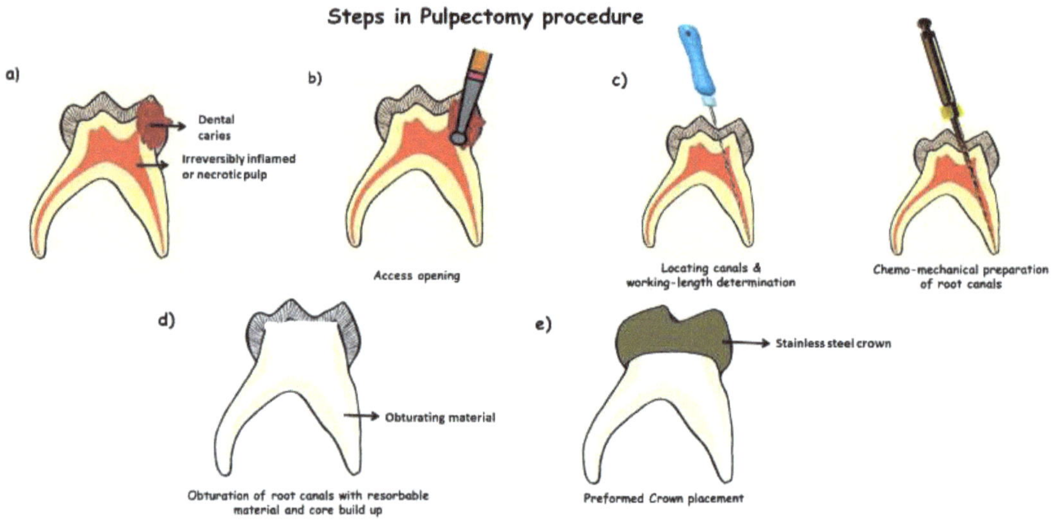

Fig. (1). Pulpectomy procedure with preformed crown placement.

With the advent of Nickel-Titanium alloys (NiTi) in endodontics, a new dimension is added to endodontic instrumentation with several NiTi file systems introduced for chemo-mechanical cleaning and shaping of the root canals providing faster, safer, and consistent root canal preparations.

Nickel-Titanium Instruments

History: George Andreasen & co. pioneered feasible studies on the potential uses of Nickel-Titanium alloys for dentistry. Andreasen and Morrow presented the mechanical properties of this alloy, especially the very low elastic modulus and very wide elastic working range of the alloy compared with stainless steel along with its notable clinical applications. Harmeet Walia thought that Nickel-Titanium (NiTi) alloy due to its very low elastic modulus might have enormous potential for endodontic files which simplifies negotiation of curved root canals with much greater ease than stainless steel instruments available at that time. Walia *et al.* developed the first prototype of NiTi hand files by machining large diameter orthodontic wires and compared it with stainless steel hand files of the same size manufactured by a similar machining process for bending and torsion, with Niti showing promising initial results. With further studies on Niti, innovative dental manufacturers began to market NiTi endodontic instruments in the 1990s. Subsequently, many other manufacturers introduced NiTi rotary instruments for endodontics. Of late studies on the properties and performance of these instruments became an intensive area for endodontic research.

Features of NiTi Endodontic Instruments

Superelasticity and shape memory: The mechanical behaviour of superelasticity and shape memory of NiTi alloys result from the nature and proportions of their microstructural phases. There are three phases in the NiTi alloys.

1. Austenitic NiTi (austenite) exists at higher temperatures and lower stress and have a complex body-centred cubic structure.

2. Martensitic NiTi (martensite) exists at lower temperatures and higher stress, and have a complex structure described as Monoclinic.

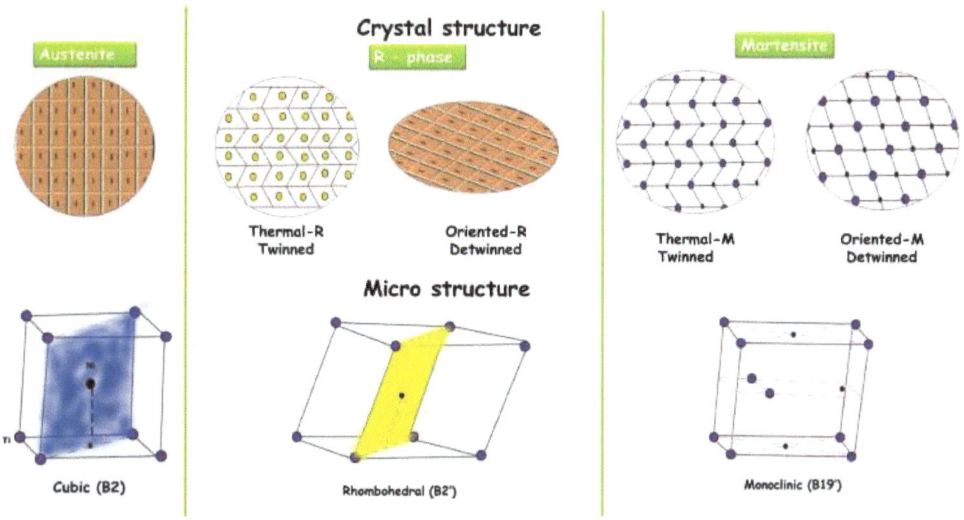

Fig. (2). Crystal and Microstructures of Nickel-Titanium alloy.

3. The R-phase is an intermediate phase that forms during the forward transformation from martensite to austenite on heating and reverses the transformation from austenite to martensite on cooling, possessing a rhombohedral structure (Fig. **2**). At the atomic level, transformation between austenite and martensite occurs by a twinning process and the reversibility of the twinning process is the origin of its shape memory (Figs. **3** and **4**) [3].

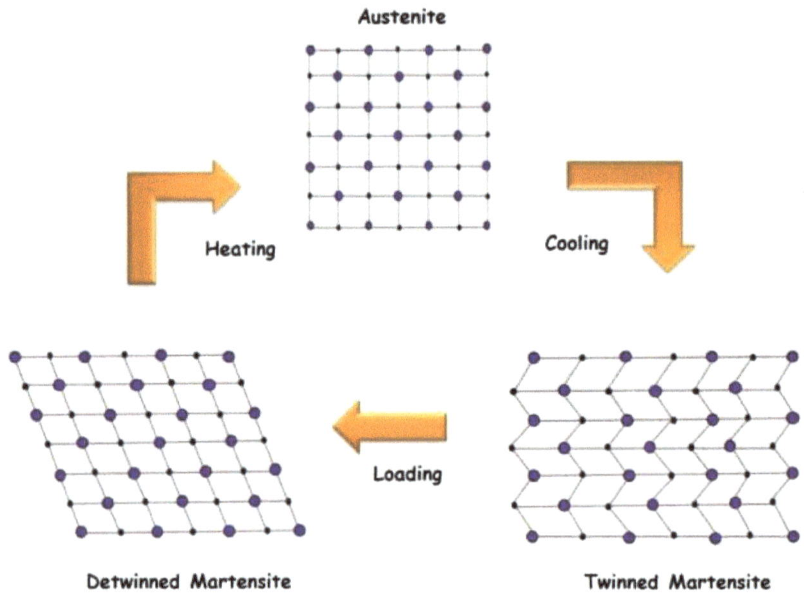

Fig. (3a). Nitinol transformations during heating/cooling and stress loading.

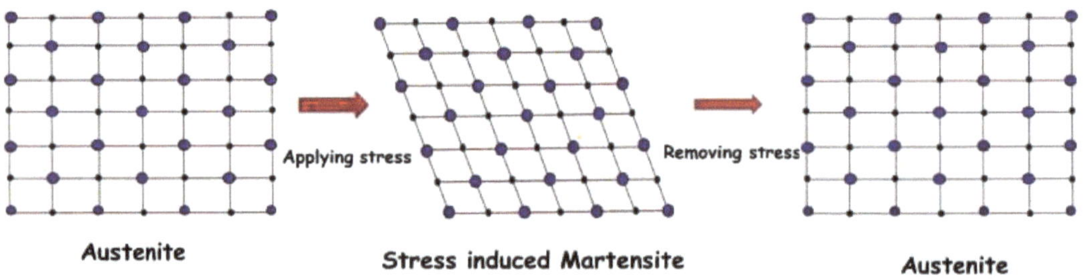

Fig. (3b). Nitinol transformations on loading and unloading of stress.

High resistance to cyclic fatigue: This property allows negotiating narrow and severely curved canals without the instrument getting fractured.

Manufacturing: Most of the NiTi endodontic instruments are manufactured by a grinding process, laser etching and others by plastic deformation under heating. Newer manufacturing methods employ casting of the alloy or stamping wire blanks. Electropolishing the machined surface, ion implantation and coating it with titanium nitride are done to improve the surface quality and enhance cutting efficiency. Heat treating the instruments during manufacturing also yields beneficial results.

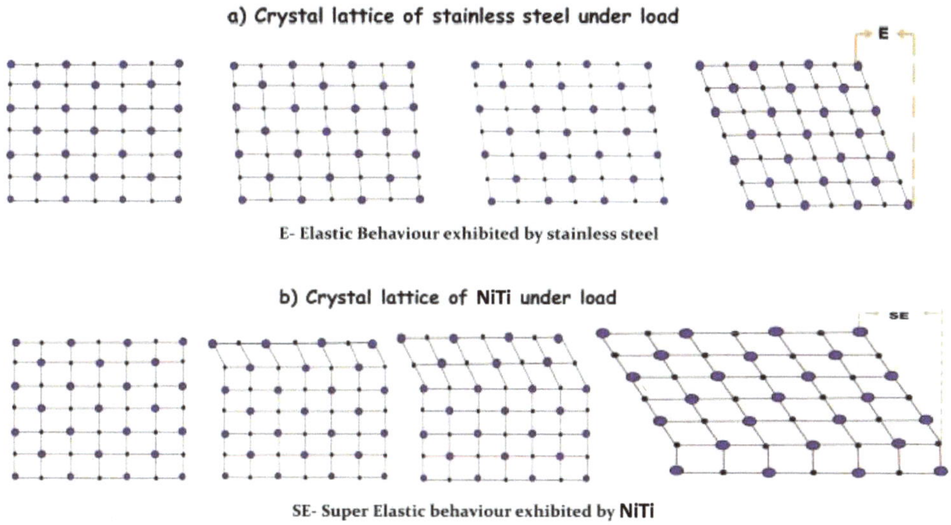

Fig. (4). Comparison of stainless steel and Nitinol crystal lattices behaviour under load.

c. Rotary NiTi files

Since the early 1990s, several NiTi instrument systems were introduced into Endodontics which vary in tip sizing, taper, cross-section, helix angle and pitch.

i. Evolution of rotary files

Each generation of files has different designs, taper, and material properties (Table **1**) [2].

Table 1. Different generations of rotary endodontic files system.

Generation	Features	File system
I^st^	• Fixed taper • Passive cutting edges • More files are required to prepare the canal	LightSpeed Quantec System GT
IInd	• Variable taper • Active cutting edges • Less no. of files is required to prepare the canal	Protaper universal Hero shaper M two
IIIrd	• Reduced cyclic fatigue • Heat-treated files • Decreased file breakage	Twisted files Hyflex cm Profile GT series X
IVth	• Bidirectional reciprocating movement • Single file concept	Self-adjusting files Reciproc

(Table 1) cont.....

Generation	Features	File system
V^{th}	• Offset design of file to minimize the engagement between the file and dentin.	Revo-S One Shape ProTaper Next

ii) Advantages of NiTi rotary files

• Several clinical problems like blocks, ledges, transportation, perforation can be reduced by using NiTi rotary instruments

• Reduced stress both to the clinician and patient as the use of rotary files easier, faster, and safe.

• Minimizes extrusion of debris.

• Spin 360^0 within the root canal space providing effective canal debridement and consistent and predictable root canal shaping.

• Instrument design and flexibility of NiTi alloy facilitate the files to closely follow the original root canal path [1, 4, 5].

Rotary NiTi files are used widely in permanent teeth, it was first introduced in paediatric endodontics by Barr *et al.* (2000) and stated that similar principles of canal debridement and shaping of canals by rotary files can be applied for deciduous teeth. Since then, many practitioners started using various rotary file systems like Profile, ProTaper, FlexMaster, Mtwo, Hero shaper, Light Speed LSX, Race, K3, twisted files and Wave One for endodontic procedures on primary teeth.

Endodontic treatment of deciduous teeth demands extra concern as they have shorter, thinner, curved roots and ribbon-shaped morphology compared to permanent teeth. Hence the use of existing rotary files which are predesigned for permanent teeth may lead to lateral perforation on the inner surface due to greater taper.

Over time, rotary file systems which can be used exclusively for deciduous teeth were introduced (Fig. **5**).

iii. Prerequisite features of paediatric rotary files

- A shortened chairside time and minimum no. of appointments.
- Minimising root canal debris extrusion which avoids postoperative complications.

- Requiring lesser series of files to achieve final cleaning and shaping the root canals.
- Shorter length of the files because of the limited mouth opening of the children.
- Efficient for the preparation of funnel-shaped canals which in turn produce uniform fill of obturating material paste [5].

d. **Differences between hand and rotary endodontics** [6, 7, 11].

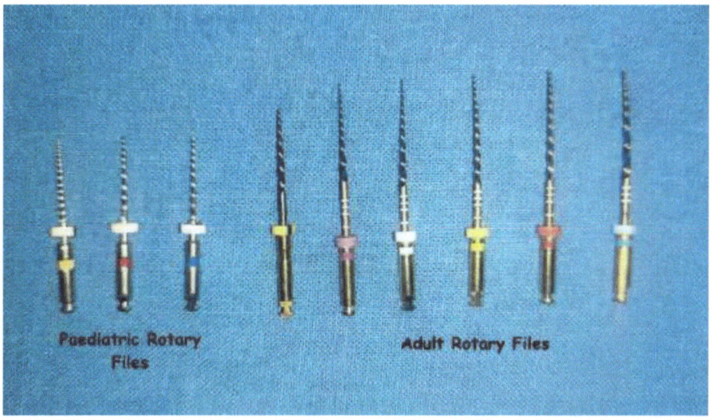

Fig. (5). Picture showing Paediatric rotary files for deciduous teeth and rotary files for permanent teeth.

Property	Hand Endodontics	Rotary Endodontics
Time	Time-consuming	Time-saving
Root dentin	Inefficient removal of the infected root dentin	Efficient cleaning of the infected root dentin
Canal Centricity	Canal Centricity is not maintained	Canal centricity is maintained
Root apex	Apex is widened	Apex is maintained narrow
Canal Taper	Insufficient taper of canals for better obturation	Sufficient taper of canals for better obturation

Various Paediatric Rotary Files Available

a. Kedo rotary files
b. PRO AF baby gold ™ files
c. Pedoflex files
d. Prime Pedo™
e. Waldent Pedoflex files
f. Fanta dental AF baby tooth files
g. Denco® Kids files
h. Neolix™
i. DXL-Pro Pedo™

Kedo Rotary Files

Kedo rotary files are the world's first rotary files exclusively for shaping primary teeth. It is designed by Dr Ganesh Jeevanandan and came into existence in 2016. The main feature of these files is Variably variable (VV) taper design which provides flexibility and efficiency to achieve consistently successful cleaning and shaping [1].

The rotary Kedo files are available as:

- Kedo-S file system (Kids endodontic shaper)
- Kedo SG
- Kedo SG blue
- Kedo-S square

Kedo-S^{TM} File System (Kids Endodontic Shaper)

- It consists of three Ni-Ti rotary files. The total length of the files is 16 mm with 12mm of working length of the files and a non-cutting tip. The files are named D1, E1, U1. All these files have a variable taper corresponding to the use in primary teeth. The taper of the instruments is designed according to the diameter of primary teeth with narrow and wide root canals [1].
- D1 red file- Used with narrow canals (mesial canals in mandibular molars and distobuccal canal in maxillary molars) and has a tip diameter of 0.25 mm with a variable taper (Fig. **6**).
- E1 blue file- Used in wider molar canals (distal canal in mandibular molars and palatal canal in maxillary molars) and has a tip diameter of 0.30 mm.
- U1 black file- Used in primary incisor teeth and has a tip diameter of 0.40 mm (Fig. **6**).

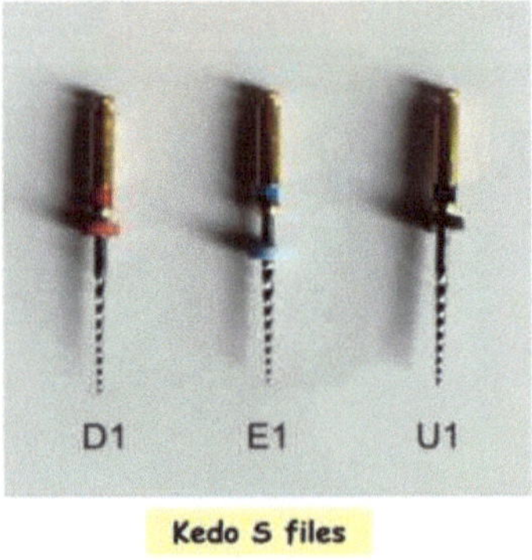

Fig. (6a). Kedo S files. D1- red colour coded with 0.25mm tip diameter, E1- blue colour coded with 0.30mm tip diameter, U1- black colour coded with tip diameter 0.40mm.

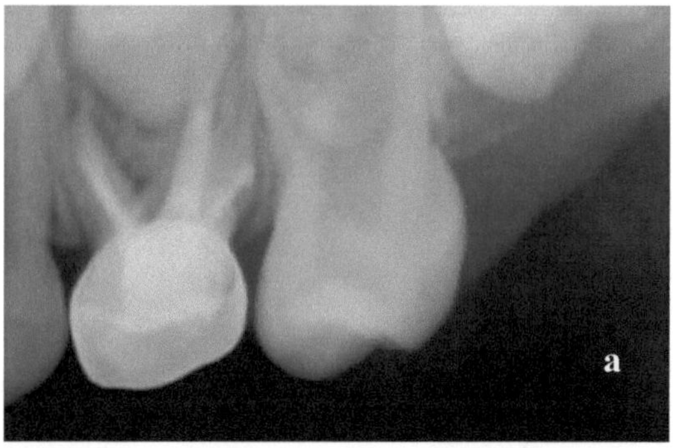

Fig. (6b). Postoperative radiograph of an obturated maxillary left first deciduous molar with root canal preparation done by Kedo S files D1& E1.

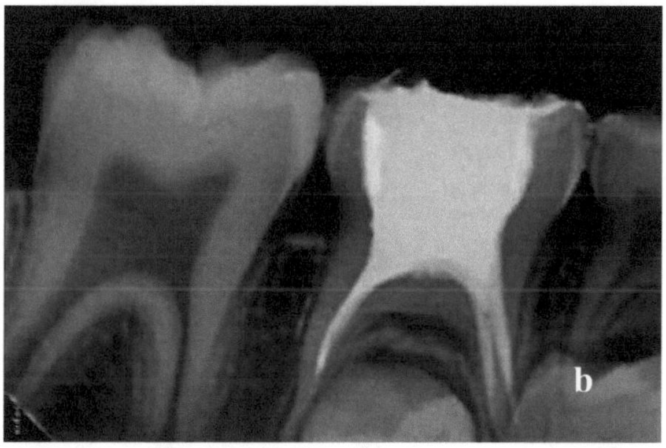

Fig. (6c). Postoperative radiograph of an obturated mandibular right second deciduous molar with root canal preparation done by Kedo S files D1& E1.

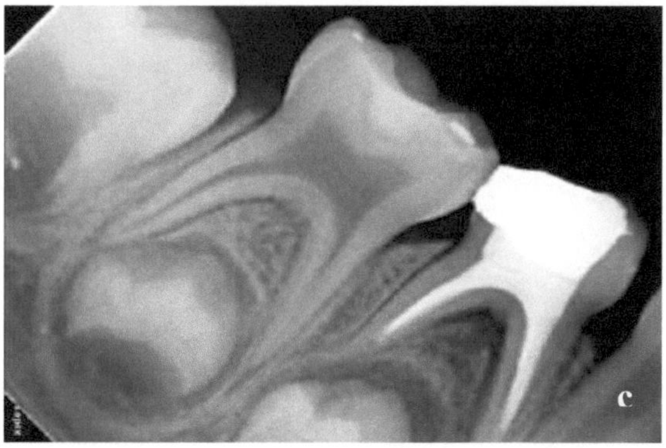

Fig. (6d). Postoperative radiograph of an obturated mandibular right first deciduous molar with root canal preparation done by Kedo S files D1& E1.

Kedo SG ™ files: They have similar features to Kedo S files, but files are heat-treated files, which have greater resistance to cyclic fatigue than Kedo S files (Fig. 7).

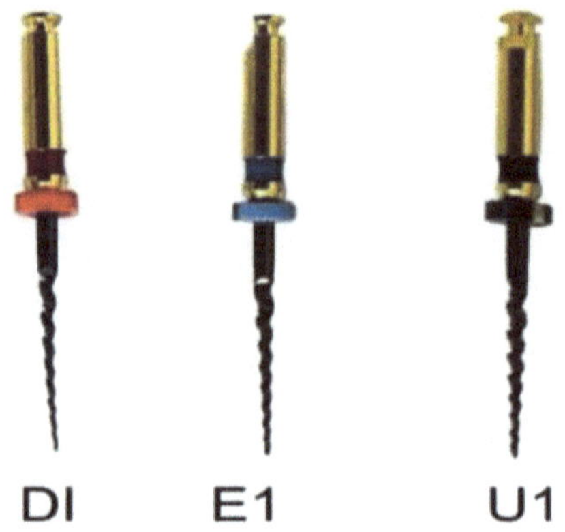

Fig. (7). Kedo SG files. D1- red colour coded with 0.25mm tip diameter, E1- blue colour coded with 0.30mm tip diameter, U1- black colour coded with tip diameter 0.40mm.

Kedo SG blue ™ files: These files are heat-treated NiTi and coated with titanium oxide which have greater resistance to cyclic fatigue and superior flexibility (Fig. **8**).

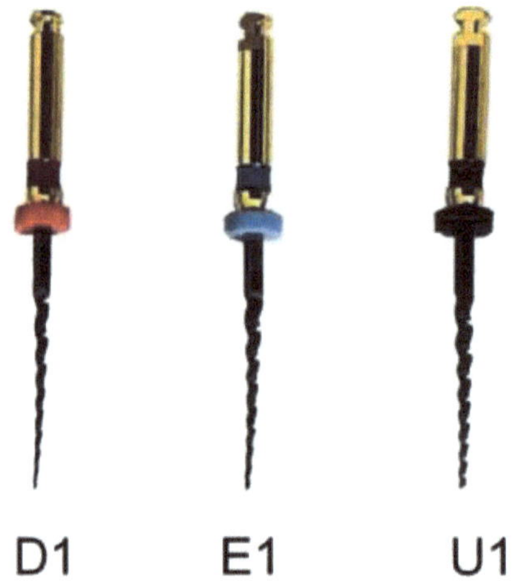

Fig. (8). Kedo SG blue files. D1- red colour coded with 0.25mm tip diameter, E1- blue colour coded with 0.30mm tip diameter, U1- black colour coded with tip diameter 0.40mm.

Kedo-S™ square files: They are truly single file systems with one file for canal preparation of complete molar. These files are heat-treated NiTi with titanium oxide coated. It has the advantage of finishing canal preparation in lesser time than current paediatric rotary files (Fig. **9**).

Available as:

P1- used for primary molars

A1 –used for primary anteriors

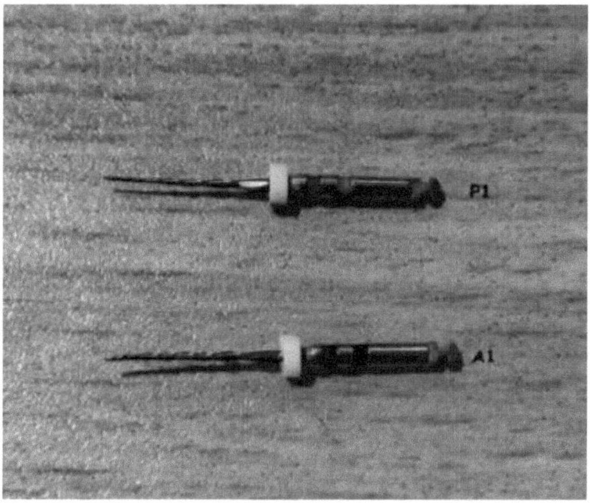

Fig. (9). Kedo- S square files. P1- used for deciduous molars, A1- used for deciduous anteriors.

Technique for Using Kedo Rotary Files

a. Torque controlled endodontic motor with 300 RPM, 2-2.4 torque to be used for the rotary files.
b. Files should be used 'in and out' action but not in brushing motion and irrigate the canal.
c. Once the working length is reached, file should be withdrawn.
d. After each step, the used file should be cleaned and checked for distortion.
e. Forceful preparation should be avoided by not applying excess pressure during the instrumentation (Fig. **10**) [7].

PRO AF BABY GOLD ™ FILES

Features

- The length of the files is 17mm
- Advanced NiTi controlled memory wire of these files has better canal centricity unlike NiTi file.
- Heat-treated files with minimal file separation in the canals.
- A sequential combination of 4% and 6% taper files improves the canal shaping.

Instrumentation protocol

Once access opening is done, canal should be negotiated with No. 10 K hand file upto working length

Determine the width of the canals using Nos. 15 K files

- If the Nos. 15 hand files have a snug fit, the canal is said to be narrower
- Nos. 15 hand files are used reciprocating back and forth motion passively and progressively until they are loose

- D1 (red) rotary file is used in the narrower canals.
- D1 is designed to cut dentin, in a crown down manner, with its controlled taper avoiding excess root dentin removal and used till the working length.
- Irrigate the canals to break up debris.

- If the Nos. 15 hand files have a loose fit, the canal is said to be wider
- Nos. 15 is used for initial enlargement

- E1 (blue) is used in the wider canals.
- For ease in preparation of the wider canals, D1 can be used first followed by E1 kedo rotary file (blue).
- Irrigate the canals to break up debris.

- U1 (black) Kedo rotary file is used in the anterior canals.
- U1 is designed to cut dentin, in a crown down manner, with its controlled taper avoiding excess root dentin removal.
- U1 files are used till the working length.
- Irrigate the canals to break up debris.

Fig. (10). Instrumentation protocol for using Kedo rotary files.

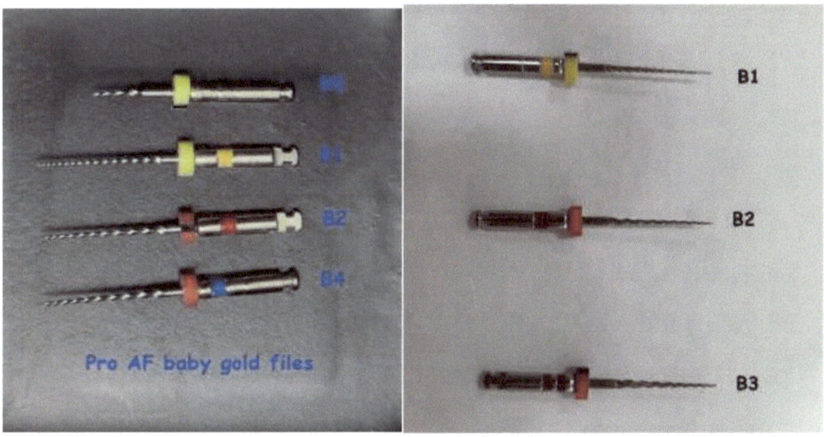

Fig. (11). PRO AF baby gold files system.

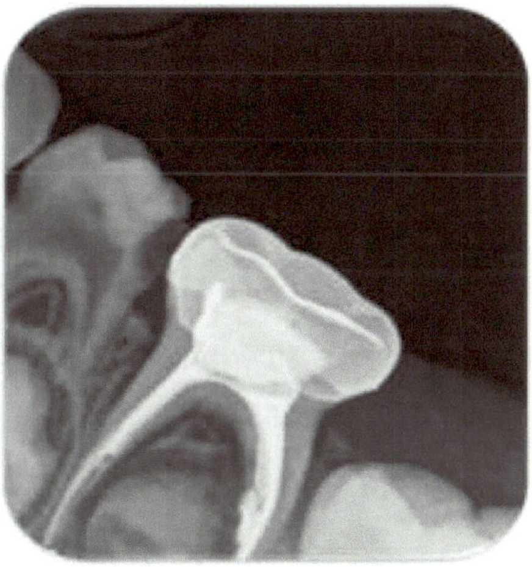

Fig. (12a). Postoperative radiograph of an obturated mandibular left second deciduous molar with root canal preparation done by PRO AF baby gold files.

Table 2. Combination of Pro AF baby gold files for different root canals.

File	Purpose
B1 and B2	Narrow canals
B2 and B3	Medium canals
B2 and B4	Wide canals
B5	For maxillary anteriors

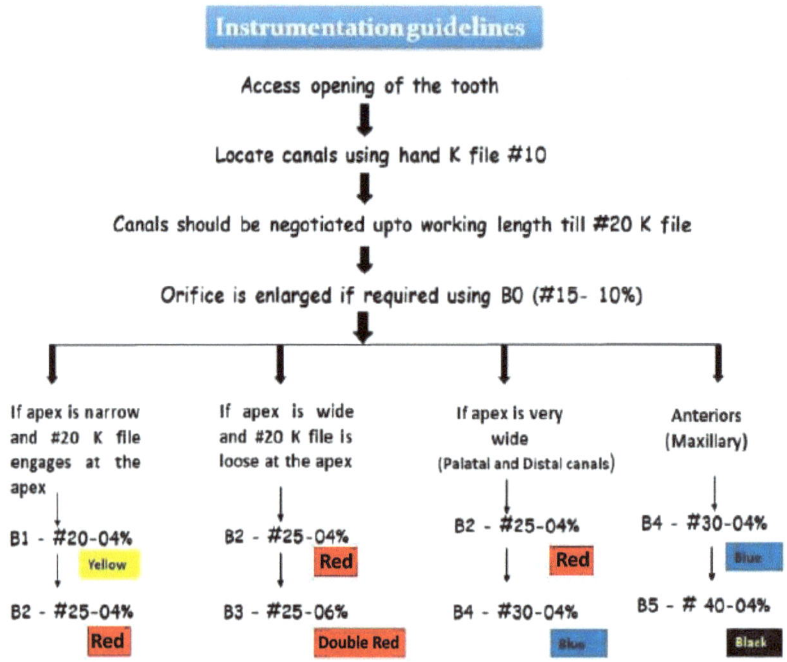

Fig. (12b). Instrumentation guidelines for PRO AF baby gold files.

Available in five file system and an orifice opener (Figs. **11** and **12**, Table **2**).

- B0 – orifice opener
- B1 - #20-04%
- B2 - #25-04%
- B3 - #25-06%
- B4 - #30-04%
- B5 - #40-04%

NEOENDO PEDOFLEX FILES

- Simple file sequence for easy & quick treatment procedure
- Unique file design with its flexibility & efficiency makes it compatible with all types of canals of primary teeth
- The total length of the file is 16mm
- Available in 3 file system (Figs. **13a**, **b**)
  - Yellow -#20, 4% taper
  - Red - #25, 4% taper
  - Blue - # 30, 4% taper

PRIME PEDO ™ FILE SYSTEM

These type of files have a triangular cross-section, are heat-treated, and have controlled memory which allow them to be centred in the curved canals of the primary molars. Heat-treated files are more resistant to deformation and follow the original anatomy of the root canals [8].

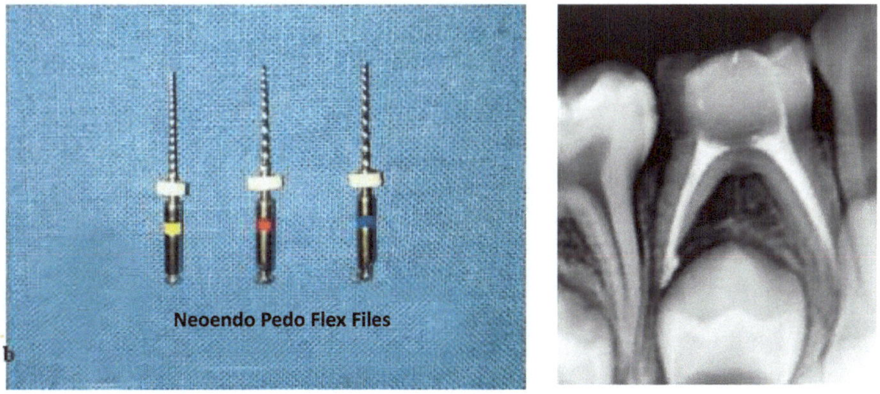

Fig. (13). a. Picture showing Neoendo Pedoflex files, **b.** Postoperative radiograph of an obturated mandibular right first deciduous molar with root canal preparation done by Neoendo Pedoflex files.

It consists of four files (Starter, P1, P2, Endosonic file).

- Starter -16mm length, 8% taper
- P1 – 18 mm 6%, no.15 (for narrow canals)
- P2 – 18mm 6%, no.25 (for standard &large canals)
- Endosonic file: 18mm 2% taper for apical 1/3rd preparation

Endosonic file with 2% taper allows for conservative apical preparation of primary molars. Files are operated at the speed of 250-400 RPM and torque 2.0-4.0 N/cm.

WALDENT PEDO- FLEX FILES

- Pedo-flex files made of Niti, durable and temperature rebound memory.
- Length of the files is 16mm available as 4 file system 4% 20, 4% 25, 4% 30, 6% 25.
- Files have a triangular cross-section, guiding non-cutting tips with sharp cutting edges.

FANTA DENTAL AF BABY TOOTH FILES

- These files are made by proprietary control memory Niti technology with greater flexibility.
- Classic cross-section and taper design preserve more dentine
- The length of the file is 16mm and available in three files

  AF1 – 4% taper 20 size

  AF2 – 4% taper 25 size

  AF3 – 4%taper 30 size

DENCO® KIDS FILES

- Short thread design, matching small roots of deciduous teeth
- The thread of the file is changed from the tip of the file to the back to facilitate chip evacuation.

  Available in four file system (Table 3)

Red - 4% 25 size, 17mm length

Red- 6% 25 size, 17mm length

Blue- 4% 30 size, 17mm length

Black- 4% 40 size, 19mm length

Table 3. Specifications of Denco Kids files.

-	Length (mm)	Size		Taper (%)	Diameter in mm
Denco files	17	Red	25#04	04	0.25
	17	Red	25#06	06	0.25
	17	Blue	30#04	04	0.30
	19	Black	40#04	04	0.40

Sterilization of Rotary Files

Files must be sterilized before use. ANSI/ADA Specification 28 recommends:

Instruments are Scrubbed with Soap and Warm Water

- Rinsed with distilled or deionized water thoroughly and is allowed to dry.
- Instruments are kept in an autoclave tray unwrapped.
- Instruments are steam autoclaved at 136^{0}C (plus or minus 2^{0}C) for 20 minutes.
- All rotary files are single patient use instruments.

- Used files are placed in Biohazard Sharps container.

Step Method (P Parashos)

1. 10 vigorous strokes in a scouring sponge soaked in 0.2% chlorhexidine solution
2. 30-minute pre-soaking in an enzymatic cleaning solution
3. 15-minute ultra-sonication in an enzymatic cleaning solution.
4. 20-second rinse in running tap water [9, 10].

Instrument Separation\ Fracture

It is one of the major concerns with the use of nickel-titanium rotary files. They have been reported to undergo unexpected fracture without warning or any visible defects of previous permanent deformation. Fracture of rotary files occurs in two distinct modes, torsional and flexural [11, 12].

- **Torsional Fracture** - instrument tip is locked in a canal while the shank continues to rotate, thereby exerting enough torque to fracture the tip. It also may occur when instrument rotation is sufficiently slowed in relation to the cross-sectional diameter (Fig. **14**).
- **Flexural fracture** - Cyclic loading leads to metal fatigue.
    a. Factors governing the potential for Niti rotary files fracture
    b. Guidelines to minimize the risk of fracture:
- Always create a glide path and patency with small (at least #10) hand files.
- Good finger rests and ensuring straight-line access to the canals.
- Use stiffer, larger, and stronger files (such as orifice shapers) to create coronal shapes before using the narrower, more fragile instruments in the apical regions.
- Use a light touch only, ensuring to never push hard on the instrument.
- Use a pecking (*i.e.,* touch-retract) action, with increments depending upon particular canal anatomy and instrument design characteristics.
- Do not hurry during the instrumentation and avoid rapid jerking movements; beware of clicking.
- Replace files sooner after use in very narrow and severely curved canals.
- Files should be examined regularly with magnification during usage.
- Files should be moved in a chamber flooded with sodium hypochlorite.
- Avoid keeping the file in one spot, especially in curved canals.
- Practice is essential when learning new techniques and new instruments [11, 12].
- Clinician's handling (most important) includes the number of times file is used, pressure on instrument, irrigation & lubrication, dynamics of instrument use.
- A combination of torsional load, bending and axial fatigue
- Manufacture process and quality
- Root canal anatomy

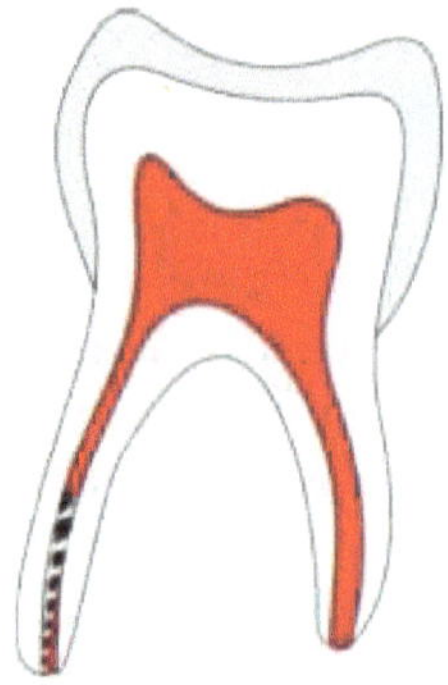

Fig. (14). Picture showing instrument separation in the root canal of deciduous tooth.

Disadvantages of the Rotary System in Deciduous Teeth

- High cost of files and low constant-torque handpiece.
- Due to a decrease in tactile sensitivity during apical preparation of the root canal compared to manual mechanical preparation, rotary preparation requires training of the operator.
- Root tip resorption is often undetectable which may lead to overfilling of canals and increased risk of perforation.
- Peculiar root canal morphology leaves unclean areas and potentially infected tissue in fins and isthmuses necessitating the use of an additional H-file along with sodium hypochlorite irrigation for the removal of loose pulp tissue. (Drukteinis and Balciuniene, 2006).
- Risk of file separation in the canal.

CONCLUSION

Rotary endodontics has taken a giant leap in paediatric endodontic procedures and has become an excellent adjunct. Less time for endodontic procedures has a greater impact on a child's chairside behaviour and cooperation. Even though the technique is simple, fast and gives excellent results, the practitioner should not be complacent and should follow the guidelines for its use. Rotary files should be used in combination with hand instruments based on the clinical situation to avoid untoward complications.

CONSENT FOR PUBLICATION

Not applicable.

CONFLICT OF INTEREST

The authors declare no conflict of interest, financial or otherwise.

ACKNOWLEDGEMENT

Declared none.

REFERENCES

[1] Jeevanandan G, Govindaraju L. Clinical comparison of Kedo-S paediatric rotary files *vs* manual instrumentation for root canal preparation in primary molars: a double blinded randomised clinical trial. Eur Arch Paediatr Dent 2018; 19(4): 273-8.
[http://dx.doi.org/10.1007/s40368-018-0356-6] [PMID: 30003514]

[2] Kuzekanani M. Nickel- Titanium Rotary Instruments: Development of the Single- File Systems. J Int Soc Prev community medicine 2018; 8(5): 386-90.

[3] Zupanc J, Vahdat-Pajouh N, Schäfer E. New thermomechanically treated NiTi alloys - a review. Int Endod J 2018; 51(10): 1088-103.
[http://dx.doi.org/10.1111/iej.12924] [PMID: 29574784]

[4] Manchanda S, Sardana D, Yiu CKY. A systematic review and meta-analysis of randomized clinical trials comparing rotary canal instrumentation techniques with manual instrumentation techniques in primary teeth. Int Endod J 2020; 53(3): 333-53.
[http://dx.doi.org/10.1111/iej.13233] [PMID: 31587323]

[5] George S, Anandaraj S, Issac JS, John SA, Harris A. Rotary endodontics in primary teeth – A review. Saudi Dent J 2016; 28(1): 12-7.
[http://dx.doi.org/10.1016/j.sdentj.2015.08.004] [PMID: 26792964]

[6] Musale P, Jain K, Kothare S. Comparative assessment of dentin removal following hand and rotary instrumentation in primary molars using cone-beam computed tomography. J Indian Soc Pedod Prev Dent 2019; 37(1): 80-6.
[http://dx.doi.org/10.4103/JISPPD.JISPPD_210_18] [PMID: 30804312]

[7] Jeevanandan G. Kedo-S paediatric rotary files for root canal preparation in primary teeth – case report. J Clin Diagn Res 2017; 11(3): ZR03-5.
[http://dx.doi.org/10.7860/JCDR/2017/25856.9508] [PMID: 28511532]

[8] Katge F, Ghadge S, Poojari M, Jain K, Patil D. Comparative evaluation of cleaning efficacy of prime Pedo™ AND DXL-Pro™ Pedo rotary files in root. J Clin Diagn Res 2019; 13(7): ZC06-9.

[9] Dioguardi M, Sovereto D, Illuzzi G, *et al.* Management of instrument sterilization workflow in endodontic: A systematic review and meta-analysis. Int J Dent 2020; 2020: 1-20.
[http://dx.doi.org/10.1155/2020/5824369] [PMID: 32148504]

[10] Parashos P, Linsuwanont P, Messer HH. A cleaning protocol for rotary nickel-titanium endodontic instruments. Aust Dent J 2004; 49(1): 20-7.
[http://dx.doi.org/10.1111/j.1834-7819.2004.tb00045.x] [PMID: 15104130]

[11] McGuigan MB, Louca C, Duncan HF. Endodontic instrument fracture: causes and prevention. Br Dent J 2013; 214(7): 341-8.
[http://dx.doi.org/10.1038/sj.bdj.2013.324] [PMID: 23579132]

[12] Tang WR, Smales RJ, Chen HF, *et al.* Prevention and management of fractured instruments in endodontic treatment. World Journal of Surgical Procedures 2015; 5(1): 82-98.
[http://dx.doi.org/10.5412/wjsp.v5.i1.82]

CHAPTER 8

Traumatic Injuries to Anterior Teeth: Introduction, Prevalence, and Classifications

Ritesh Kalaskar[1,*] and **Abdulkadeer M. Jetpurwala**[2]

[1] *Department of Pediatric Dentistry, Government Dental College and Hospital, Nagpur, India*

[2] *Department of Pediatric Dentistry, Nair Hospital Dental College, Mumbai, India*

Abstract: Smile with beautiful natural teeth is one of the greatest assets of a person. Untreated fractured teeth can affect day to day activities of children in school which can have a psychological impact on children. Apart from dental caries and periodontal diseases, a traumatic dental injury is the third most common cause of tooth loss. Violence, accidents, falls and sport-related activities are the leading causes of traumatic dental injuries, that majorly involve anterior teeth. Epidemiological studies indicate that dental trauma is a significant problem in young people and that soon, it will be a major dental health care requirement. Prevalence of traumatic dental injury in primary and permanent dentition ranges from 9.4-41.6% and 1% to 58.6%, respectively. The management of traumatic injuries to anterior teeth is also changing with advances in materials sciences and understanding of the mechanism of traumatic injuries.

Keywords: Classification of dental trauma, Prevalence of trauma, Traumatic dental injury.

INTRODUCTION

Oral injuries are most frequent during the first ten years of life, decreasing gradually with age, and are very rare after the age of thirty. Although the oral region comprises a small area of 1% of the total body area, it accounts for 5% of all bodily injuries. In preschool children, oral injuries make up as much as 17% of all bodily injuries, with injuries to the head being the most common. This contrasts with later in life when injuries to hands and feet are the most common. Of all patients seeking consultation or treatment for injuries to the oral region, dental injuries are the most common and are seen in as many as 92% of patients presenting with oral injuries, whereas soft-tissue injuries to the same patients are seen in 28%, often simultaneously with dental injuries. Therefore, mass awareness has to be created in society amongst the children, parents and school teachers who

* **Corresponding author Ritesh Kalaskar:** Department of Pediatric Dentistry, Government Dental College and Hospital, Nagpur, India; E-mail: riteshpedo@gmail.com

are often the first responders, and they have to be educated in terms of preventing and managing traumatic dental injury [1, 2].

Prevalence of Traumatic Dental Injury

In current terminology, the use of the word trauma implies a reasonable severe, non-physiological lesion to any part of the body. Any thermal, chemical or mechanical insult that affects the dentition should be analyzed as a dental trauma and its effect, as a traumatic dental injury. Interpersonal altercations, road traffic accidents, accidental falls, sports activities and non-accidental injuries, have been identified as the major causes that contribute to dental trauma and pose a significant public health problem. These causes especially emerge as an increasingly significant threat to the dental health of children and adolescents. It has been claimed that the volume represented by dental trauma and its sequelae within the near future will probably exceed dental caries and periodontal disease in the young population. Various studies have been conducted to ascertain the prevalence of traumatic dental injuries in different age groups including primary and permanent teeth. These studies have reported a range of prevalence rates. The great variation in reported rates can be attributed to a number of factors, including types of study, classification of trauma used for assessment, methodology, study size and population, geographical location and differences in cultural behavior [3, 4].

The region-wise distribution of traumatic dental injuries has been summarized in the following tables (Tables **1** - **4**) [1, 2].

Table 1. WHO-region wise distribution of prevalence of traumatic dental injury to permanent teeth.

WHO Region	Number of Subjects	Prevalence (%)
World	268755	15.2
European Region	62 389	14.0
Region of the Americas	53 080	19.1
Western Pacific Region	79 177	9.9
South-East Asia Region	41 922	12.2
Eastern Mediterranean Region	17 392	16.0
African Region	14 795	11.1

Table 2. WHO-region wise distribution of prevalence of traumatic dental injury to primary teeth.

WHO Region	Number of Subjects	Prevalence (%)
World	59 436	22.7
European Region	21 869	14.2
Region of the Americas	28 736	26.5
Western Pacific Region	–	–
South-East Asia Region	3312	27.0
Eastern Mediterranean Region	2052	22.7
African Region	3467	22.7

Table 3. WHO-region wise distribution of prevalence of traumatic dental injury to permanent teeth among 12 years old children.

WHO Region	Number of Subjects	Prevalence (%)
World	33 829	18.1
European Region	1693	13.5
Region of the Americas	14 968	22.1
Western Pacific Region	1630	13.3
South-East Asia Region	8133	15.8
Eastern Mediterranean Region	2269	14.9
African Region	5136	13.2

Table 4. Traumatic dental injuries.

Region	Author	Country	Year	Age	Sample Size	Incidence (per 1000/year)
Australia	-	-	-	-	-	-
-	Stockwell	Australia	1988	6-12	66500	17
Europe	-	-	-	-	-	-
-	Hamilton, Hill and Holloway	United Kingdom	1997	11-14	2022	34
-	Skaare, Peterson and Jacobson	Norway	2005	1-8	20000	13
-	Ravn	Denmark	1974	7-16	50000	30
-	Glendor, Hailing Anderson, Eilert-Peterson	Sweden	1996	0-19	Unspecified	13

(Table 4) cont.....

Region	Author	Country	Year	Age	Sample Size	Incidence (per 1000/year)
-	Borssen and Holm	Sweden	2015	1-16	3007	28
-	Oldin, Lundgren, Nilsson, Noren, Robertson	Sweden	2015	0-17	889	28
-	Andreasen and Ravn	Denmark	1972	0-14	487	40
Asia	-	-	-	-	-	-
-	Basha, Mohammad and Swamy	India	2015	13	782	30.1
South America	-	-	-	-	-	-
-	Ramos-Jorge *et al*	Brazil	2008	11-13	208	1.2
-	Ramos-Jorge *et al*	Brazil	2008	11.13	208	5.72
-	Cecconella and Traebert	Brazil	2007	Unspecified	176	44

The prevalence of traumatic injuries accordingly to the region of the world has been summarized as [5]:

Classification of Traumatic Injuries

Traumatic injuries can be classified as:

I. Based on the type of tissue involved
    1. Hard tissue
    2. Soft tissue
        a. Contusion
        b. Abrasion
        c. Laceration
        d. Incision
        e. Stab
        f. Puncture
II. Based on type of injury
    1. Direct trauma
    2. Indirect trauma
III. Based on shape of impacting object
    1. Blunt injury
    2. Sharp injury
IV. Based on vector of forces
    1. Acceleration injury

2. Deceleration injury

The damage to the tissues is specific according to the type of traumatic incident.

Classification of Traumatic Dental Injury [6, 7]

Classification of Anterior Teeth Trauma by Sweets (1955)

It is mainly based on the anatomy and morphology of the tooth structure. The disadvantages of this classification are that no stress has been laid on injuries to supporting soft tissue structures and bone. It indicates more towards the permanent teeth than primary teeth as injury to periodontium is more common in primary teeth as compared to permanent ones (Table **5**).

Table 5. Classification of anterior teeth trauma by Sweets.

Class	Fracture	Class	Fracture
Class I	A simple fracture of the crown exposing no dentition	**Class V**	Complete fracture of crown exposing pulp
Class II	A parallel fracture of the crown involving little dentin	**Class VI**	Fracture of root with or without loss of crown structure
Class III	Extensive fracture of crown involving more dentin but no pulp exposure	**Class VII**	Tooth loss as a result of trauma
Class IV	Extensive fracture of crown exposing pulp	-	-

Andreasen's Classification

It is a descriptive classification of traumatic dental injuries and incorporates the different tissues involved with trauma (Table **6**). However, it is not easy for communication and cannot be used in regular practice.

Table 6. Classification by Andreasen (1981).

Injuries to Structure	Type of Injury	Injury Number	Clinical Observation
Injuries to the hard dental tissues and pulp	Crown infarction	N873.60	An incomplete fracture (crack) of the enamel without loss of the tooth substance
	Uncomplicated crown fracture	N 873 N 873.61	A fracture contained to the enamel OR Fracture involving enamel and dentin, but not exposing the pulp
	Complicated crown fracture	N 873.62	A fracture involving enamel and dentin and exposing the pulp
	Uncomplicated crown root fracture	N 873.64	A fracture involving enamel, dentin and cementum but not involving the pulp
	Uncomplicated crown root fracture	N 873.64	A fracture involving enamel, dentin and cementum but not involving the pulp
	Root fracture	N 873	A fracture involving dentin, cementum, and the pulp
Injuries to the periodontal tissues	Concussion	N 873.66	An injury to the tooth supporting structures without abnormal loosening or displacement of the tooth, but with marked reaction to percussion.
	Subluxation	N 873.66	An injury to the tooth supporting structures with abnormal loosening but without displacement of the teeth.
	Intrusive Luxation (central dislocation)	N 873.66.	Displacement of the tooth into the alveolar bone. This injury is accompanied by comminution or fracture of the alveolar socket.
	Extrusive luxation (peripheral dislocation partial avulsion)	N873.66	Partial displacement of the tooth out of its socket.
	Lateral Luxation	N873.66	Displacement of the tooth in a direction other than axially. This is accompanied by comminution or fracture of the alveolar socket.
	Ex-articulation (complete avulsion)	N873.68	Complete displacement of the tooth out of its socket.

(Table 6) cont.....

Injuries to Structure	Type of Injury	Injury Number	Clinical Observation
Injuries of the supporting bone	Comminution of alveolar socket	Mandible- N 802.20, Maxilla- 802.40	Crushing and compression of the alveolar socket. This condition is found together with intrusive and lateral luxation
	Fracture of the alveolar socket wall	Mandible- N 802.20, Maxilla- N802.40	A fracture contained to the facial or lingual socket wall.
	Fracture of the alveolar process	Mandible- N802.20, Maxilla - N802.40	A fracture of the alveolar process, which may or may not involve the alveolar socket.
	Fracture of the Mandible and Maxilla	Mandible - N802.21, Maxilla- N802.42	A fracture involving the base of the mandible or maxilla and often the alveolar process (jaw fracture). The fracture may or may not involve the alveolar socket.
Injuries to gingiva or oral mucosa.	Laceration of gingiva or oral mucosa	N873.69	A shallow or deep wound in the mucosa resulting from a tear and usually produced by a sharp object.
	Contusion of gingiva or oral mucosa	N 902.00	A bruise usually produced by an impact from a blunt object and not accompanied by a break of the continuity in the mucosa, causing submucosal hemorrhage
	Abrasion of gingiva or oral mucosa	N 910.00	A superficial wound produced by rubbing or scraping of the mucosa leaving a raw bleeding surface

Galea's Classification

The traumatic injuries are divided into broad classes as shown in Table 7.

Table 7. Classification by Galea (1984).

Crown facture without pulp exposure	Subluxation	Fracture of the alveolar socket
Crown facture with pulp exposure	Subluxation with intrusion	Dento- alveolar fracture
Crown –Root fractures	Subluxation with extrusion	Fractures to the maxilla and mandible
Root fractures	Luxation	Injuries to the soft tissues
-	-	Other injuries.

Classification by Fried and Erickson

It is based on six classes based on the amount of tooth structure lost, presence of pulp exposure and root surface involvement (Table **8**). It does not include luxation injuries.

Table 8. Classification of dental trauma of primary teeth by Fried and Erickson (1995).

<table>
<tr><th colspan="2">Classification of Hard Tissue Fractures</th><th>Trauma Affecting the Periodontium</th></tr>
<tr><td>Class I</td><td>Simple fracture of enamel only</td><td>Concussion - Sensitivity of the tooth to trauma without abnormal loosening or mobility</td></tr>
<tr><td>Class II</td><td>Fracture involving enamel and dentin</td><td>Subluxation - Loosening of the tooth without mobility</td></tr>
<tr><td>Class III</td><td>Fracture extends farther into the tooth, with a small pulpal exposure</td><td rowspan="4">Luxation - Displacement of the traumatized teeth.</td></tr>
<tr><td>Class IV</td><td>Fracture involves a significant amount of pulpal exposure</td></tr>
<tr><td>Class V</td><td>Complete loss of the tooth</td></tr>
<tr><td>Class VI</td><td>Fracture of the root</td></tr>
</table>

WHO Classification

It is adapted from Andreasen's classification and described in Table **9**.

Table 9. WHO classification of traumatic dental injury.

<table>
<tr><th>Type of Injury</th><th>WHO Code</th><th>Type of Injury</th><th>WHO Code</th><th>Type of Injury</th><th>WHO Code</th><th>Type of Injury</th><th>WHO Code</th></tr>
<tr><th colspan="2">Injuries to the hard dental tissues and the pulp</th><th colspan="2">Injuries to the periodontal tissues</th><th colspan="2">Injuries to supporting bone</th><th colspan="2">Injuries to gingiva or oral mucosa</th></tr>
<tr><td>Enamel infraction</td><td>N 502.50</td><td>Concussion</td><td>N 503.20</td><td>Comminution of the axillary alveolar socket</td><td>N 502.40</td><td>Laceration of gingiva or oral mucosa</td><td>S 01.50</td></tr>
<tr><td>Enamel fracture</td><td>N 502.50</td><td>Subluxation</td><td>N 503.20</td><td>Comminution of the mandibular alveolar socket</td><td>N 502.60</td><td>Contusion of gingiva or oral mucosa</td><td>S 00.50</td></tr>
<tr><td>Enamel- dentin fracture</td><td>N 502.51</td><td>Extrusive luxation</td><td>N 503.20</td><td>Fracture of the maxillary alveolar socket</td><td>N 502.40</td><td>Abrasion of gingiva or oral mucosa</td><td>S 00.50</td></tr>
<tr><td>Complicated crown fracture</td><td>N 502.52</td><td>Lateral luxation</td><td>N 503.20</td><td>Fracture of the mandibular alveolar socket</td><td>N 502.60</td><td>-</td><td>-</td></tr>
</table>

(Table 9) cont.....

Type of Injury	WHO Code	Type of Injury	WHO Code	Type of Injury	WHO Code	Type of Injury	WHO Code
Uncomplicated crown- root fracture	N 502.54	Intrusive luxation	N 503.20	Fracture of the maxillary alveolar process	N 502.40	-	-
Complicated crown-root fracture	N 502.54	Avulsion	N 503.20	Fracture of the mandibular alveolar process	N 502.60	-	-
Root fracture	N 502.53	-	-	-	-	-	-

Classification by Spinas

It is a based on the extent of tooth structure loss and divides traumatic dental injuries in four classes (Table **10**).

Table 10. Classification by Spinas (2002).

Class	Clinical Presentation	Sub Class	Clinical Presentation
Class A	All the simple enamel lesions, which involve a mesial or distal crown angle, or only the incisal edge	-	-
Class B	All the enamel dentin lesions, involve a mesial or distal angle and the incisal edge.	b1	When a pulp exposition exists defined as a subclass
Class C	All the enamel dentin lesions, involve the incisal edge and at least a third of the crown surface.	c1	In case of pulp exposure defined as subclass
Class D	All the enamel dentin lesions, involve a mesial or distal crown angle and the incisal or palatal surface, with root cement involvement (crown root fracture)	d1	In case of pulpal exposure defined as subclass

Benett's Classification (1963)

Benett's classification is according to injuries to periodontium and alveolus considering the anatomy and morphology of the teeth which can be applied partially for primary and permanent teeth (Fig. **1**).

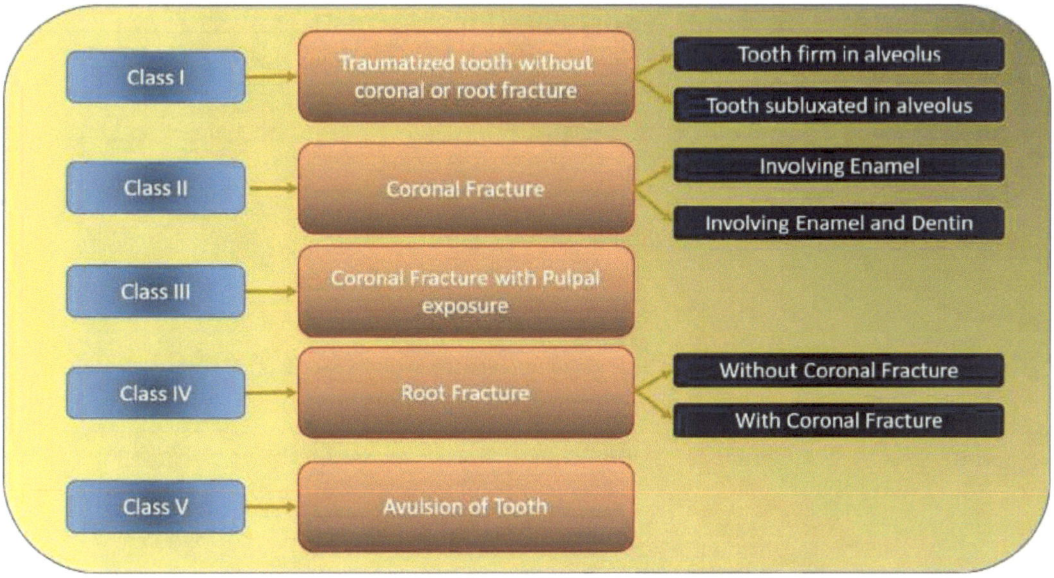

Fig. (1). Benett's classification.

Classification by Rabinowitch

Classifies dental trauma in six groups as shown in Fig. (**2**).

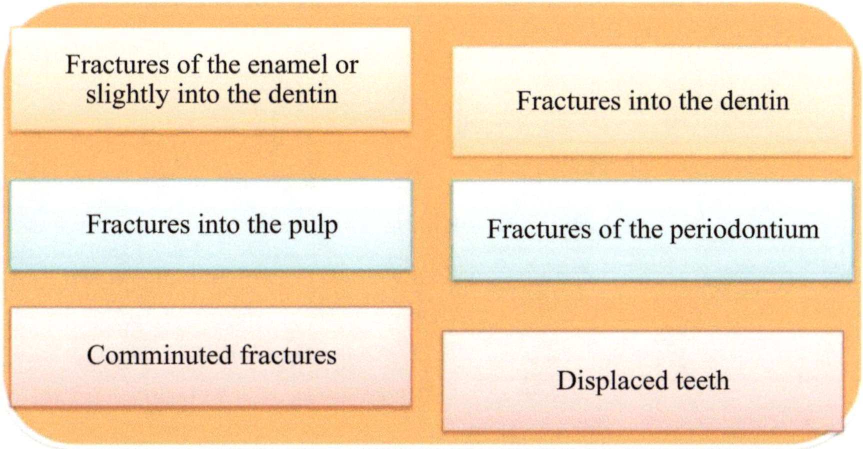

Fig. (2). Classification by Rabinowitch.

Classification by Ellis and Davey (1970) (Figs. 3 and 4)

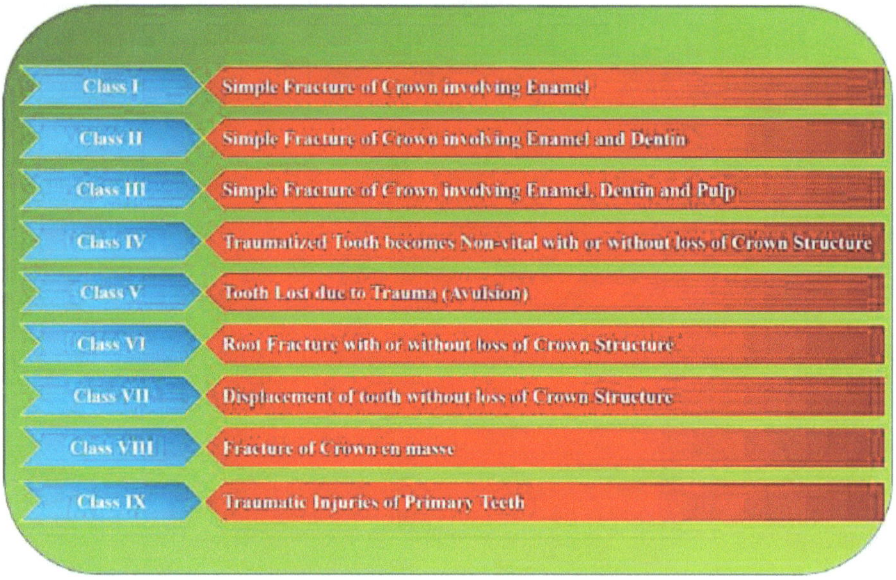

Fig. (3). Classification by Ellis and Davey.

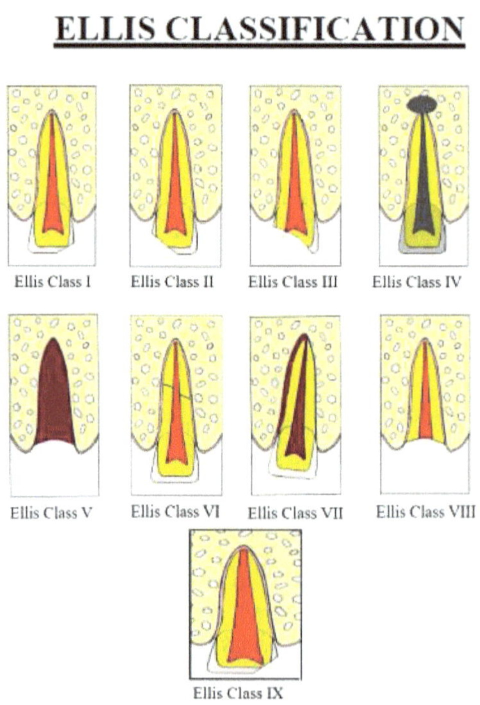

Fig. (4). Ellis and Davis classification.

It is a simplified classification, which groups many injuries and allows for subjcctivc intcrprctation by including broad terms such as simple or extensive or extensive fractures. It is the most frequently used classification. However, it has certain disadvantages like the absence of clarification of luxation injuries in subtypes. And all deciduous teeth traumatic injuries are grouped as a single class.

Classification by Garcia Godoy (Fig. 5)

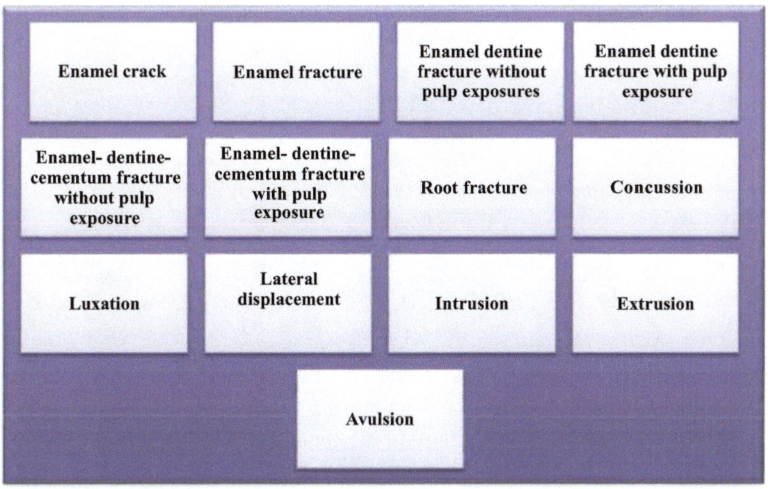

Fig. (5). Garcia – Godoy classification-1981.

Stock well's Classification

It is shown in Fig. (6). It has a unique class for the representation of recurrent traumatic injuries to previously affected teeth.

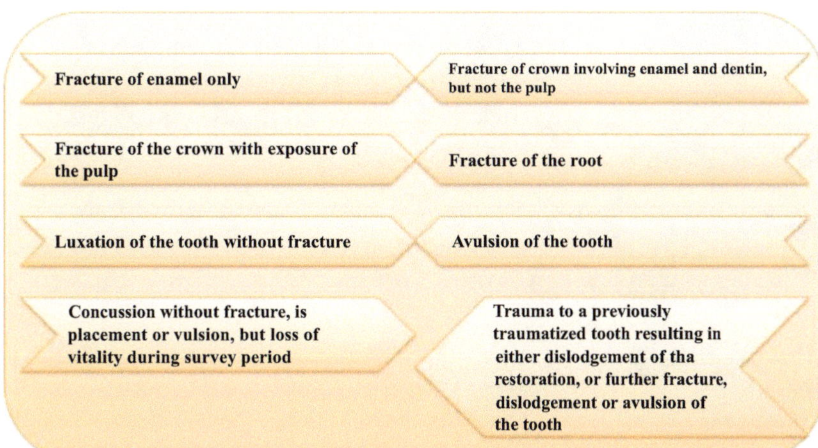

Fig. (6). Stockwell classification-1988.

Classification put forth by: Lee-Knight (1986), Hunter (1990), Forsberg and Tedestam (1990) is also vital in deciding the proper treatment plan, however comparing to ellis and Dewey this classification is not popular (Fig. **7**).

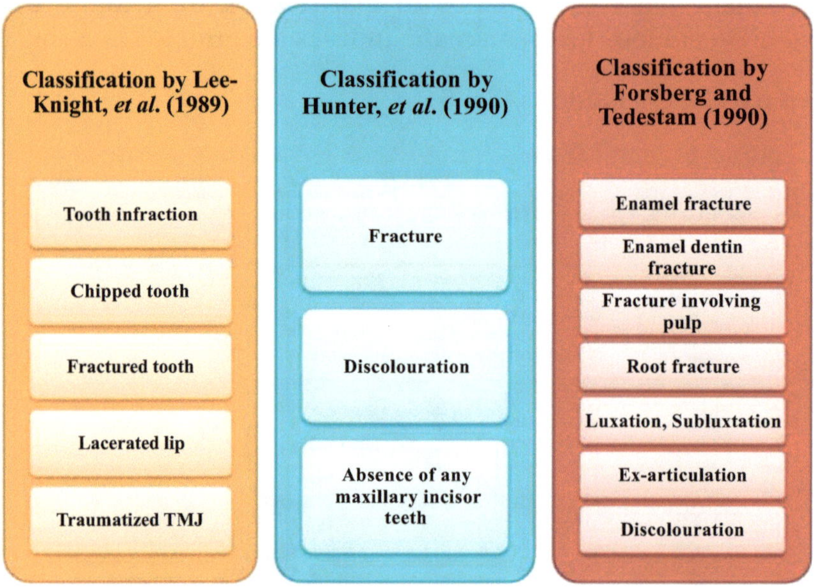

Fig. (7). Classification by: Lee-Knight (1986), Hunter (1990), Forsberg and Tedestam (1990).

McDonald's Classification

It is a concise classification and quick clinical assessment of traumatized teeth. it does not include injuries to teeth supporting structures (Fig. **8**).

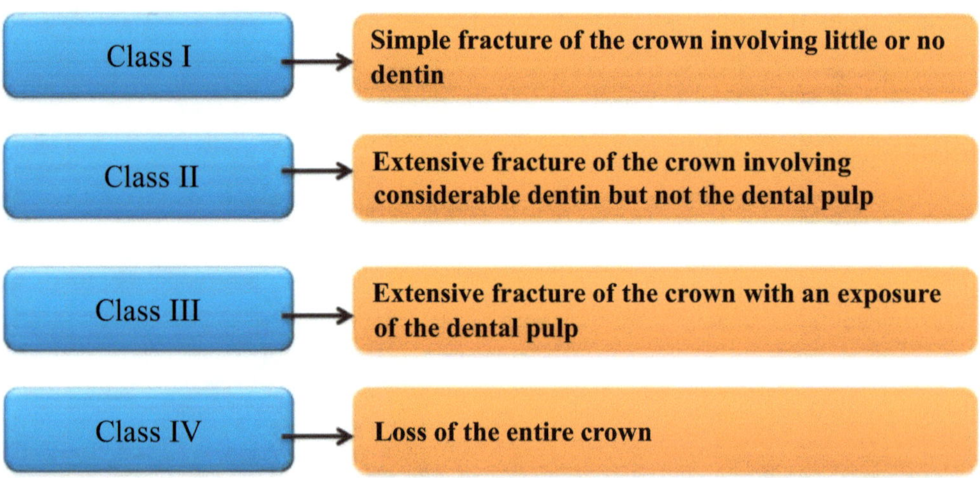

Fig. (8). Classification by McDonald (2004).

Hargreaves Classification

Similar to McDonald's classification but includes root fracture also (Fig. **9**).

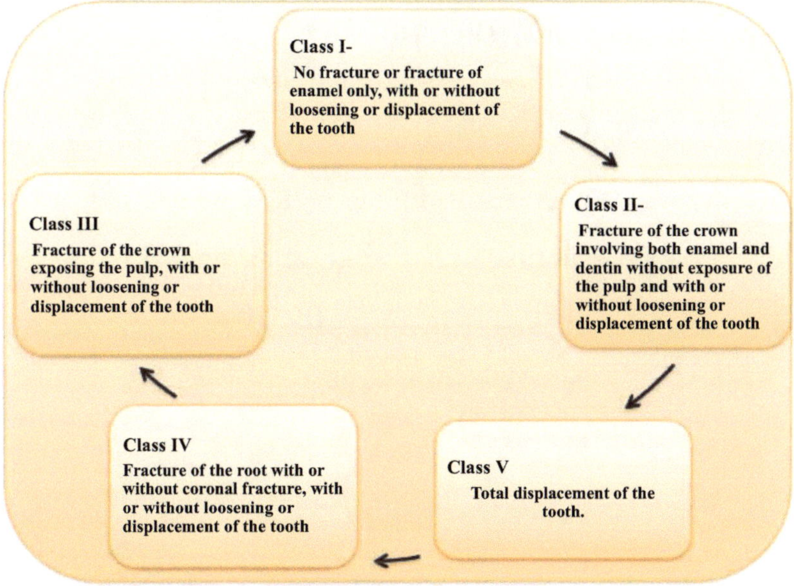

Fig. (9). Classification by Hargreaves and Craig (1970).

Classification by Ulfohn (1969)

Ulfohn examines a classification of crown fracture from a clinical endodontic point of view based on three fundamental aspects.

- The possibility of identifying the clinical state of the pulp.
- The absolute conviction that it is impossible to view the dentin and the pulp as separate organs and that they constitute one organ. Considering this, any attack on the dentin represents indirect damage to the pulp.
- Determination of treatment.

This classification tends to simplification. It does not take into account large or small amount of indirect pulp exposure.

Crown Fractures

- of enamel
- with indirect pulp exposure through the dentin.
- with direct pulp exposure

The shape of the fracture may encompass an incisal angle or more part of the crown. The pulp may be clinically normal, hyperemic, inflamed, or dead. The apical foramina may or may not have completed its physiologic calcification.

Classification by Basrani (1982), (Fig. 10)

- **Crown fracture**
  - **Fracture of the enamel**
  - **Fracture of the enamel and dentin**
    - **Without pulp exposure**
    - **With pulp exposure**
- **Root fractures**
- **Crown-root fractures**

Fig. (10). Basrani's Classification of traumatic dental injuries.

It is based on the anatomy of the teeth

Pulver's Classification of Traumatic Injuries (1982)

It is descriptive system which partially deals with the aspect of combination traumas.

Class I

- Division I No external fracture, no displacement
- Division II No fracture but displacement
- Division III Fracture of enamel only, no displacement
- Division IV Fracture of enamel and displacement

Class II

- Division I Fracture of enamel and dentin only, no displacement
- Division II Fracture of enamel and dentin only with displacement

Class III

- Division I Fracture (with exposure of pulp), no displacement

•Division II Fracture (with exposure of pulp) and displacement

Class IV

•Division I Fracture of root

Class V

•Division I Intrusion
•Division II Partial avulsion
•Division III Complete avulsion

CONCLUSION

Classification of traumatic injuries helps to record and communicate the patient's condition in a simple and understandable way between professional colleagues. It also allows the operator to design a treatment plan based on various guidelines that have been laid down for traumatic injury management. The classifications which are too extensive are difficult to remember while the simple classifications do not cover all the injuries encountered in clinical practice. There is no universal classification of dental traumatic injuries, though the Ellis and Davis classification is the most commonly used classification in the dental literature.

CONSENT FOR PUBLICATION

Not applicable.

CONFLICT OF INTEREST

The authors declare no conflict of interest, financial or otherwise.

ACKNOWLEDGEMENT

Declared none.

REFERENCES

[1] Petti S, Glendor U, Andersson L. World traumatic dental injury prevalence and incidence, a meta-analysis-One billion living people have had traumatic dental injuries. Dent Traumatol 2018; 34(2): 71-86.
[http://dx.doi.org/10.1111/edt.12389] [PMID: 29455471]

[2] Richards D. One billion people have experienced a traumatic dental injury. Evid Based Dent 2018; 19(2): 34-5.
[http://dx.doi.org/10.1038/sj.ebd.6401297] [PMID: 29930374]

[3] Naidoo S, Sheiham A, Tsakos G. Traumatic dental injuries of permanent incisors in 11- to 13-year-old South African schoolchildren. Dent Traumatol 2009; 25(2): 224-8.
[http://dx.doi.org/10.1111/j.1600-9657.2008.00749.x] [PMID: 19290905]

[4] Bratteberg M, Thelen DS, Klock KS, Bårdsen A. Traumatic dental injuries-Prevalence and severity among 16-year-old pupils in western Norway. Dent Traumatol 2018; 34(3): 144-50. [http://dx.doi.org/10.1111/edt.12399] [PMID: 29569840]

[5] Lam R. Epidemiology and outcomes of traumatic dental injuries: a review of the literature. Aust Dent J 2016; 61(1) (Suppl. 1): 4-20. [http://dx.doi.org/10.1111/adj.12395] [PMID: 26923445]

[6] Pagadala S, Tadikonda DC. An overview of classification of dental trauma. a. Intl Arch Integ Med 2015; 2(9): 157-64.

[7] Andreasen JO, Andreasen FM, Andersson L. Textbook and Color Atlas of Traumatic Injuries to the Teeth. 5th Edition, Wiley-Blackwell, Hoboken, 2018. https://www.wiley.com/en-us/Textbook

CHAPTER 9

Traumatic Injuries to Anterior Teeth: Etiology, Predisposing Factors and Examination

Abdulkadeer M. Jetpurwala[1,*], **Nilesh Rathi**[2] and **Ritesh Kalaskar**[3]

[1] *Department of Pediatric Dentistry, Nair Hospital Dental College, Mumbai, India*

[2] *Department of Pediatric Dentistry, DY Patil Dental College and Hospital, Pimpri, Pune, India*

[3] *Department of Pedodontic and Preventive Dentistry, Government Dental College & Hospital, Nagpur, India*

Abstract: Traumatic injuries are commonly seen in children. There are various causes and factors that make an individual or a particular tooth more susceptible to traumatic injury. Owing to factors like early fine motor development of infants and toddlers, participation in sports and other physical activities, accidental and non-accidental injuries or common reasons, children may suffer from dental trauma. Many facial types like convex facial profiles, class malocclusions and malposition of teeth also make the teeth prone to trauma. This section describes the etiologic and predisposing factors and sketches an outline for a detailed examination of traumatic dental injuries.

Keywords: Etiology of dental trauma, Examination of dental trauma.

RISK FACTORS AFFECTING TDI

Nature and severity of traumatic dental injury and its treatment outcomes are influenced by various risk factors that are described in Figs. (**1** and **2**).

ETIOLOGY

While compassion and love are a part of human nature, anger and violence form the other negative end of human behavior. Violence has increased in severity during the past few decades and its role has been underestimated when looking at intentional vs unintentional Traumatic Dental Injuries (TDIs). The WHO Healthy Cities and WHO Health Promoting Schools programs offer a broad solution for dental trauma as a public health problem in an age group which is most vulnerable to trauma.

* **Corresponding author Abdulkadeer M. Jetpurwala:** Dept. of Pediatric Dentistry, Nair Hospital Dental College, Mumbai, India; E-mail: 24deemes@gmail.com

Satyawan Damle, Ritesh Kalaskar & Dhanashree Sakhare (Eds.)

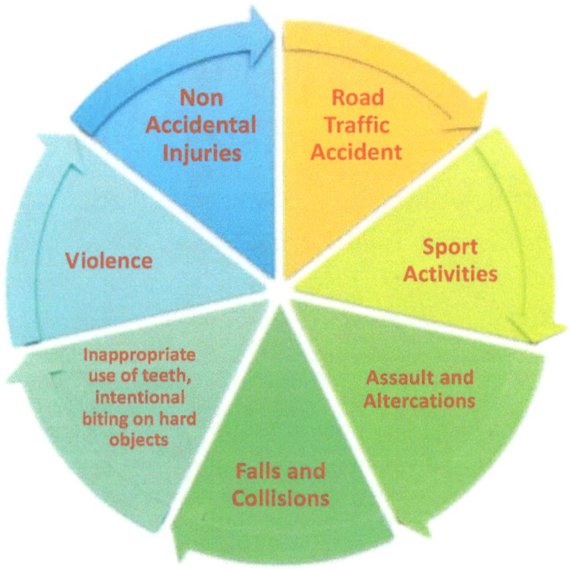
Non Accidental Injuries
Road Traffic Accident
Sport Activities
Assault and Altercations
Falls and Collisions
Inappropriate use of teeth, intentional biting on hard objects
Violence

Fig. (1). Causes of traumatic dental injury.

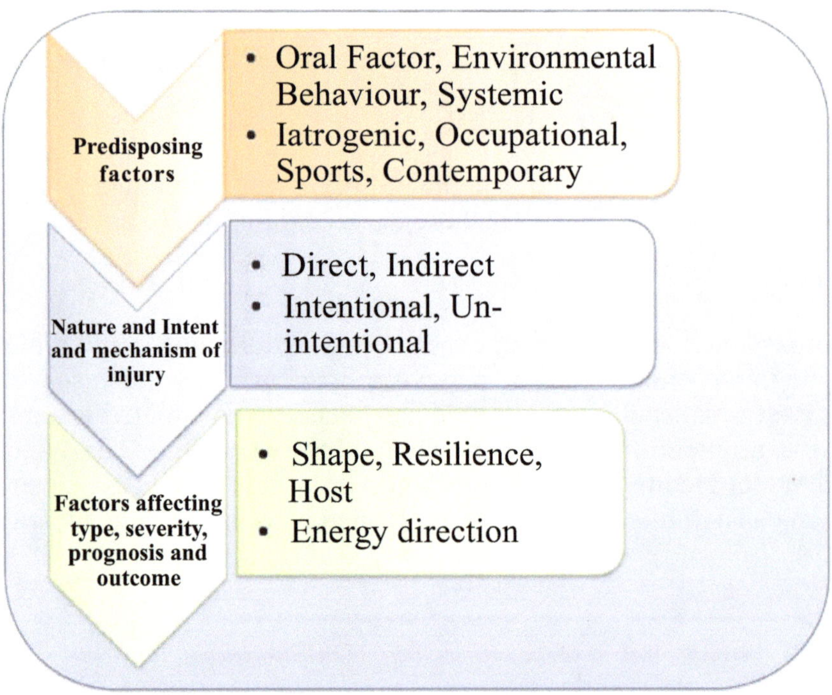

Fig. (2). Etiological of trauma to anterior tooth.

It was revealed that falls were the main common cause of traumatic dental injuries (from 31.7 to 64.2%) followed by sport activities (up to 40.2%), bicycling accidents (up to 19.5%), traffic accidents (up to 7.8%), and physical violence (up to 6.6%). Amongst all the causes, traffic accidents constitute a special group of traumas due to predominant multiple injuries including head injuries and trauma to supporting tissues. Moreover, new types of facial trauma occur from airbag explosion in cars during traffic accidents. Bicycling accidents are a common cause of dental trauma in schoolchildren. Various studies conducted throughout the world confirm that wearing a helmet during bicycle ride can minimise or reduces the incidence by 65 percent [1, 2].

Sport activities are one of the main causes of dental trauma, they are classified as contact sport and non-contact sports. The contact sports are further divided according to their risk categories: high-risk (boxing, soccer, American football, hockey, martial sports, rugby, cycling and skating) and medium-risk sports (cricket, baseball, basketball, handball, diving, squash, and gymnastics) (Table **1**).

Table 1. Types of sporting activities.

High Risk Sports	Medium Risk Sports
Boxing	Cricket
Soccer	Baseball
American Football	Basketball
Hockey	Handball
Martial sports	Diving
Rugby	Squash
Cycling	Tennis
Skating	Gymnastics

The tendency of increase in the severity of violence among individuals concerning traumatic dental injuries is an alarming factor. It is important to emphasize that dentists could be the first ones to detect children who had suffered physical abuse and non-accidental injuries. In the united states, the findings reveal that nearly 30 per cent of dentists had a suspicion about child abuse however only 9 to 14 per cent reported it.

Compared to non-oral accidents, bicycle-related oral injuries seem to be more frequent up to the age of 14 years. Biting a pen, opening soda bottles, hair clips, food packages, attempting to repair electrical devices or replacing batteries, cutting or carrying items, and opening screw top bottles are among the most frequent improper uses of teeth mentioned in the literature. TDI can also occur in children with learning difficulty and special health care needs like epilepsy, cerebral palsy, anaemia and dizziness. Causes of oral injuries in some children are exhibited in battered child syndrome (or non-accidental injuries), a condition in which an infant has undergone serious physical abuse [3].

Some traumatic dental injuries are of iatrogenic nature and occur during the intubation procedure during general anesthesia. This type of trauma constitutes 0.04% to 12% of all cases. In UK, this complication during anesthesia is reported to constitute approximately one-third of all medicolegal claims. Dental traumas related to iatrogenic reasons are mainly fractures of crowns and roots and luxation injuries including avulsions.

Piercing of tongue and lips presents a new category of traumatic dental injuries and may lead to fracturing of teeth and restorations, pulp damage, and cracked tooth syndrome. The prevalence of chipped teeth among individuals with tongue piercing constitutes 19.2%.

The impact of socioeconomic status reveals two questionable opinions. One of them states that children with low socioeconomic background are more likely to have traumatic dental injuries due to greater exposure to violence, while another study reports children from high socioeconomic background have a higher risk for dental trauma due to their greater access to leisure activities [4].

PRE-DISPOSING FACTORS

Class II division malocclusion with excessive overjet, environmental determinants (material deprivation), and human behavior (risk-taking children, children being bullied, emotionally stressful conditions, obesity and attention-deficit hyperactivity disorder) are found to increase the risk for TDIs. Other factors increasing the risk for TDIs are the presence of illness, learning difficulties, physical limitations, teeth weakened due to dental caries or hypoplasia, professional risk (*e.g.*, sportspersons, electricians, laborer's) and inappropriate use of teeth. A new cause of TDIs that is of particular interest is oral piercing. In road traffic accidents, the facial injury was similar in unrestrained occupants (no seat belts) and occupants restrained only with an air bag. The ideal protection was reported when both seat belts and airbags were present. Amateur athletes have been found to suffer from TDIs more often than professional athletes. Falls and collisions mask intentional TDIs, such as physical abuse, assaults and torture.

Children with class II division 1 malocclusion were more often reported (70%) to have traumatic dental injuries than children with other types of occlusion. The most commonly reported factors are large overjet (>3.0 mm), incompetent lips and absence of mouthguards while playing sports. Children with an overjet with size greater than 3.0 mm were 5.4 times more likely to present with a dental injury than children with an overjet size equal to or lower than 3.0 mm. Rotated teeth and ectopic teeth erupting out of the arch form are also at higher risk to fractures.

School children with incompetent lips presented a higher risk of traumatic dental injuries up to 3.4 times more compared to children with competent lips.

Children during the formative years when learning to crawl, stand and walk are reported to have higher incidence of traumatic injuries to deciduous teeth. Concomitant medical problems like neuro-Musculo-skeletal disorders impairing locomotion and seizure disorders also pose a higher risk of TDI [5].

FACTORS AFFECTING TYPE, SEVERITY, PROGNOSIS, AND OUTCOME OF TDIS [3, 5]

Energy of the Impact

The energy of impact is a product of mass and acceleration. It is an important factor that might influence the outcome of a traumatic dental injury. Mass and velocity can have different pattern, for example high velocity and low mass (gunshot) or high mass and low velocity (playground injury). High velocity blows do not damage the supporting or surrounding structures, on the contrary, low-velocity blow can largely destroy the surrounding structures.

Resiliency of Bone

The resiliency of impacted bone is correlated with fracture or displacement. If the Bone is more resilient the displacement of the tooth will be more (in children bone is more resilient), however in adults, the bone is less resilient, hence trauma is associated with fracture of teeth.

Shape of Impacting Object

Sharp and blunt objects can create more impact in influencing the injuries. In case of a sharp object, energy is distributed rapidly over a limited area so the displacement of the tooth is less but it is associated with crown fracture. In case of blunt object injury, energy is distributed over larger area and is transmitted to the apical region. Therefore, root fracture and displacement of teeth are more common than crown fracture.

Vector of Force

Direction of the impact or force *i.e.*, parallel, or perpendicular will also play an important role in the type and severity of injury. The force or impact can meet the tooth in a different angle, most often hitting the tooth facially perpendicular to the long axis of the root. By assessing the fracture properties of enamel and dentin, it is seen that enamel is the weakest when parallel to the enamel rods and dentin is fractured easily, perpendicular to the dentinal tubules.

Direct Trauma

When an object or surface directly strikes the tooth or dentoalveolar apparatus, the resultant trauma is a direct trauma. Such trauma results in dento-alveolar type of injuries to anterior teeth.

In-direct Trauma

In this case, the object or surface does not directly strike the fractured part. The force is transmitted to the fracture site from the other part of the injury. For example, a blow to the chin results in the fracture of the condyle or crown root fracture of premolar or molars. In this case, the fracture of the condyle or crown root fracture of premolars is due to indirect trauma [6].

Sharp Injury

The shape of the impacting object is also important to allow the distribution of the forces. A sharp injury to the teeth may be in for on a bat, edge of a table, rock, *etc.* The forces concentrated at the edge of the object are transferred to the tooth in a small area and usually results to the fracture of teeth.

Blunt Injury

Objects such as a ball or fist would allow for the forces to be distributed over a larger area and lead to soft tissue and displacement type of injuries including damage to the supporting structures of the teeth. It leads to concussion, subluxation, luxation, and avulsion of teeth [5].

EXAMINATION OF TRAUMATIZED TEETH

Accurate history taking and clinical examination are the keys to successful management of traumatized tissues. The following features are thus important to determine the type and impact of the trauma [6 - 9]:

1. The direction of impact (its relationship to the occlusal plane)
2. Possible lip/soft tissue involvement
3. Resilience of the periodontal structures

HISTORY

1. **Demographic Details:** These details are a necessity for communication and legal measures. In addition to this, it provides a hint to possible cerebral involvement or general mental status.
2. **Head Injury:** A thorough history of loss of consciousness, vomiting dizziness and bleeding or discharge of fluids from the nose or ear should be taken to rule out possible head injury.
3. **Medical History:** Numerous conditions can influence the emergency and routine management of traumatized structures. *e.g.*, allergic reactions, epilepsy, or bleeding disorders such as hemophilia.
4. **General Examination:** The vital signs should be checked and in case of soft tissue injuries, a history of time required for and ease of bleeding control and tetanus prophylaxis taken by the patient should be recorded
5. **When:** The time lapsed after the injury significantly influences the treatment plan and subsequently the result of replantation of avulsed teeth.

Conditions affected by delayed treatment:

- Luxated teeth
- Crown fractures with and without pulp exposures
- Bone fractures
- **Where:** The area or the region of the accident may indicate a need for appropriate disinfection procedures, vaccinations, and medications. *e.g.*: tetanus and antibiotics.
- **How:** The type of injury to be expected can be determined easily by understanding the etiology. *e.g.*, An injury to the chin will often cause fracture at the mandibular symphysis or condylar region as well as crown-root fractures in the premolar and molar regions. Understanding the direction of the forces of the object allows the clinician to correlate the severity of the injury. At times, the history of injury may not match with the clinical presentation thereby raising doubts about non accidental injuries or child abuse.
- **History of treatment:** Before providing any further treatment, past history of immobilization, reduction, or replantation of teeth, should be considered.

Transport Media: It is vital to ascertain how the avulsed tooth was stored, *e.g.*, tap water, sterilizing solutions or dry.

- **Past history of Trauma:** Any history of repeated injuries to their teeth, can influence pulpal sensibility tests and the recuperative capacity of the pulp and/or periodontium. Repeated history of trauma allows the clinician to rate the degree of susceptibility of future incidents and helps in counseling the parents towards preventive measures.

- In addition to this, the following enquiries and inferences as shown in Table **2**, should be conducted:

Table 2. History taking for traumatic injuries.

Condition	Inference
History of amnesia, unconsciousness, drowsiness, vomiting or headache post trauma	• The presence of these symptoms may require intensive medical care. • However, chairside dental stabilization may be done.
Presence and spontaneity of pain from the teeth	• Damage to the tooth-supporting structures *e.g.*, hyperemia or extravasation of blood into the periodontal ligament. • Damage to the pulp
Sensitivity on consumption of hot or cold, sweet, or sour foods	Pulp hyperemia, exposed dentin, or pulp
Tenderness of teeth on touching/ biting/ chewing	Injuries such as extrusive or lateral luxation, alveolar or jaw fractures, or crown-root fractures should be suspected
Changes in the bite or occlusion	

CLINICAL EXAMINATION

In order to pinpoint treatment needs, examination should progress from the facial surface into the oral cavity.

- Recording of extraoral wounds and palpation of the facial skeleton:
    - The location of the wound indicates the possibility of the type and intensity of the dental injuries.
    - A wound located under the chin correlates to:
        - Findings in the premolar and molar regions possibly in combination with a concomitant fracture or TMJ changes in the form of clicking of deviation on opening or closing movements of the mandibular condyle and/or symphysis [10].
    - Factures of the facial skeleton:
        - May present with hematomas, contusions, lacerations of soft tissues.
        - Palpation is vital for the identification of jaw fractures.
        - Jaw fractures of the maxilla and mandible have distinct patterns
- Maxillary fracture
    - Dentoalveolar
    - LeFort I

    - LeFort II
    - LcFort III
- Mandibular fracture
    - Dentoalveolar
    - Symphysis
    - Para symphysis
    - Body mandible
    - Ramus
    - Angle of Mandible
    - Condylar
- Recording of injuries to the oral mucosa or gingiva:
    - The tissues must be carefully examined in a bloodless field, to identify the extent of the lesions. *e.g.*: The bleeding obscures the displacement of the mucoperiosteum into the buccal sulcus.
    - The possibility of embedded tooth fragments must be considered as these remnant pieces cause chronic infections. Identification of fractured tooth segments, and foreign bodies embedded in the soft tissues can be done by palpation and soft tissue radiography.
        - Careful radiographic examination must be done to confirm the presence and removal of such objects.
- Examination of the crowns of teeth for the presence and extent of fractures, pulp exposures or changes in colour:
    - The tooth should be examined for ascertaining the extent of damage and defining the involvement of enamel, dentin, and pulp
    - The tooth should be checked under good lighting to check for enamel cracks and abfractions.
    - The fracture surface should be carefully examined for pulp exposures; if present, the size and location and size of exposure should be recorded.
    - It is necessary to examine occlusal fissures of all molars and premolars to confirm the presence or absence of possible fractures.
    - Vertical crown fractures or very fine fracture lines can be detected by gently biting on rubber discs or using dyes.
    - A pinkish tinge may be imparted to the dentin due to its reduced thickness following the fracture.
    - Colour of the traumatized tooth likely to change in the post-injury period. These are prominently appreciated at the cingulum of the crown. The best method for identification is by transillumination which shows varying opacities in traumatized teeth, indicating non-vitality.

- Examination of the tooth-supporting structures:
  - Check for bleeding or occult blood along the gingival margin, usually seen in subluxation cases.
  - Abnormal mobility and tenderness on percussion should be recorded.
  - Recording of displacement of teeth (*i.e.*, intrusion, extrusion, lateral displacement, or avulsion):
  - Examine the occlusion as well as radiographs taken at various angulations.
  - The possibility of aspiration or swallowing teeth at the time of injury should always be considered
- Disturbances in occlusion:
  - The direction of the dislocation can sometimes be determined by palpation.
- Abnormal mobility of teeth or alveolar fragments:
  - Test for abnormal mobility, both horizontally and axially
    - No mobility may also mean ankylosis. Hence upon percussion, the type of sound may be indicative of the type of injury.
    - Axial mobility may be indicative of disruption of the vascular supply to the pulp.
    - Movement of adjacent teeth when the mobility of a single tooth is evaluated is a typical sign of dento-alveolar fracture.
- Palpation of the alveolar process:
  - The direction of the dislocation can be determined by palpation.
  - Uneven contours of the alveolar process may indicate a bony fracture.
- Tenderness of teeth to percussion and change in percussion (ankylosis):
  - Conducted by using the handle of a mouth mirror and gently tapping the teeth in the verticals as well as the horizontal direction.
  - Injuries to the periodontal ligament will result in pain.
  - A hard, metallic sound upon percussion in a horizontal direction, is indicative of the tooth ankylosis.
  - A dull sound indicates subluxation or extrusive luxation.
- Examination for root fractures:
  - Root fractures are difficult to identify by clinical examination alone and need radiographs from different angles to check for fracture lines.
  - The tooth may show abnormal mobility
- Reaction of teeth to pulpal sensibility testing:
  - Pulpal sensibility testing at the time of injury is important for establishing a point of reference for evaluating pulpal status at later follow□up examinations.
  - The tests have been summarized as follows.

Pulp Testing

Pulp testing can be done by:

1) Transmitting stimuli to the sensory receptors of the dental pulp and registering thc rcaction.

2) Certain appliances record the status of the vascular component in the pulp canal.

Ideally, the requirements for a method assessing pulpal health must be:

- Simple
- Objective
- Valid
- Reliable
- Reproducible
- Inexpensive
- Not painful or injurious

Principles of pulp testing for traumatic injuries are as follows:

- The pulp is in a state of shock immediately after trauma and results of pulp vitality should be considered with caution.
- Care should be taken that further pulp damage does not take place.
- The stimulus should not be placed over exposed dentin or directly over any cracks of enamel.
- Baseline vitality results help to compare the pulp status in the future and should be recorded on the case paper.
- Vitality tests should be done at baseline, after one month and regularly at six-month intervals over longer periods upto three years after trauma.
- The pulp vitality test may show changes over a period of time.

THERMAL TESTS [11]

This depends on the "threshold effect," which refers to the point that a non-response by a patient is considered to be positive. The threshold responses to the cold and heat tests vary from a maximum of 18 seconds of cold and hot stimuli application to the coronal third of a permanent tooth, to 10 seconds for primary teeth. Hence, the stimuli should not be in contact with the tooth for short duration of approximately 5 seconds but should not exceed the threshold limit

Agents used

Cold tests: Propane-butane mixture, carbon di-oxide snow, dichloro tetrafluoroethene, ethyl chloride, ice sticks

Heat Tests: Heated gutta percha or ball burnisher, warm water

These tests rely on the subjective response of a patient. Hence, false-positive, and false-negative responses are commonly encountered with such tests specially in children who are anxious and are unable to elicit proper responses. This is seen especially when the involved teeth have immature apices or have temporarily disabled sensory nervous supply, due to the impact of the trauma.

To overcome this, the concept of 'wait and see' was devised which may last up to 6 months, rendering pulp sensibility tests inaccurate. The treatment protocol advocates that root canal treatment should not be initiated until at least one additional sign of pulp necrosis has developed. This could include sinus tracts, discoloration of the crown or peri-radicular radiolucency.

ELECTRICAL PULP TESTING [12]

The electric pulp test (EPT) was found to be more reliable in detecting teeth with healthy pulpal tissue when compared to diseased pulp.

- There is evidence of higher reliability of EPT when compared to the thermal tests. However, certain cases of false positive results are encountered which could be explained by a failure to establish adequate isolation using a rubber dam or celluloid strips.
- Case of false negative results may also be seen due inadequate contact of the electrode with the tooth, higher pain threshold of the patients, calcifications, *etc.*
- In case of the heavily restored and crowned teeth, they tend to transmit electric current to adjacent teeth and gingiva without appropriate isolation.

TESTS EVALUATING THE VASCULAR SUPPLY

Relatively objective reading of the pulp's blood oxygen saturation and pulpal blood flow, respectively.

Pulse Oximetry

The pulse oximeter measures the percentage of hemoglobin in the arterial blood that is saturated with oxygen. Oxygenated blood is bright red in color while deoxygenated blood has a darker, red-blue shade. A light-emitting diode (LED) transmits light which measures the color difference. This determines the oxygen saturation of arterial blood.

Recently, customized smaller sensors have been developed to suit the dental morphology and can be effectively used for pulp vitality testing.

Laser Doppler Flowmetry (LDF)

- The LDF test has the ability to directly assess the presence or absence of blood flow within the dental pulp.
- A computerized record that describes the pulpal condition can be read and saved for future reference.
- Advantages:
  - Objective
  - Non-invasive
  - Accurately assesses the pulpal health of teeth following traumatic injuries

Using the EPT along with CO_2 snow or Endo-Ice was more accurate than when the techniques were used alone. Hence, a combination of all the methods with clinical correlation has been recommended for assessing the pulpal health of teeth.

RADIOGRAPHIC EXAMINATION [13]

Conventional or digital intraoral techniques are reliable in the detection of dentoalveolar fractures. Exposures from different angles must be carried out to pinpoint the exact location of the fracture lines.

TECHNIQUES

- **Intra Oral Peri-Apical (IOPA) Radiograph**

It is the most commonly used form of imaging for assessment of trauma to teeth and supporting structures. It can be obtained on a film or as a digital image by RVG, xeroradiography or PSP techniques. It may be required to take multiple images from different angles to assess the tooth, especially in root fractures and displacement injuries. It is also useful for taking soft tissue images during location of foreign bodies or tooth fragments.

- **Orthopantomogram (OPG)**

An OPG is indicated in cases where a jaw fracture is suspected or a temporomandibular joint (TMJ) problem is expected. However, the sensitivity and specificity values of this technique have not yet been studied in relation to dental trauma.

- **Cone Beam Computed Tomography (CBCT)**

CBCT, also called digital volume tomography (DVT), produces 3D digital imaging at a reduced cost and with less radiation for the patient when compared with traditional spiral CT scans. It delivers a faster and easier image acquisition. Additionally, since no film and/or material are introduced inside the patient's mouth, the technique might be suitable even for patients presenting with different levels of fear and anxiety or behavioral problems.

- **Micro-CT**

Conventional dental and panorama images have limited diagnostic ability due to their 2D characteristics. Recently, a micro-CT scanner has been developed and its clinical efficacy in detecting the nuances in dental traumatic injuries have been proven.

CONCLUSION

Traumatic injuries of teeth are true emergencies in dental practice. The patients report in a sense of distress and alleviated anxiety. The dental surgeon needs to maintain a calm and composed demeanor and assure the patients and parents at the same time. Taking a thorough history of the incident is an important part in the beginning of examination. Step wise and meticulous checking of the oral and para oral soft and hard tissues provides substantial insights to understand the extent of trauma thereby allowing the examiner to manage the different injuries effectively.

Examination should be followed by necessary investigation which are corroborated with clinical examination, and a customized treatment plan is formulated for the patient.

CONSENT FOR PUBLICATION

Not applicable.

CONFLICT OF INTEREST

The authors declare no conflict of interest, financial or otherwise.

ACKNOWLEDGEMENT

Declared none.

REFERENCES

[1] Naidoo S, Sheiham A, Tsakos G. Traumatic dental injuries of permanent incisors in 11- to 13-year-old South African schoolchildren. Dent Traumatol 2009; 25(2): 224-8. [http://dx.doi.org/10.1111/j.1600-9657.2008.00749.x] [PMID: 19290905]

[2] Bratteberg M, Thelen DS, Klock KS, Bårdsen A. Traumatic dental injuries-Prevalence and severity

among 16-year-old pupils in western Norway. Dent Traumatol 2018; 34(3): 144-50. [http://dx.doi.org/10.1111/edt.12399] [PMID: 29569840]

[3] Azami-Aghdash S, Ebadifard Azar F, Pournaghi Azar F, *et al.* Prevalence, etiology, and types of dental trauma in children and adolescents: systematic review and meta-analysis. Med J Islam Repub Iran 2015; 29(4): 234. [PMID: 26793672]

[4] Zaleckiene V, Peciuliene V, Brukiene V, Drukteinis S. Traumatic dental injuries: etiology, prevalence and possible outcomes. Stomatologija 2014; 16(1): 7-14. [PMID: 24824054]

[5] Andersson L. Epidemiology of traumatic dental injuries. J Endod 2013; 39(3) (Suppl.): S2-5. [http://dx.doi.org/10.1016/j.joen.2012.11.021] [PMID: 23439040]

[6] Bakland LK, Andreasen JO. Dental traumatology: essential diagnosis and treatment planning. Endod Topics 2004; 7(1): 14-34. [http://dx.doi.org/10.1111/j.1601-1546.2004.00059.x]

[7] Andreasen FM, Kahler B. Diagnosis of acute dental trauma: the importance of standardized documentation: a review. Dent Traumatol 2015; 31(5): 340-9. [http://dx.doi.org/10.1111/edt.12187] [PMID: 26058528]

[8] Moule A, Cohenca N. Emergency assessment and treatment planning for traumatic dental injuries. Aust Dent J 2016; 61 (Suppl. 1): 21-38. [http://dx.doi.org/10.1111/adj.12396] [PMID: 26923446]

[9] McCann PJ, Sweeney MP, Gibson J, Bagg J. Training in oral disease, diagnosis and treatment for medical students and doctors in the United Kingdom. Br J Oral Maxillofac Surg 2005; 43(1): 61-4. [http://dx.doi.org/10.1016/j.bjoms.2004.08.023] [PMID: 15620777]

[10] Lee CS, McCullom C III, Blaustein D. Pediatric chin injury: Occult condylar fractures of the mandible. Pediatr Emerg Care 1991; 7(3): 160-2. [http://dx.doi.org/10.1097/00006565-199106000-00009] [PMID: 1876507]

[11] Gopikrishna V, Tinagupta K, Kandaswamy D. Comparison of electrical, thermal, and pulse oximetry methods for assessing pulp vitality in recently traumatized teeth. J Endod 2007; 33(5): 531-5. [http://dx.doi.org/10.1016/j.joen.2007.01.014] [PMID: 17437866]

[12] Fuss Z, Trowbridge H, Bender IB, Rickoff B, Sorin S. Assessment of reliability of electrical and thermal pulp testing agents. J Endod 1986; 12(7): 301-5. [http://dx.doi.org/10.1016/S0099-2399(86)80112-1] [PMID: 3461119]

[13] Cohenca N, Simon JH, Roges R, Morag Y, Malfaz JM. Clinical indications for digital imaging in dento-alveolar trauma. Part 1: traumatic injuries. Dent Traumatol 2007; 23(2): 95-104. [http://dx.doi.org/10.1111/j.1600-9657.2006.00509.x] [PMID: 17367457]

CHAPTER 10

Traumatic Injuries to Anterior Teeth: Management of Trauma

Satyawan Damle[1,*], **Abdulkadeer M. Jetpurwala**[1] and **Dhanashree Sakhare**[2]

[1] *Department of Pediatric Dentistry, Nair Hospital Dental College, Mumbai, India*

[2] *Founder, Lavanika Dental Academy, Melbourne, Australia*

Abstract: Management of traumatic dental injuries has remained a problem for the dental surgeons due to the wide range of clinical presentations and the unpredictable nature of the pulpal response. Combined with the anxiety and fear at the time of the trauma. Trauma also makes the children apprehensive about any treatment. The approach to the management of traumatic dental injuries, must be customized according to age, general vital signs, systemic conditions, growth potential, and type of trauma to the individual tooth or supporting structures. Each type of traumatic injury has a unique approach and the evidence for their management is updated from time to time. Hence it is important to keep the latest recommendations in mind while adhering to the traditional time-tested methods in the management of traumatic injuries in children.

Keywords: Avulsion, Luxation, Management, Pediatric Dental Trauma, Splinting of Teeth, Traumatic Dental Injuries.

MANAGEMENT

Any traumatic injury to the dentition has a psychological bearing on the mind of the child and parents. Esthetic value of anterior teeth becomes a primary factor in the "psychological well-being" of a person. An unacceptable or improper restoration of fractured tooth often leads to a sense of inferiority, which may be a direct factor in the social acceptance of the child in future. In this situation, efficient treatment planning becomes crucial for successful management of these cases. Even a small fracture of the enamel edge may make a child conscious about their appearance and alter their patterns of social skill development including smiling as they may not be comfortable to display their broken teeth [1].

* **Corresponding author Satyawan Damle:** Department of Pediatric Dentistry, Nair Hospital Dental College, Mumbai, India; E-mail: sgdamble@gmail.com

Satyawan Damle, Ritesh Kalaskar & Dhanashree Sakhare (Eds.)

***Emergency treatment*:** Immediate treatment must be rendered in case of trauma for the clearance of the airway passage and control of bleeding. When there is suspicion of neurological involvement or medical emergency, physician/surgeon should be communicated, or patient should be shifted to tertiary care center. Any loose fragments of tooth should be accounted for and aspiration or embedment of these fragments in soft tissues should be ruled out.

***Emergency treatment of soft tissue injury*:** soft tissue wounds should be cleaned and debrided carefully. Control of bleeding should be of paramount importance. All efforts should be directed towards control of bleeding before dental examination is contemplated. If abrasion is shallow debridement may be the only treatment required. In deeper wounds care should be taken to ensure that no tooth fragment or foreign body like gravel are embedded in the tissue. The dentist must recognize the possibility of the development of tetanus after the injury and must carry out adequate first aid measures. Soft tissue injuries are associated with swelling and distortion of tissues. This leads to a panicky situation for the parents as they are worried about the extensive swelling. Soft tissue swelling should also be evaluated from the perspective of airway obstruction [1 - 3].

MANAGEMENT OF DENTAL TRAUMA [4, 5]

Ellis Class I Fracture (Fig. 1)

Clinical Features

Loss of enamel is observed in form of fractured incisal edge or angle. No sign of dentin or pulpal involvement is present. Pain if present is secondary to any other associated TDI as root fracture or luxation.

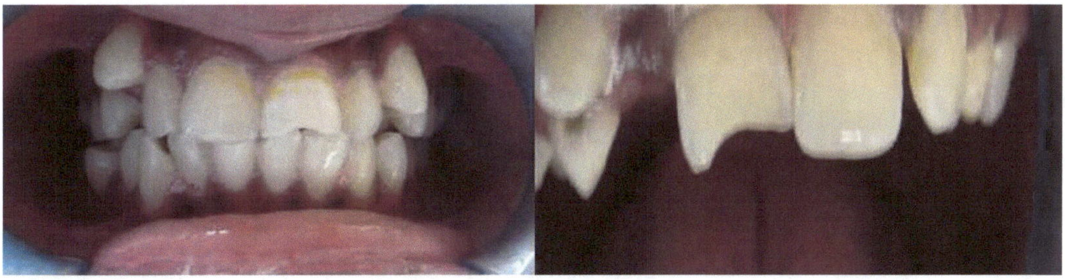

Fig (1). Ellis class I trauma involving enamel only.

Investigations

Ellis class I trauma require IOPA radiographs and pulp testing. Radiographs are helpful in ruling out any root fracture while the pup testing establishes a baseline observation against which future comparisons can be made. In cases of soft tissue lacerations concomitant with enamel fractures, it must be radiographed to search for broken tooth fragment.

Treatment (Fig. 2)

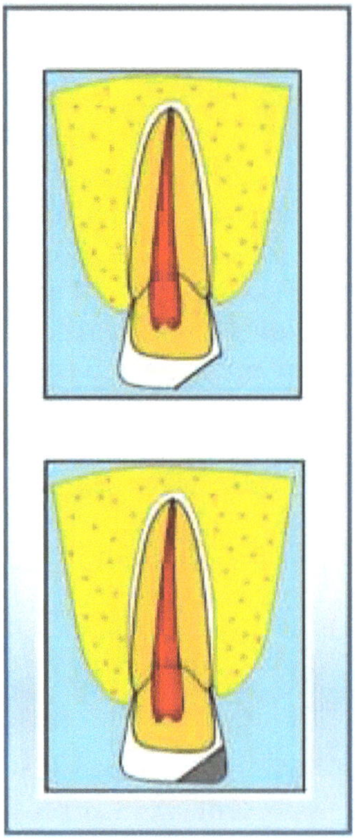

Fig (2). Ellis class I treatment.

a. Re-contour injured tooth
b. Apply fluoride varnish to prevent sensitivity (Duraphat 5% / Fluorprotector 1%)
c. Treatment of choice is "Fragment Reattachment" if patient reports with the fractured part. The method of reattachment is simple and requires stability during composite bonding. If the patient does not have the fragment, composite resin restoration and contouring are done. Care must be taken to seal the entire fracture line for better prognosis.

Follow up

A follow up of 6-8 weeks and 1 year later with clinical and radiographic evaluation has been recommended in these cases.

Prognosis

Enamel fractures, if not associated with any other TDI, have a good prognosis with no adverse clinical symptoms and maintenance of pulp vitality at follow ups. However undetected TDI, other associated traumas and Multiple Dental Trauma Episodes (MDTE) can lead to loss of vitality, discoloration and apical periodontitis which require stage appropriate endodontic management.

Ellis class II fracture (Fig. 3) [4, 5]

Clinical Features

In Ellis class II cases there is considerable exposure of dentin. Patient often reports a loss of crown structure with/without transient sensitivity to cold. The associated TDI can result in increased tenderness on palpation percussion. The young permanent teeth have large pulp chambers and exhibit severe sensitivity after enamel dentin fractures. Due to the wider dentinal tubules of young permanent teeth, there is greater ingress of noxious substances towards the pulp chamber and hence emphasis should be laid towards covering the dentinal tubules as early as possible after trauma.

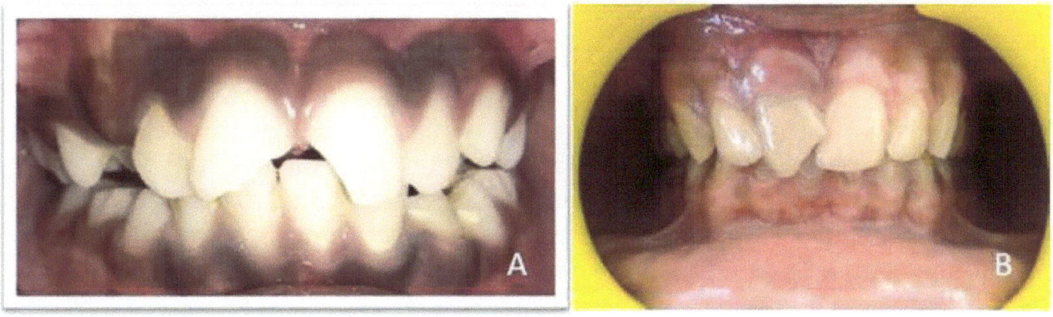

Fig (3). A-Ellis class II trauma involving 11 and 21; B-Ellis class II trauma with 11.

Investigations

Radiographs are needed in cases with marginal loss of crown structure and without any other TDI. Large fractures bordering dental pulp, require IOPA radiograph to assess the proximity of fracture line to pulp. IOPA radiograph of soft tissue injury in the vicinity might be needed to rule out the embedded fractured fragment. Pulp testing might be required if patient reports after a gap and there are signs of discoloration.

Treatment- (Fig. 4)

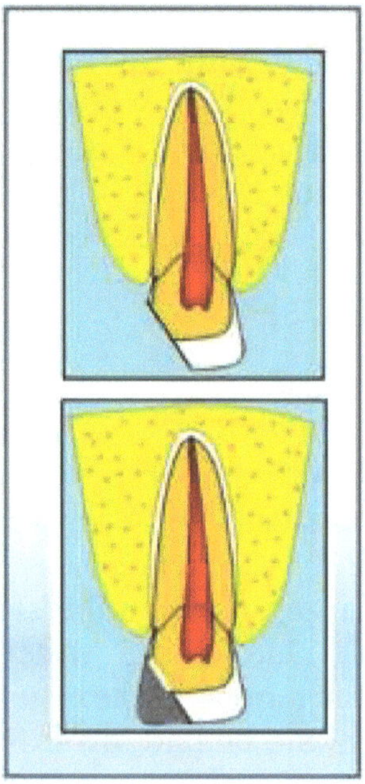

Fig (4). Ellis class II treatment restoration of tooth with calcium hydroxide base.

The primary objective is to prevent injury to the pulp. The traditional restoration of fracture exposing dentin includes the application of hard setting calcium hydroxide paste over the exposed dentinal surface before restoring it with composite resin. If early definitive restoration is not possible due to the presenting condition of the patient or need for more urgent attention towards other teeth affected by trauma, a glass ionomer cement, bandage restoration should be placed to cover the dentinal tubules temporarily.

The stepwise procedure is as follows:

- Anesthetize the area
- Cleaning of the fractured tooth, gentle irrigation with water
- Drying the tooth with air syringe
- Rubber dam isolation
- Placing calcium hydroxide paste over the exposed dentin followed by GIC base.
- Preparing the enamel with 37% phosphoric acid, rinsing with water, drying
- Applying bonding agent
- Restoring the tooth with composite resin.
- If the fractured segment is available, reattachment can also be tried

Follow up

A follow up of 6-8 weeks and later 1 year with clinical and radiographic evaluation has been recommended in these cases.

Prognosis

Enamel-dentin fractures, if not associated with any other TDI, have a good prognosis with no adverse clinical symptoms and maintenance of pulp vitality at follow ups. However undetected TDI, other associated traumas and Multiple Dental Trauma Episodes (MDTE) can lead to loss of vitality, discoloration and apical periodontitis which require stage appropriate endodontic management.

Ellis Class III Fracture (Fig. 5) [4, 5]

Clinical Features

Patients present with fractured tooth with visible or demonstrable pulp exposure. There may be provoked or spontaneous pain and tenderness due to exposed pulp. An associated luxation injury can further complicate their management and prognosis. Age and stage of development are also important for its treatment planning. A thorough history should be taken, duration elapsed between trauma and reporting to dental clinic is important to note. The size of the pulp exposure should be recorded.

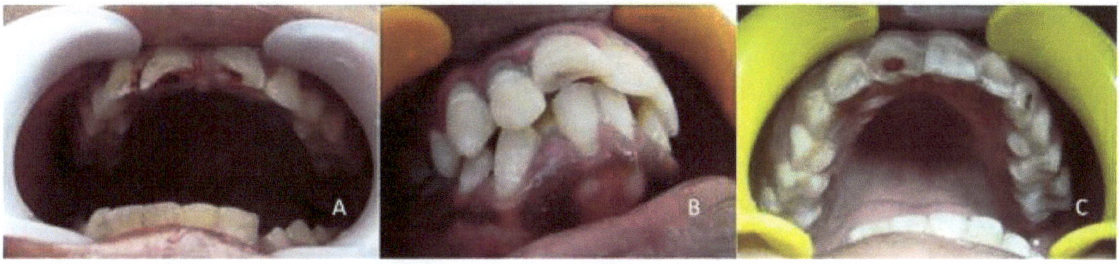

Fig (5). Ellis class III with A-#11, #21; B- #11; C--#11 showing different sizes of pulp exposure.

Investigations

These traumatic injuries require IOPA radiographs from different angulations for determining the fracture line, extent of the damage and stage of root development. Pulp sensibility testing is carried out in trauma with treatment delay.

Treatment-(Fig. 6)

The management strategy is guided by three main variables. Duration since trauma, size of exposure site, and stage of root development. Teeth with pulpal exposure may require pulp capping/ pulpotomy/ apexification / root canal therapy depending on afore said variables and nature of reversibility of pulpal inflammation and the development of the root apex. The primary aim is to preserve the vital, non-inflamed pulp surrounded by hard tissue.

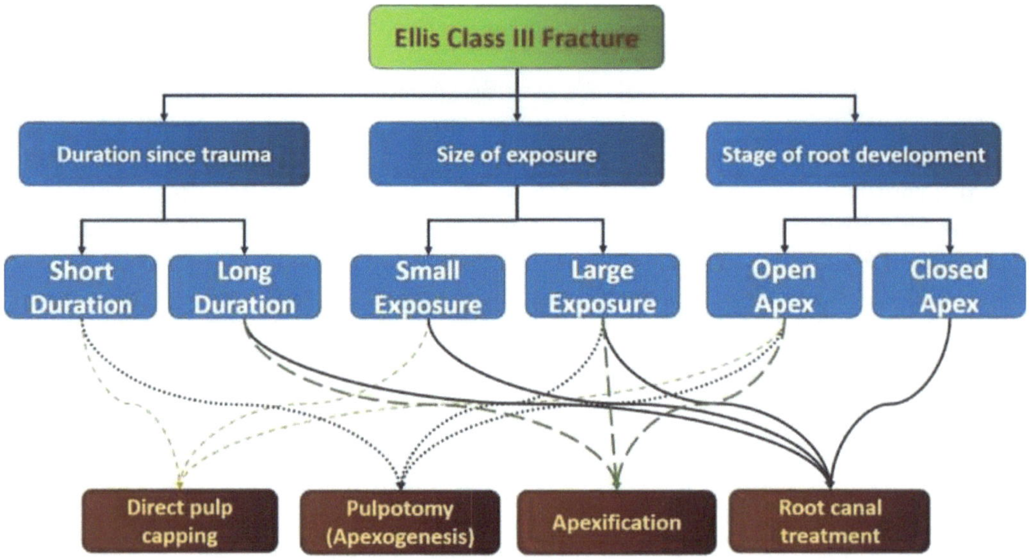

Fig (6). Treatment of Ellis class II traumatic injuries.

Immature Permanent Tooth With Open Apex [6]

Immature teeth possess wide open apices called as "blunderbuss apices." When there is a traumatic injury to teeth with open apices, it is not possible to obturate these teeth by conventional methods using gutta percha and a sealer because there is absence of hard barrier against which the filing can be condensed apically. The management of these teeth is a challenging task.

In the teeth with vital pulp and open apices, apexogenesis is the treatment of choice. Apexogenesis describes the continued physiologic development and formation of the root's apex in vital young permanent teeth. It can be achieved by implementing the appropriate vital pulp therapy techniques. It can be achieved by:

A. ***Pulp capping*:** Pulp capping is recommended only for small exposures that can be treated immediately after the injury. Preservation of vitality is attempted at the outset with direct pulp capping (pinpoint exposure, clean field) using hard setting calcium hydroxide and partial pulpotomy with calcium hydroxide followed by GIC restoration are recommended treatments. Calcium hydroxide has been widely used for vital pulp therapy. Its strong alkalinity contributes to its action. It provides a bactericidal environment in which subsequent repair and hard tissue bridge can occur. Mineral trioxide aggregate (MTA) and Biodentine® has shown to be an effective pulp capping material, which produces a hard tissue barrier. It has a high sealing ability and can set in a moist environment. During the setting reaction, calcium hydroxide ions are released, and high alkalinity is present in the exposed area. At present, MTA appears to be a promising material as an alternative to calcium hydroxide.

B. ***Pulpotomy:*** It is indicated when the coronal portion of the pulp is inflamed, and the radicular pulp is healthy (Fig. 7).

According to American Academy of Pediatric Dentistry (AAPD) guidelines, partial pulpotomy for traumatic exposures is a procedure, in which the inflamed pulp tissue beneath an exposure is removed to a depth of 1-3 mm or more to reach the deeper healthy tissue. The main objective of partial pulpotomy is to preserve the pulp vitality so that teeth with immature roots show continued normal root development and apexogenesis [7].

Various materials have been used as pulpotomy agents; calcium hydroxide has been the mainstay of pulpotomy procedures in permanent teeth for a long time. It acts by providing an alkaline pH which promotes the formation of a dentin bridge and thus seals off the healthy pulp from the external environment. However, various reports of gradual disintegration and formation of tunnel defects in the newly formed dentin have been commonly witnessed with calcium hydroxide when followed-up for longer times.

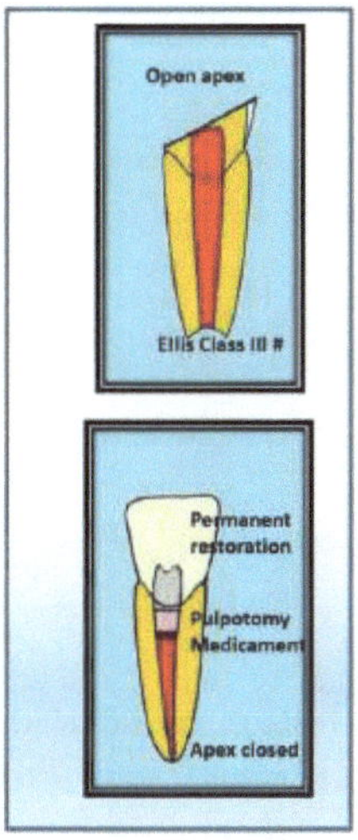

Fig (7). Pulpotomy procedure.

Lasers offer a conservative and biological alternative to other pulpotomy agents due to the regenerative or reparative effect of laser energy and exposure site sterilization. Various lasers have been reported to be used for pulpotomy including carbon dioxide (CO_2), neodymium: Yttrium-aluminum-garnet, erbium: Yttrium-aluminum-garnet (Er:YAG), erbium-chromium: Yttrium scandium gadolinium garnet and diode lasers.

Mature Permanent Tooth With Closed Apex

Root Canal Therapy: It is carried out in a tooth with closed apex when the entire pulp inflamed due to long duration after trauma. The apical closure provides a satisfactory situation for obtaining a fluid – tight seal after obturation of canal space with gutta percha in conjunction with a sealer (Fig. **8**).

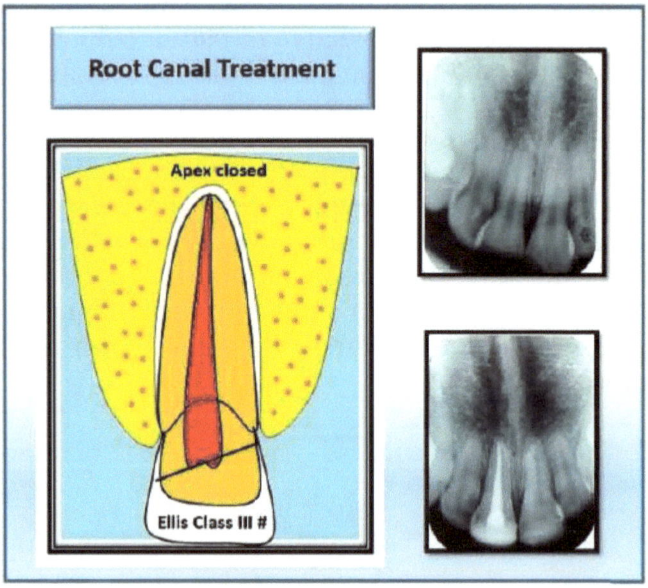

Fig (8). Root canal treatment of traumatized tooth.

Ellis class IV fracture (Fig. 9) [4, 5]

Clinical Features

Ellis class IV trauma indicates that the pulp has become non vital. There may or may not be concurrent loss of crown structure. Signs and symptoms associated with necrotic pulps may be associated with the affected tooth. The tooth may show signs of pain, grey discoloration, periapical abscess, tenderness to percussion or even extra oral swellings on the lips and fascial spaces.

Investigations

The pulp sensitivity tests will be negative and IOPA may show peri-apical radiolucency, widening of periodontal ligament space and loss of lamina dura. It is important to note when there is a long-standing history of trauma with non-vital pulp, the pulp chamber and root canal space of the affected tooth will be wider in children due to cessation of dentinal deposition in the affected tooth compared the unaffected tooth.

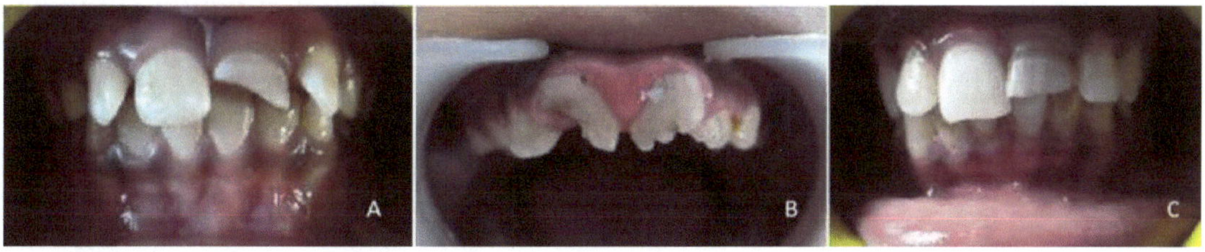

Fig (9). Ellis class IV A- #21; B-#11; C-#21.

Treatment (Fig. 10)

The treatment of teeth with Ellis class IV fracture depends on the stage of root development. If the affected tooth presents with an open apex, apexification or revascularization should be initiated; if the apex is closed then conventional root canal therapy can be done [8].

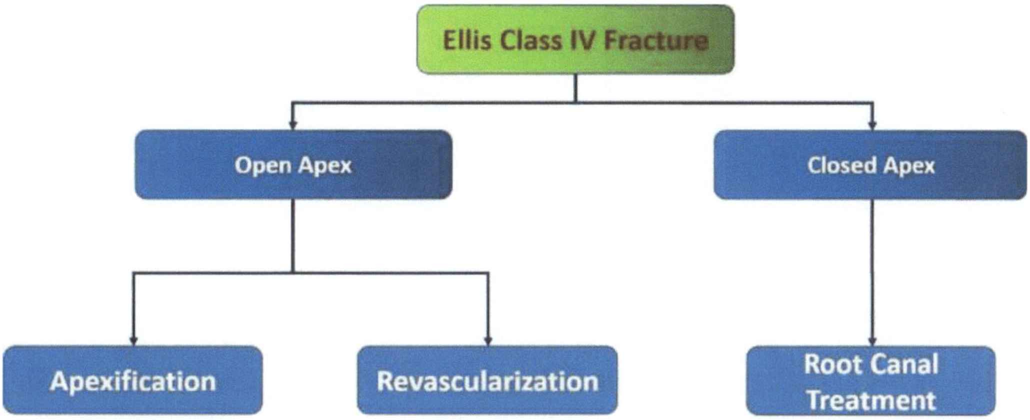

Fig (10). -Management of Ellis class IV trauma.

When discoloration of the tooth is signification simultaneous intrinsic bleaching of the tooth with 30% hydrogen peroxide should be initiated to improve the esthetic value of the tooth.

Immature Permanent Tooth with Open Apex

In the teeth with non-vital pulp and open apices, Apexification and Revascularization are the treatment of choice.

A. Revascularization (Fig. **11**)

Pulp revascularization is a treatment of choice for non-vital immature permanent teeth. The goal is to stimulate regeneration of a functional pulp-dentin complex. Pulp revascularization is a relatively new treatment modality for non-vital necrotic immature permanent teeth that allows continued root development, thickening of dentinal walls and apical closure [9].

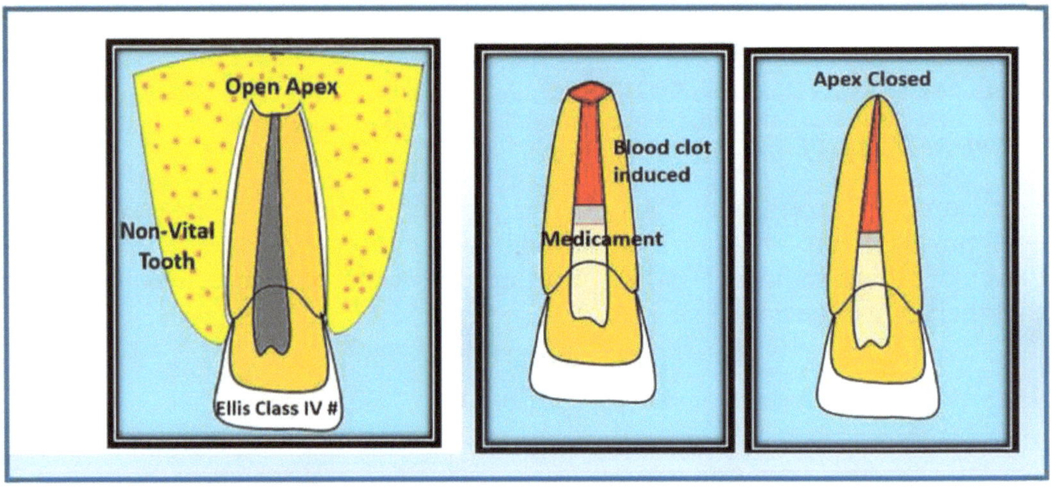

Fig (11). – revascularization of non-vital traumatized tooth.

B. Apexification (Fig. **12**)

It is a method of inducing apical closure by use of a suitable medicament, like calcium hydroxide, MTA, Biodentine® [8]. Formation of osteocementum or a similar hard tissue or the continued development of the roots of an incompletely formed tooth in which the pulp is no longer vital.

Mature Permanent Tooth With Closed Apex

Root canal therapy: It is carried out in a tooth with closed apex when the entire pulp inflamed due to long duration after trauma (Fig. **8**).

- ***Follow up***

The recommended schedule for follow up is a clinical-radiographic examination after 6-8 weeks. Tooth must further be examined clinically and with radiographs after 1 year.

- ***Prognosis***

Failure to seek early treatment after trauma often results in loss of vitality in these teeth, requiring endodontic intervention. Successful pulp therapy maintains the tooth asymptomatic, helps in continuing root development. In failure cases and those complicated by other TDI, apical periodontitis results and tooth becomes non vital.

***Ellis Class V Fracture Treatment* [4, 10]**

Clinical Features (Fig. 13)

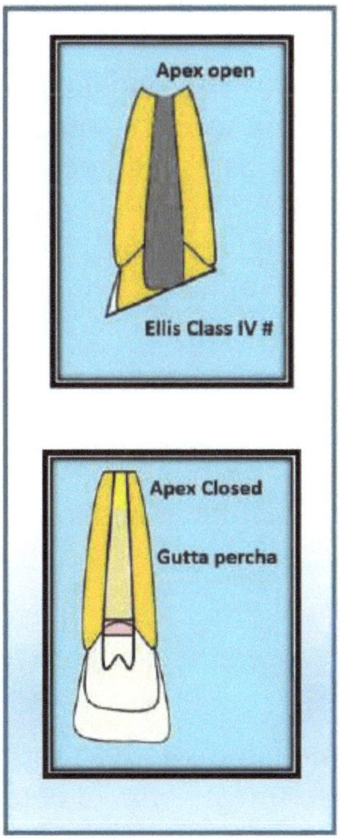

Fig 12. Apexification.

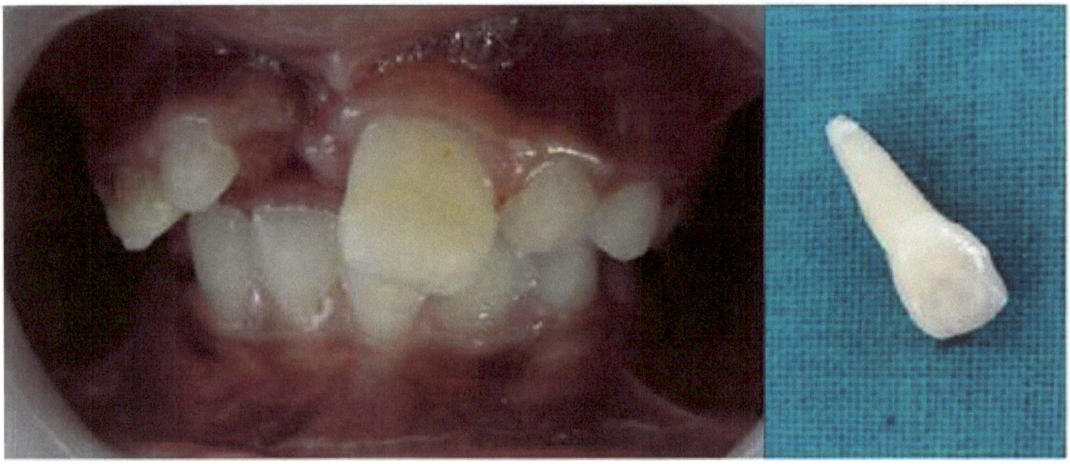

Fig (13). – Ellis class V trauma to #11 with avulsed tooth.

Patient reports with the chief complaint of loss of tooth after traumatic episode. It may be associated with other traumatic dental injuries and maxillofacial injuries. Occasionally the patient brings the avulsed teeth stored in various media or in a dry condition. Due to the gross nature of avulsions and its high frequency in road traffic accidents, emergency care is usually sought even in developing nations. Time delay has been emphasized as the biggest factor affecting prognosis of avulsed teeth [11]. Low level of awareness has been observed among parents, schoolteachers, emergency care givers and medical practitioners regarding avulsion management- immediate replantation or storage of avulsed tooth [12 - 14].

Investigations

IOPA's are essential to rule out any possibility of dento-alveolar fracture and explore the extent of damage to attachment apparatus.

Treatment

The success of the replantation procedure is related to:

- The time elapsed after the avulsion of the tooth and its replacement in the socket. Shorter the extraoral dry time results in better prognosis of avulsed tooth. It has been observed that with extraoral time less than 30 min there is 10% resorption of the tooth structure, whereas more than 90 min results in 90% resorption.
- The condition of the tooth and the periodontal ligament

Management can by divided into:

A. Management at site of injury
B. Management in the dental office

   A. ***Management at site of injury*:** Replant immediately. Rinse with water or normal saline if available before replanting if the tooth is contaminated. When immediate replantation is not possible, place tooth in the best transport medium available (Fig. **14**) [9].

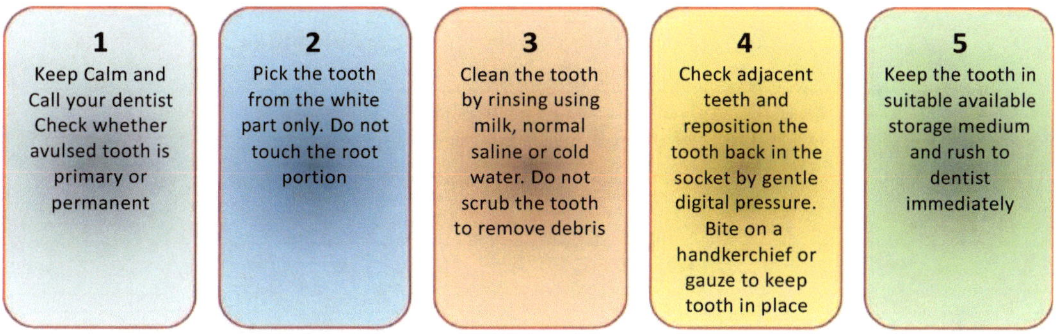

Fig (14). Management of avulsed tooth at site of injury.

Storage Media (Table 1)

Tap water is the worst storage medium because it causes rapid cell lysis however it may be preferable to dry storage. Saliva, for a small period is effective, but contains microorganisms and it has low osmolality, which adversely affects the viability of cells in the periodontal ligament. Saline solution does not have essential ions and does not provide cell nutrients. Contact lenses solutions showed no advantages over other means. Milk is significantly better than other storage media, but it only prevents cell death and does not restore the normal cell morphology.

An avulsed tooth transport system called “SAVE A TOOTH” containing Hank’s balanced salt solution (HBSS), a pH preserving fluid and trauma reducing suspension apparatus is available (Fig. **15**, Table **2**). It may be used in serious accidents that relegate replantation to secondary importance and hence replanted when crisis is over.

Table 1. Various transport media for an avulsed tooth.

Interim medium	Characteristics
Tap water	Hypotonic osmolarity. Cellular lysis
Saline Isotonic	Not conductive to periodontal ligament cell metabolism
Saliva	Readily available. Non-physiologic osmolarity and contamination
Milk	Efficacy equivalent to Hanks Balanced Salt Solution Longer duration of storage (chilled milk) Presence of antigens
Hank's Balanced Salt Solution (HBSS)	Considered as gold standard Physiologic-isotonic solution Maintain cellular vitality for extended period of storage
ViaSpan	Long-term media Inaccessible
Propolis	Maintain cellular viability for extended duration
Culture media	Maintain cellular viability for extended period Aid in periodontal ligament regeneration Can be supplemented with growth factors
Coconut water	Biological-isotonic fluid. Contrasting results regarding efficacy
Powdered milk	High protein content and water Lack of microbial contamination Maintain viability only up to four hours
Egg albumin	Equivalent cellular viability as HBSS
Salvia officinalis	Natural substance. Antioxidant Short-term storage
Morus rubra	Natural substance. Antioxidant and anti-bacterial Extended storage
Emdogain (Enamel Matrix Derivative, EMD)	Doubtful efficacy in replanted and auto-transplanted teeth
Green tea extract	antibacterial, antioxidative and anti-inflammatory can keep the PDL cells alive for 15 hours
Tooth rescue box	Contains amino acids, vitamins and glucose. Maintains the vitality and viability of PDL cells at room temperature for at least 48 hours. Avulsed teeth stored in a rescue box for 15 minutes have exhibited functional healing irrespective of storage duration

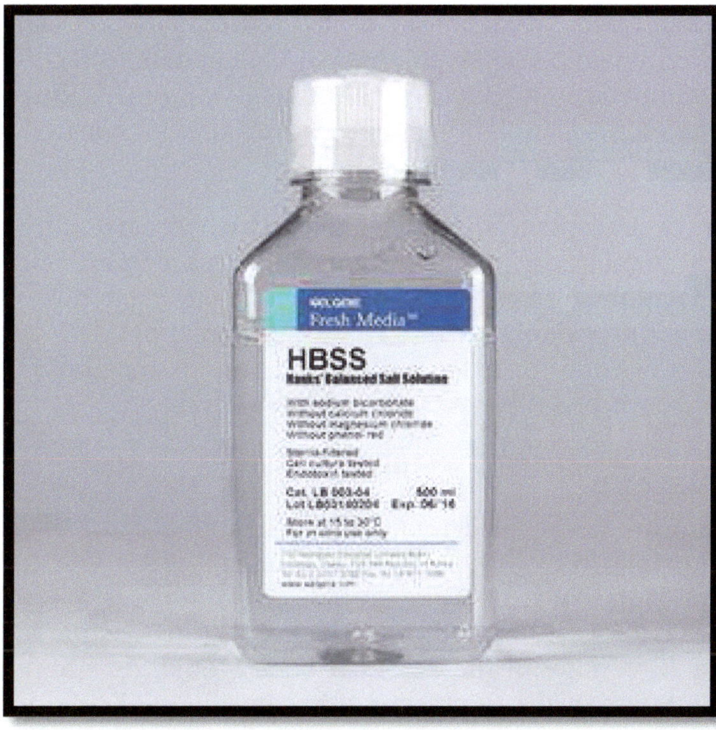

Fig (15). "SAVE A TOOTH" - Hank's balanced salt solution (HBSS).

Table 2. Composition of Hank's Balanced Salt Solution.

Ingredients	Concentration
Sodium Chloride	8 gm/L
d-Glucose	0.4 gm/L
Potassium Chloride	0.4 gm/L
Sodium Bicarbonate	0.35 gm/L
Sodium Phosphate	0.09 gm/L
Potassium Phosphate	0.14 gm/L
Calcium Chloride	0.14 gm/L
Magnesium Chloride	0.1 gm/L
Anhydrous Magnesium Sulphate	0.1 gm/L
Water	To constitute

Hanks' balanced salt solution with a pH of 7.2 and osmolality of 270–290 osm/kg is a non-toxic and biocompatible standard saline solution. The presence of glucose, calcium, and magnesium sustains and reconstitutes the depleted cellular components of PDL cells. It has a long shelf life of 2 years and does not require refrigeration. A removable suspension basket with handle to receive the avulsed tooth permits atraumatic storage and handling, thus minimizes the trauma to cells during transportation. Its osmolality and pH are ideal, but the medium is not easily available in India yet.

Viaspan, an organ transplant storage media, which dramatically prolongs the storage time of human organs has showed decrease the incidence of root resorption after replantation and is considered a better medium than milk and HBSS. Viaspan has an osmolality of 320 mosm/kg and pH of 7.4 which is ideal for cell growth. It is good for extended storage periods for 72-96 hrs. However, disadvantages are cost, and it is also not readily available.

Management in the Dental Office [10]

The management of the avulsed tooth in the dental office follows a complex algorithm of previous prevailing conditions under which the tooth has been presented to the dental surgeon (Fig. **16**). If the tooth is already repositioned, check whether it is properly placed or not, correct if necessary. If the extra oral time is less than 20 minutes or the tooth has been brought in a transport medium, immediate replantation of the tooth should be considered. With increase in extra oral time, the prognosis of the tooth becomes questionable due to loss of viability of periodontal ligament cells. When periodontal ligament cell viablity is questionable, the root surface should be prepared to reduce the rate of post operative replacement resorption.

i. Management of the root surface:
   - Always keep the tooth moist.
   - Do not touch the root surface (hold tooth by the crown).
   - Do not scrape or brush the root surface or remove the tip of the root.
   - If the root appears clean, replant as it is, after rinsing with saline.
   - If the root surface is contaminated, rinse with Hank's balanced salt solution (HBSS)or saline (use tap water if above are not available). If persistent debris remains on root surface, gently use cotton pellet or wet sponge to remove remaining debris.
   - If the periodontal cells are non-viable, the avulsed tooth should be soaked for 5 min in sodium fluoride solution before replantation, as it reduces resorption. According to Andreasen, 1.0%-2.4% topical Sodium fluoride solution can be used.

ii. Management of the Socket (Fig. **17**).
   - Do not curette the socket. If a clot is present, use light irrigation with saline

- Do not make a surgical flap unless bony fragments prevent replantation.
- If the alveolar bone is collapsed and prevents replantation, carefully insert a blunt instrument into the socket to reposition the bone to its original position. After replantation, manually compress facial and lingual bony plates.

iii. Management of Soft Tissues:

- Suture any soft tissue lacerations, particularly in the cervical region.
    i. Replantation of tooth (Figs. **18 - 20**)

Permanent Teeth with Closed Apex [10]

Patient Reports with Replanted Tooth

1. The tooth is not disturbed from its socket.
2. The area is cleaned using water, saline, or chlorhexidine. Bleeding is stopped using pressure and suturing of lacerations. Its position is verified and stabilized using flexible splint for 2 weeks.
3. Systemic antibiotics, analgesics and tetanus immunization must be instituted.
4. Pressure habits of the patient and occlusal contact must be checked at the time of splinting.
5. Root canal treatment is initiated at 7-10 days after replantation.

Extra Oral Dry Time Less than 60 Minutes and Tooth Stored in Physiologic Medium

1. The root surface and apex are cleaned with stream of saline to remove debris and dead cells.
2. Socket is irrigated after administering local anesthesia and alveolar fracture is repositioned with suitable instrument
3. Coagulum is removed and tooth is replanted gently with digital pressure without forcing it, verified by radiograph, and stabilized by flexible splint for 2 weeks. Gingival laceration is managed by suturing.
4. Pressure habits of the patient and occlusal contact must be checked at the time of splinting.
5. Root canal treatment is initiated at 7-10 days after replantation.

Extra Oral Dry Time more than 60 Minutes or other Reasons Suggesting Non-viable Cells- (Fig. 19)

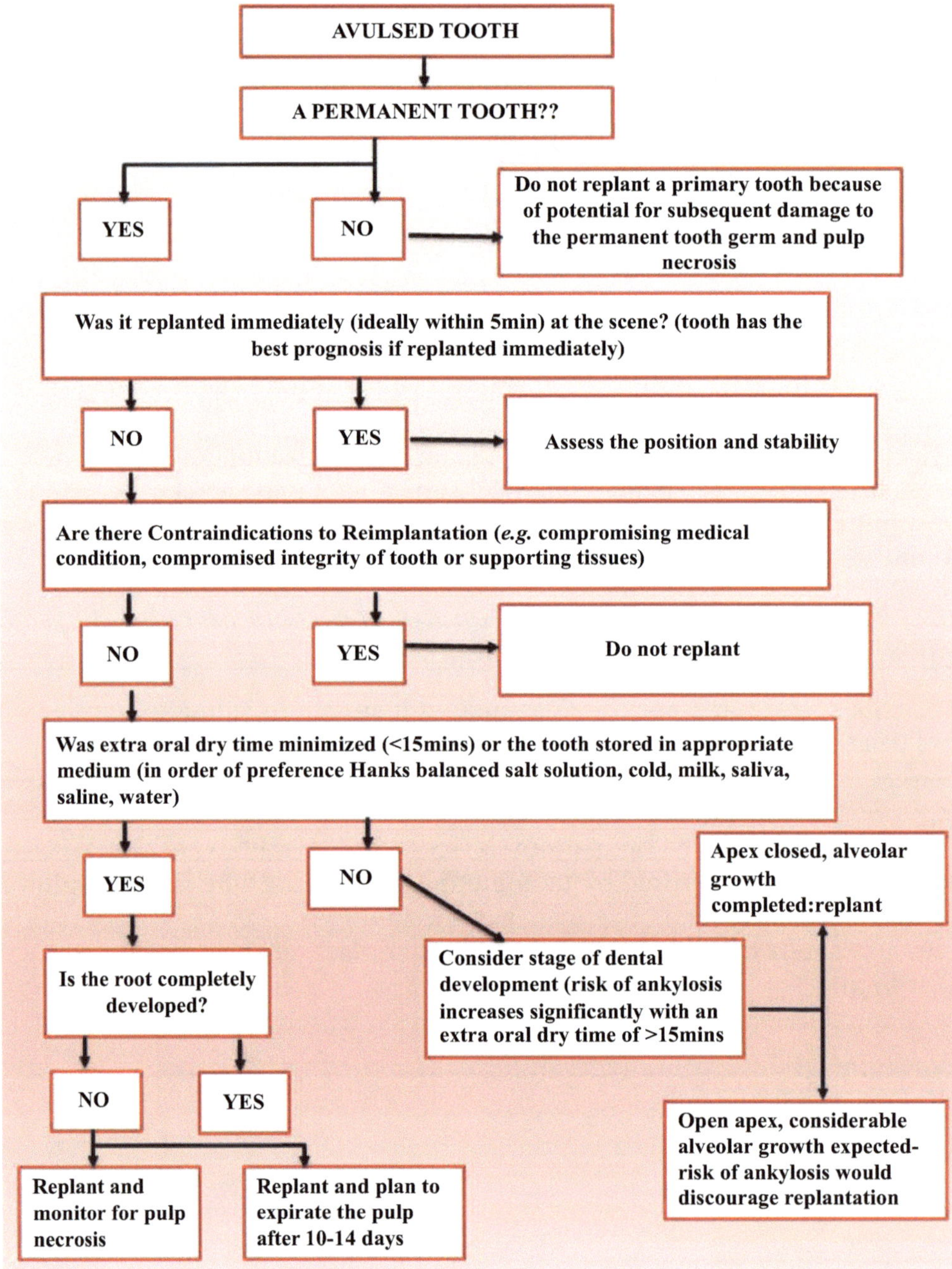

Fig (16). Decision tree for management of avulsed tooth in dental office.

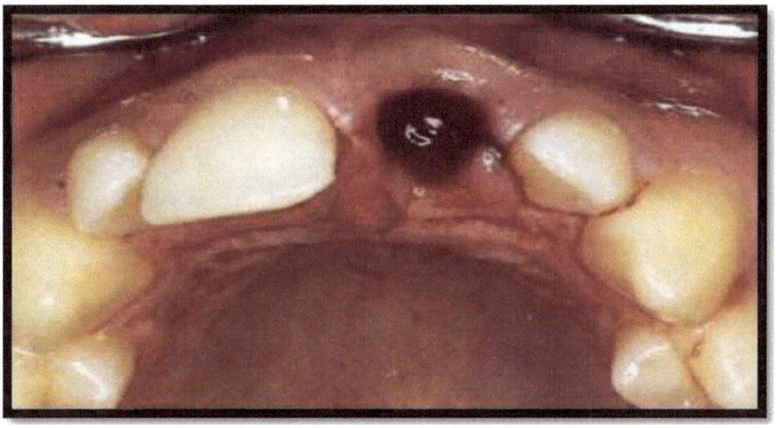

Fig (17). Examine socket and irrigate with sterile saline.

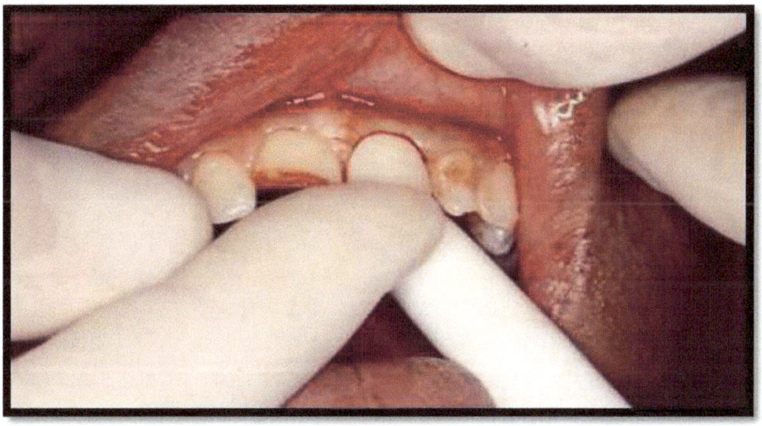

Fig (18). Replant tooth using light digital pressure.

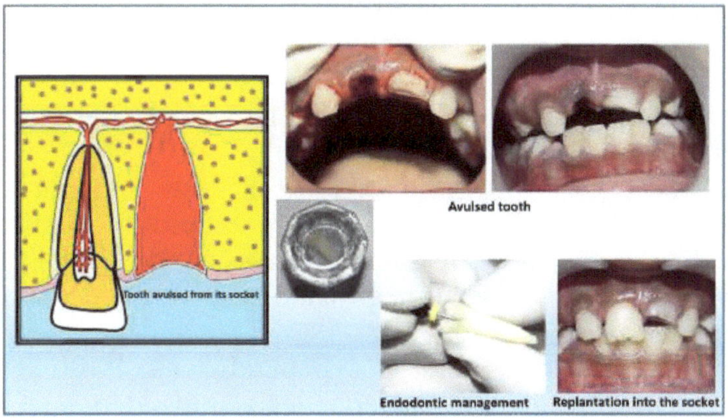

Fig (19). Management of tooth with avulsion and extra oral dry time > 60 minutes.

Delayed replantation has a poor long-term prognosis. The periodontal ligament will be necrotic and not expected to heal. In addition to restoring the tooth for aesthetic, functional and psychological reasons, the goal in delayed replantation is to maintain alveolar bone contour. However, the expected eventual outcome is ankylosis and resorption of the root and the tooth might be lost. The parents must be counseled, and five-year survival rate of the tooth should be discussed based on presenting condition.

- The attached non-viable soft tissue is carefully removed with gauze, periodontal curette or scalpel from the root surface and apex is cleaned with stream of saline to remove debris and dead cells.
- Extra oral endodontic treatment should be completed
- Various authors have suggested immersion of the tooth in Doxycycline, 10% citric acid, Sodium fluoride solutions for 5 minutes each to reduce the rated of replacement resorption.
- The rest of the procedure is same as for tooth with extra oral time less than 60 minutes.

Permanent Teeth with Open Apex (immature teeth)- [10]

Patient Reports with Replanted Tooth

1. Procedure is same as that for teeth with closed apex
2. The goal of replanting immature permanent teeth is to allow for possible reestablishment of pulp vitality. If it does not occur, stage appropriate endodontic treatment- apexification (MTA or Calcium hydroxide) & revascularization has been recommended.

Extra Oral Dry Time Less than 60 Minutes and Tooth Stored in Physiologic Medium

1. The root surface and apex are cleaned with stream of saline to remove debris and dead cells, if needed.
2. Caution must be exercised to minimize the dry time without disturbing the attached periodontal ligament. Soaking in antibiotic solution (preferably doxycycline) has been shown to promote revascularization.
3. Socket is irrigated after administering local anesthesia and alveolar fracture is repositioned with suitable instrument.
4. Coagulum is removed and tooth is replanted gently with digital pressure without forcing it, verified by radiograph, and stabilized by flexible splint for 2 weeks.
5. Gingival laceration is managed by suturing. Systemic antibiotics, analgesics

and tetanus immunization must be instituted.

6. Pressure habits of the patient and occlusal contact must be checked at the time of splinting. The goal of replanting immature permanent teeth is to allow for possible reestablishment of pulp vitality.
7. The risk of infection and root resorption should be weighed against the chances of vitality reestablishment.
8. If it does not occur, stage appropriate endodontic treatment- apexification (MTA or Calcium hydroxide) & revascularization has been recommended.

Extra Oral Dry Time more than 60 Minutes or other Reasons Suggesting Non-viable Cells

The procedure is same as that for tooth with extra oral time less than 60 minutes. However, the expected eventual outcome is ankylosis and resorption of the root and the tooth might be lost as the periodontal ligament will be necrotic and not expected to heal. In addition to restoring the tooth for aesthetic, functional and psychological reasons, the goal in delayed replantation is to maintain alveolar bone contour. If the tooth with open apex is not replanted in a short time after trauma, extra oral retrograde filling of the root apex may also be considered prior to repositioning.

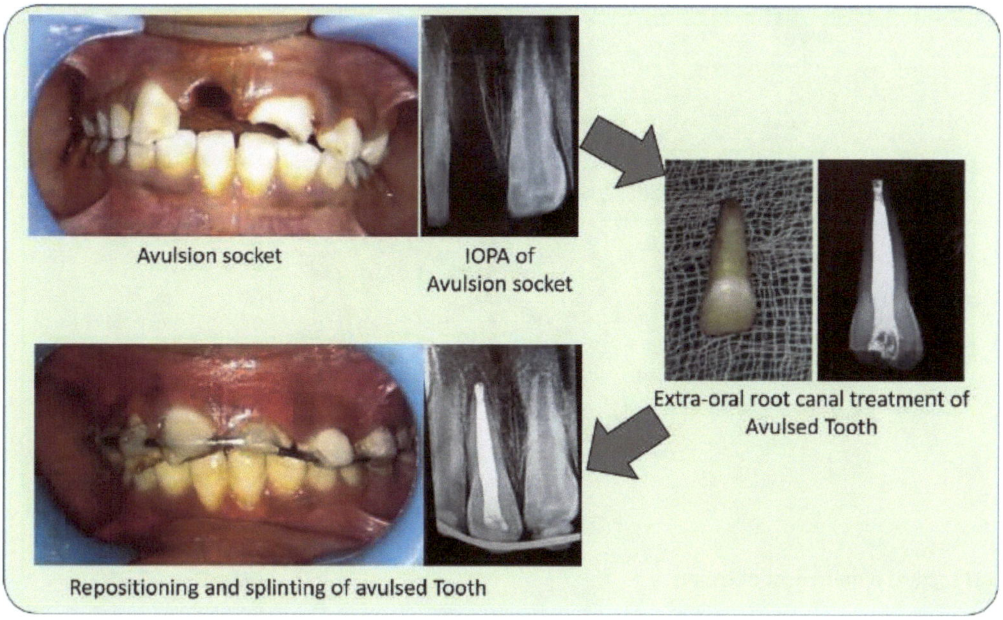

Fig (20). Replantation of avulsed tooth.

Splinting [15] (Fig. 21)

- Use acid-etch resin alone or with soft arch wire or use orthodontic brackets with passive arch wire (described below).
- Suture in place only if alternative splinting methods are unavailable. (Circumferential wire splints are contraindicated).
- Splint should remain in place for 7-10 days. However, if tooth demonstrates excessive mobility, splint should be maintained until mobility reduces.
- Bone sresulting in mobility usually require longer splinting periods (2-8 weeks).

Home care instructions for patients during splinting period include:

- Do not bite on splinted teeth
- Soft diet
- Maintenance of proper oral hygiene

A splinting technique should allow physiologic movement of the tooth during healing and should be in place for a minimal time which will result in a decreased incidence of ankyloses. The splint should allow movement of the tooth and should not impinge on the gingiva and should not prevent maintenance of oral hygiene in the area.

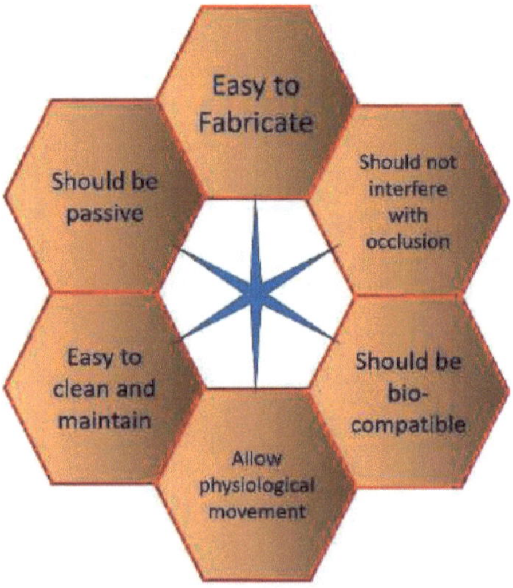

Fig (21). Ideal requirement of splints.

Types of Splints

Various types of splints have been tried for immobilization of teeth some of them are (Fig. **22**).

1. Bonded wire composite splint
2. Arch wire bonded splint
3. Acid etched nylon monofilament splint
4. Nylon fishing wire splint
5. Sutures
6. Titanium trauma splint
7. Brackets with passive orthodontic arch wire

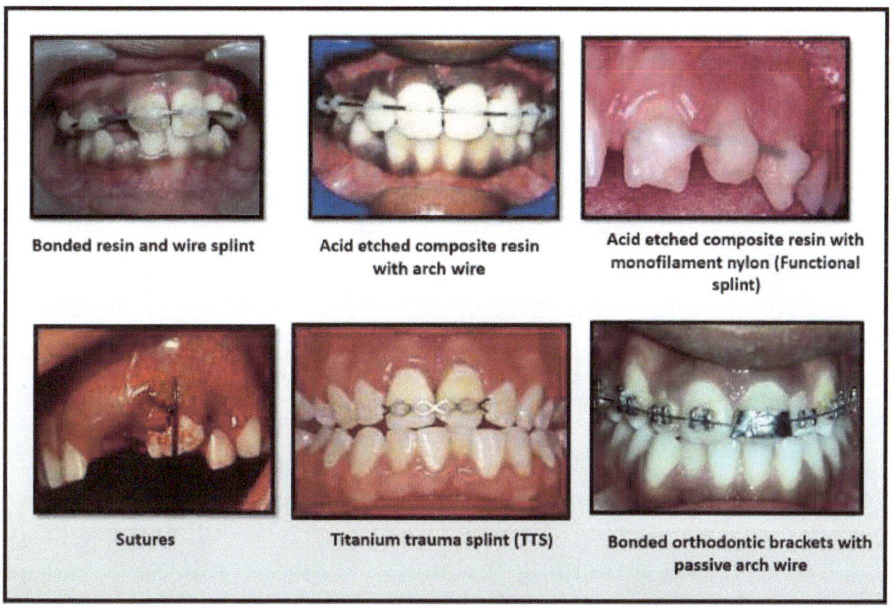

Fig (22). Types of splints.

Many splints satisfy the requirements of an acceptable splint, with a new titanium trauma splint (TTS) proved to be effective. It is made of pure titanium and has thickness of 0.2mm hence can be easily adapted to the contour of the dental arch. Pliers and other bending instruments are not required as it can be bent with fingers. It has a rhomboidal mesh structure which makes it flexible which allows physiologic tooth movement without transmitting orthodontic forces to the tooth.

After the splint is in place, a radiograph should be taken to verify the positioning of the tooth and as a preoperative reference for further treatment and follow-up. When the tooth is in the best possible position, it is important to adjust the bite to ensure that it has not been splinted in a position that will cause traumatic occlusion. Two weeks are sufficient for periodontal support and to maintain the avulsed tooth in position, therefore, the splint should be removed within two weeks. The only exception to this is when avulsion occurs in conjunction with alveolar fractures or horizontal root fracture, in such cases it is suggested that the tooth should be splinted for a period of 2–8 weeks (Table **3**).

Adjunctive Drug Therapy

- Oral/systemic antibiotics
- Referral to physician for tetanus prophylaxis within 48 hours.
- Chlorhexidine rinses
- Analgesics

Table 3. Duration of splinting according to injury.

Type of injury	Duration of splinting
Subluxation	(optional) 7-10 days
Avulsion	7-10 days
Extrusion	3 weeks
Lateral Luxation	3 weeks, additional 3-4 days if marginal bone fracture is present
Crown root fracture	3 weeks
Root fracture	3-4 weeks
Dento-alveolar fractures	2-8 weeks

Tetracycline is antibacterial and has proven anti-resorptive properties that would limit the area of root surface damaged by inhibiting collagenase activity and osteoclast function, thus promoting favorable healing. Tetracycline also promotes fibroblast and connective tissue attachment thereby enhancing regeneration of periodontal attachment, which could be beneficial to a replanted tooth. Corticosteroids have been widely used to reduce inflammatory responses and osteoclastic bone resorption. Alendronate is a third-generation bisphosphonate and is currently being used to inhibit pathologic osteoclast-mediated hard tissue resorption in disease states such as osteoporosis.

Follow Up

Replanted teeth should be clinically and radiographically monitored after 4 weeks, 3 months, 6 months, one year and yearly thereafter. Clinical and radiographic examination will provide information to determine outcome. Splint removal is done at 2 weeks for immature and mature permanent teeth with immediate replantation and extraoral dry time <60 minutes. Teeth with extra oral dry time >60 minutes are followed for splint removal after 4 weeks. Initial intra canal placement of calcium hydroxide has been recommended during splinted period, when prognosis of pulp is questionable.

Prognosis

The best prognosis has been stated in immature permanent teeth which have been replanted immediately after avulsion. These teeth continue with their apex formation and positive response to pulp sensibility testing. Better survival of pulp and periodontium is also observed in mature permanent teeth with immediate replantation.

The long extra oral dry time (>60 minutes & beyond), inadequate storage, no media, hypotonic and hypertonic media, infection, and complex maxillofacial trauma lead to poor prognosis. The periodontal cell viability is a key element in success of replantation. Teeth loose vitality and exhibit ankylosis and resorption (inflammatory, infection related and replacement resorption).

Ankylosed teeth present with infra position of replanted tooth and a metallic sound on percussion. Radiographic evidence of loss of periodontal space is seen. On the other hand, resorption leads to increased mobility and loss of replanted tooth. Increased peri radicular radiolucency and resorption lacunae are observed as well.

Although ankylosis, loss of vitality and resorption are major risks involved with replantation, researchers have advised it as a method to maintain adequate bone height even in failure cases.

Complications (Fig. 23)

The response of the periodontal ligament to a replanted tooth into the socket will be one of the following- Surface resorption/ Replacement resorption/ Inflammatory resorption, which influences the future outcome of the tooth.

Potential complications of replantation are (Fig. **24**):

1. Inflammatory resorption
2. Replacement resorption
3. Ankylosis
4. Tooth Submergence

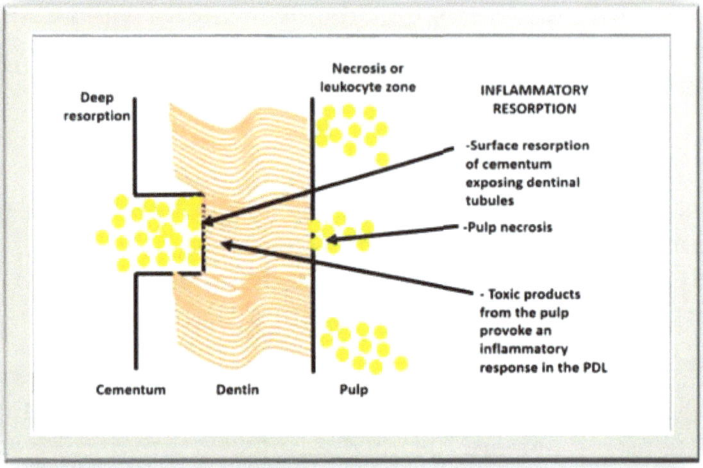

Fig (23). Complications of replantation.

Ellis Class VI fracture (Fig. 24) [16, 17]

• *Clinical Features*

Patients report with pain and mobility of tooth/crown and bleeding from gingival sulcus. The fracture line is usually below the gingival margin and makes chewing difficult. Spontaneous pain due to pulp exposure can be seen in complicated crown root fractures.

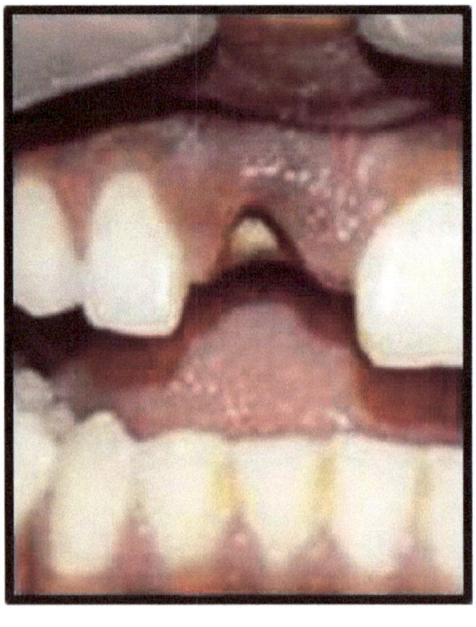

Fig (24). Ellis Class VI fracture.

- ***Investigations***

Multiple angulations of IOPA radiographs aid in visualization of sub-gingival fracture line (Fig. **25**). Pulp sensibility can be checked if there is a gap in reporting to dental surgeon.

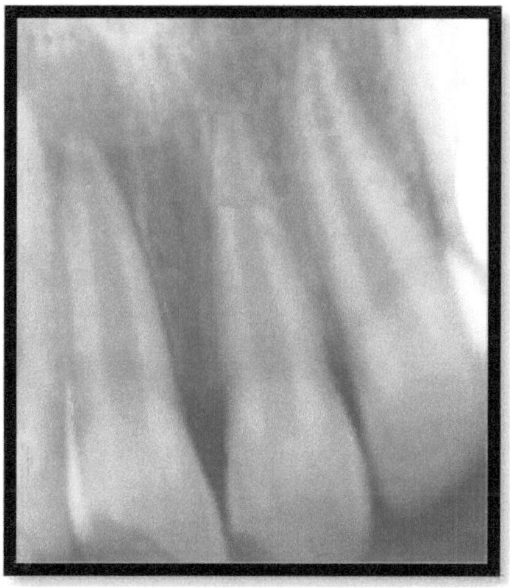

Fig (25). Radiographic image of Ellis Class VI fracture.

Root fracture can be either vertical or transverse. Four factors are important in treatment of transverse root fractures which are:

1- Position of the tooth after it has fractured

2- Mobility of the coronal segment

3- Status of the pulp

4- Position of the fracture line

- ***Treatment*** (Figs. **26 & 27**)

The position of the fracture lines an important factor in determining the treatment outcome.

Since mobile fragment is the main source of pain and infection, temporary stabilization is an emergency measure. Anterior stainless-steel crown, bands or bonding materials have been tried for stabilization. Mobile portion can also be fixed using neighboring teeth. This further aids in preservation of vitality of pulp.

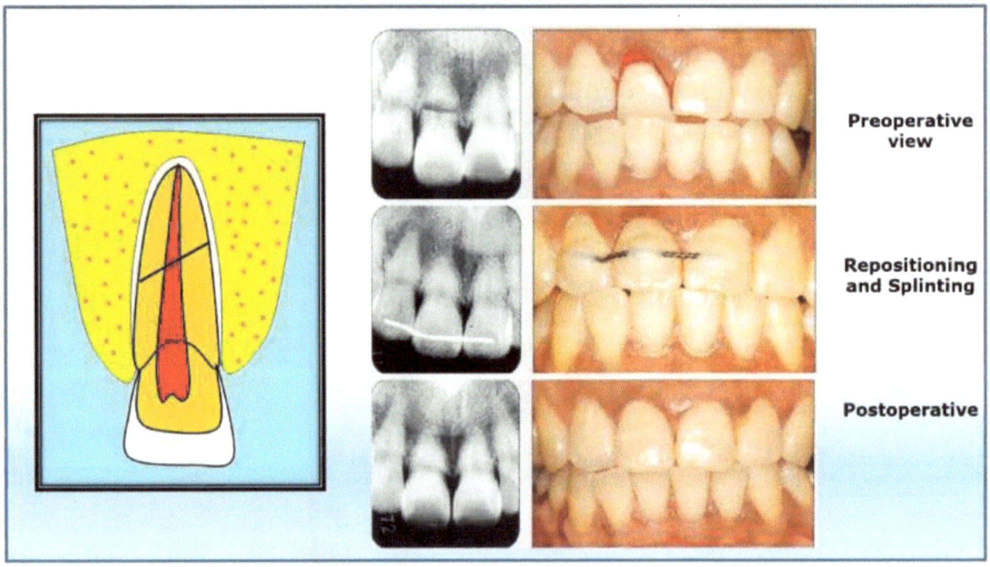

Fig (26). Treatment of Class VI fracture.

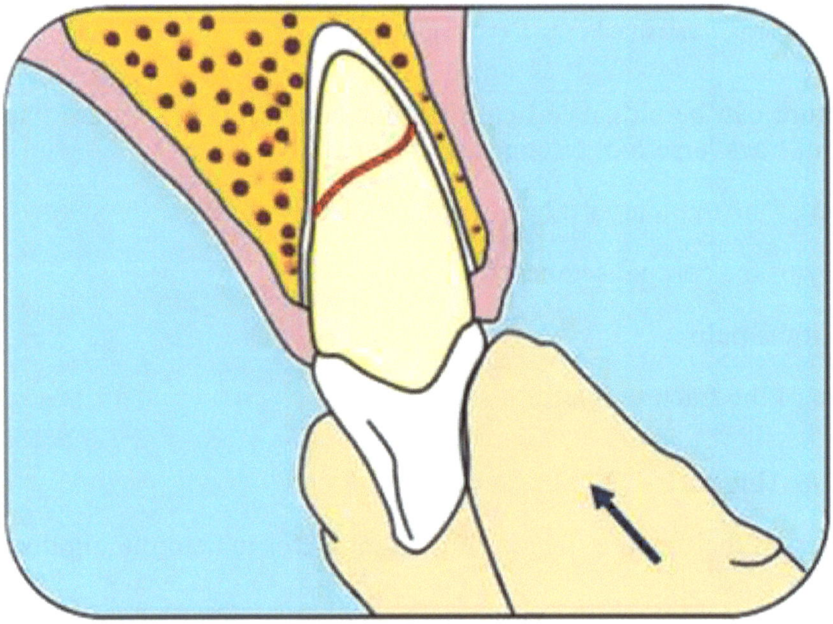

Fig (27). Repositioning of coronal fragment.

When fracture line goes deep inside the socket, removal of crown portion is followed by gingivectomy (with/without ostectomy & osteoplasty) to lengthen the crown for subsequent endodontic treatment and post retained crown. Subgingival custom ccramic cores have also been attempted in past. Another viable option in these cases is orthodontic extrusion (Fig. **28**) of apical fragment after endodontic treatment and later a post retained crown. Less preferable option is surgical extrusion and repositioning. Root submergence is done if future implant rehabilitation is planned. Extraction is least desirable treatment option but becomes necessary in extremely deep fracture lines and vertical fractures. The management of immature teeth is attempted in the same way as with complicated crown fracture.

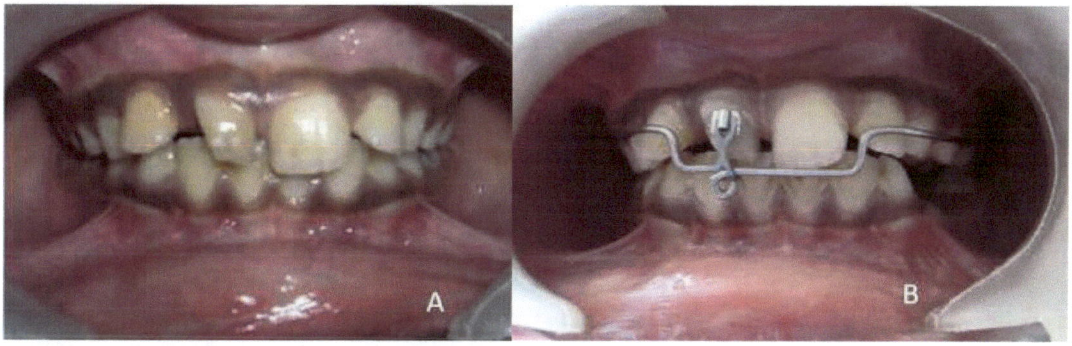

Fig (28). A- #11 showing crown root fracture extending below the gingival margin **B-** Orthodontic extrusion of tooth.

- ***Follow up***

The recommended schedule for follow up is a clinical-radiographic examination after 6-8 weeks. Tooth must further be examined clinically and with radiographs after 1 year.

- ***Prognosis***

Complicated crown root fractures with subgingival fracture lines in cervical third of root have better prognosis than the deep ones. Vertical fractures have worst prognosis. Failure to seek treatment often results in loss of vitality in these teeth, requiring endodontic intervention. Successful vital pulp therapy maintains the tooth in asymptomatic state and helps in continuing root development. In failure cases and those complicated by other TDI, apical periodontitis results and tooth becomes non vital.

- ***Healing***

Healing of fractures site can occur by 4 modalities (Fig. **29**).

- Healing with calcified tissue, which is characterized by a uniting callus or hard tissue that may consist of dentin, osteodentin or cementum
- Healing with interposition of connective tissue
- Healing with interposition of bone and connective tissue
- Healing with granulation tissue

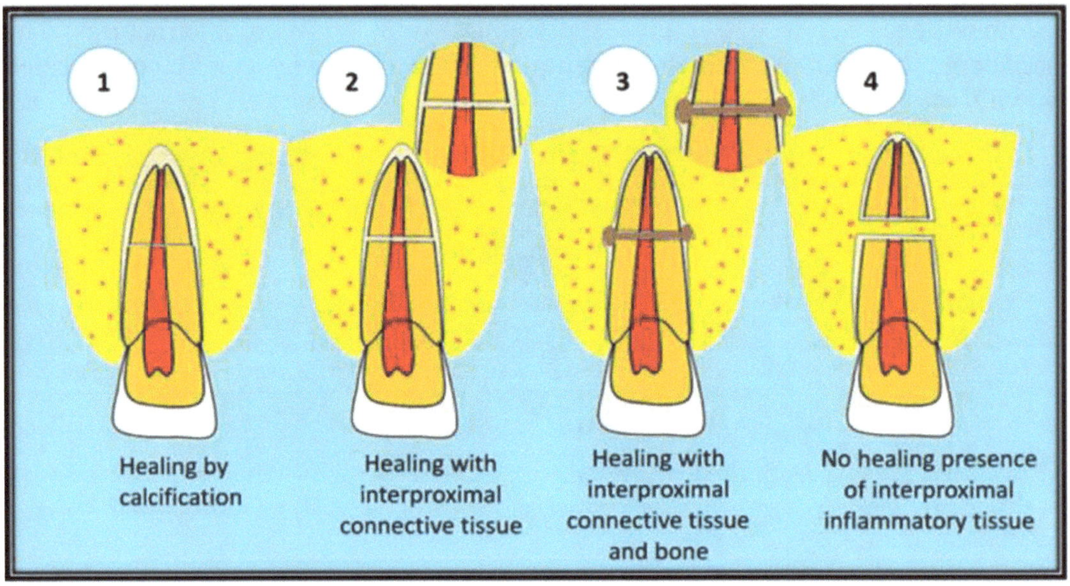

Fig (29). Sequelae of Root Fracture.

Follow up radiographs and pulp tests are necessary at interval.

Ellis Class VII Fracture [4]

An injury to the attachment apparatus of the teeth supporting structure that may lead to the loosening or displacement of the tooth without any damage to the tooth structure in included in Ellis class VII trauma. It can range from minor damage to the periodontal ligament fibers in the form of concussion to more severe displacement of teeth (Fig. **30**).

Concussion (Fig. 31)

An injury to the tooth-supporting structures without abnormal loosening or displacement of the tooth, but with increased response to percussion.

Clinical Features

Patient presents with highly tender tooth with no displacement or mobility. Palpation of teeth injured by concussion should be done carefully to avoid discomfort to the patient.

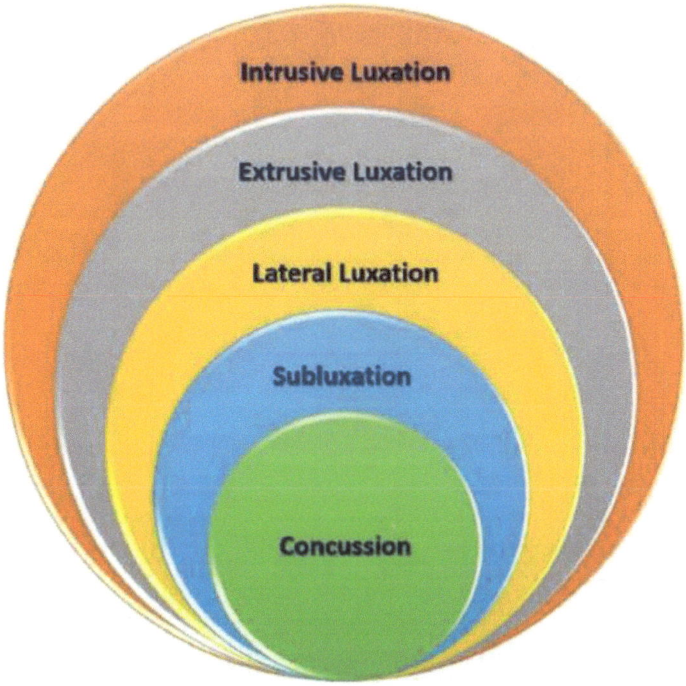

Fig (30). Types of Ellis class VII trauma.

Investigations

Radiographic abnormalities are not present, but it is generally advised to rule out any other type of injury. Same is the case with pulp sensibility test, which usually give positive results.

Treatment

No treatment is needed except for periodical follow up. Any unusual occlusal contact must be checked and relieved along with pressure habits. Instructions for soft diet are helpful.

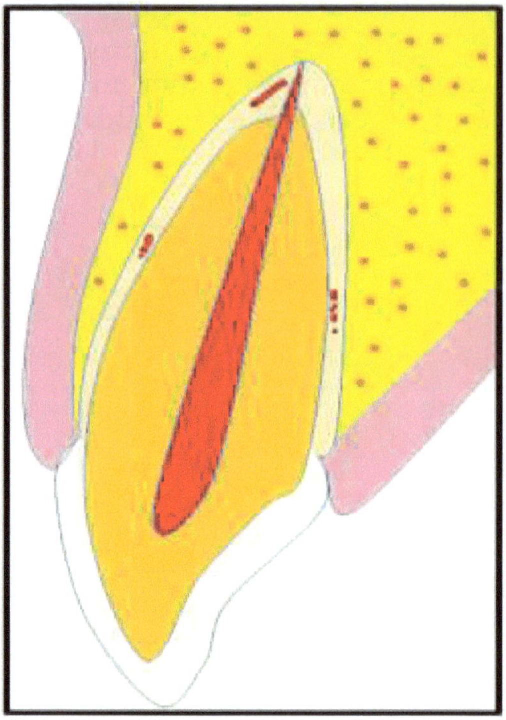

Fig (31). Concussion injury to periodontal ligament.

Follow up

A follow up schedule of 4 weeks, 6-8 weeks and 1 year is given for clinical and radiographic examination. Pulp tests are also conducted to monitor pulpal status in the period.

Prognosis

Concussion injuries must always be regularly monitored. Though a good prognosis has been reported, any sign of loss of vitality warrants appropriate endodontic therapy.

Subluxation (Fig. 32)

An injury to the tooth supporting structures with abnormal loosening but without displacement of the tooth.

Clinical Features

Patient presents with highly tender tooth with increased mobility but no displacement. Bleeding can be observed from gingival crevice.

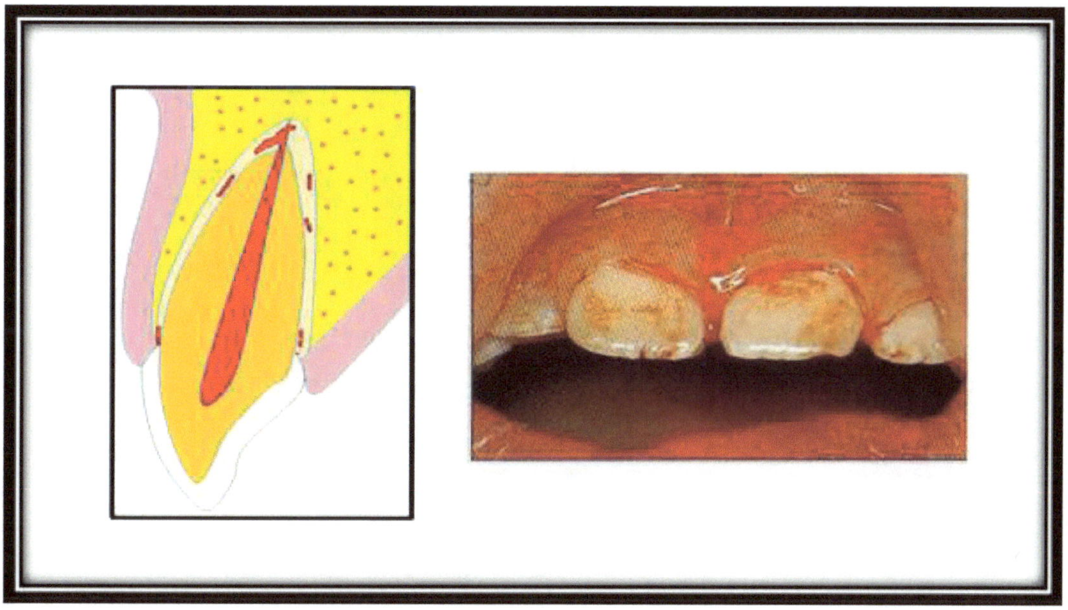

Fig (32). Subluxation injury to periodontal ligament.

Investigations

Radiographic abnormalities are not present, but it is generally advised to rule out any other type of TDI. A radiograph is recommended to rule out any root fracture. It also serves as a baseline for comparing follow up features. Pulp sensibility testing is usually negative initially indicting transient pulp damage. This must be repeated periodically so that a definitive pulpal diagnosis can be made.

Treatment

No treatment is needed except for periodical follow up. Any unusual occlusal contact must be checked and relieved along with pressure habits. Patient is instructed to follow a soft diet. Flexible splint to stabilize the tooth for patient comfort can be used for up to 2 weeks. Use of mouthwash and maintenance of oral hygiene is helpful. If the pulp status on follow-up visit is unfavorable, with signs of pulpal inflammation or periapical changes on radiographs, endodontic treatment needs to be initiated (Fig. **33**).

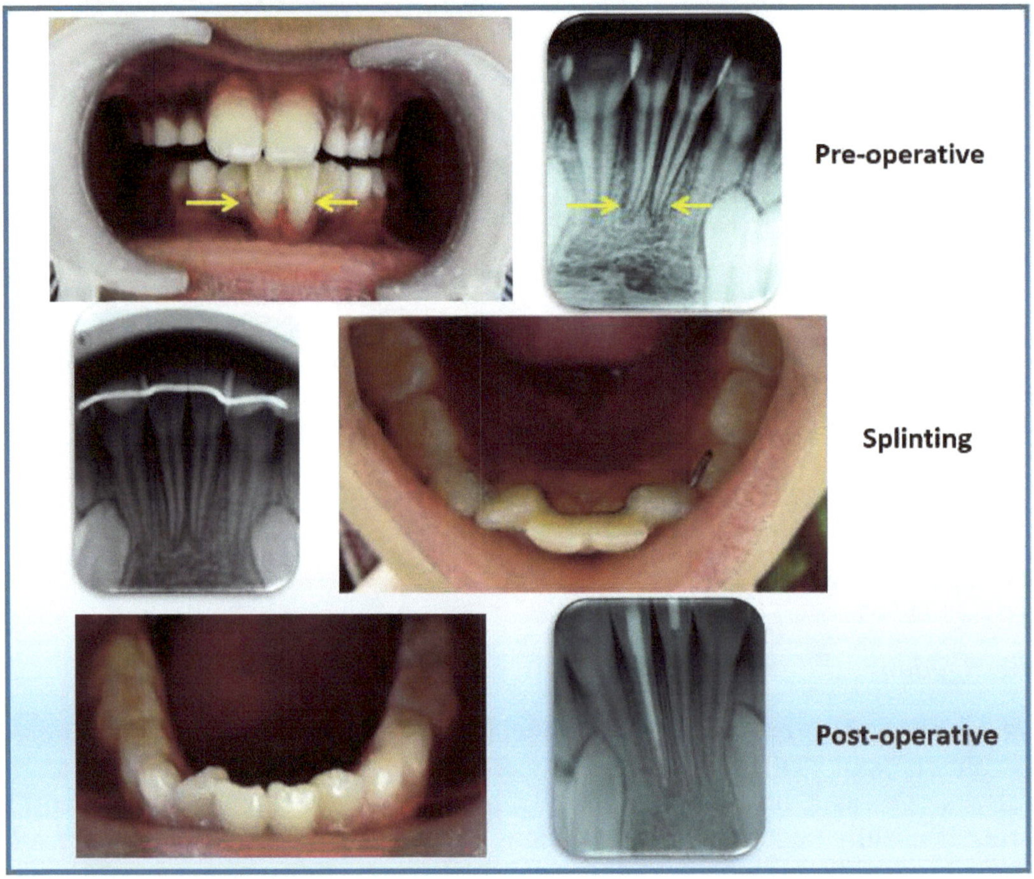

Fig (33). Treatment of Subluxation.

Follow up

First follow up at 2 weeks is for splint removal and clinical-radiographic examination. Further a schedule of 4 weeks, 6-8 weeks, 6 months and 1 year is given for clinical and radiographic examination. Pulp tests are also conducted to monitor pulpal status.

Prognosis

Subluxation injury must always be regularly monitored for loss of vitality and/or external root resorption. Though a good prognosis has been reported, any sign of loss of vitality warrants stage appropriate endodontic therapy.

Lateral Luxation: Displacement of the tooth in a direction other than axially. This is accompanied by comminution or fracture of the alveolar socket. (Fig. 34, 35)

Clinical Features

Patient presents with highly tender and immobile tooth with mild to moderate displacement, usually in labial or palatal direction. Slight deviations in mesio-distal directions can also be present. Gingival injury and bleeding can be observed. A high, metallic (ankylotic) sound can be elicited on percussion. It is commonly associated with other luxation injuries and alveolar fracture.

Investigations

Tooth appears to be out of its socket with radiolucent area apical to it on IOPA radiographs. Multiple angulations are required to rule out associated traumatic dental injuries and alveolar fracture. Occlusal exposure demonstrates increased periodontal space apically and position of displaced tooth. Role of pulp sensibility tests is negligible in diagnosis but important in follow up.

Treatment (Fig. 34)

Treatment of permanent tooth lateral luxation is based on the degree of displacement, occlusal interference, and root formation. Gentle re-positioning to original position, either by finger pressure or after disengaging the tooth from bony lock has been recommended. After verifying the accurate position teeth are stabilized using flexible splint for 4 weeks. Any loss of vitality of pulp is treated by age-appropriate endodontic procedure (Fig. **35**).

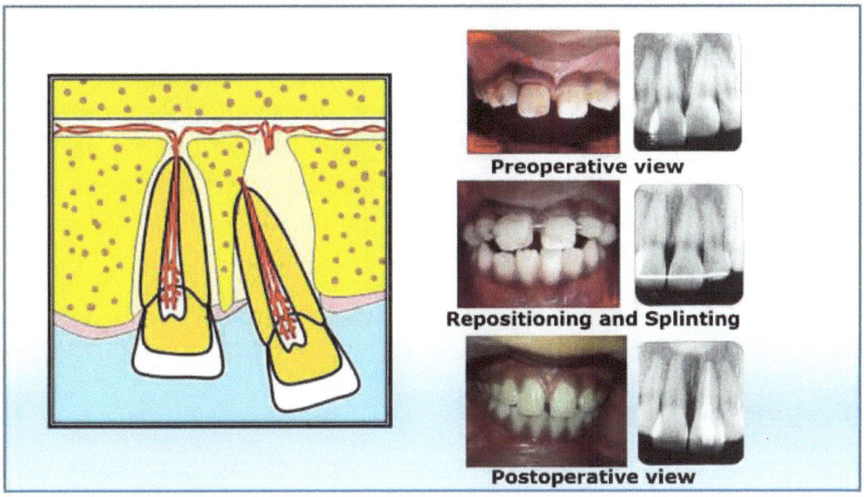

Fig (34). Treatment of Lateral Luxation.

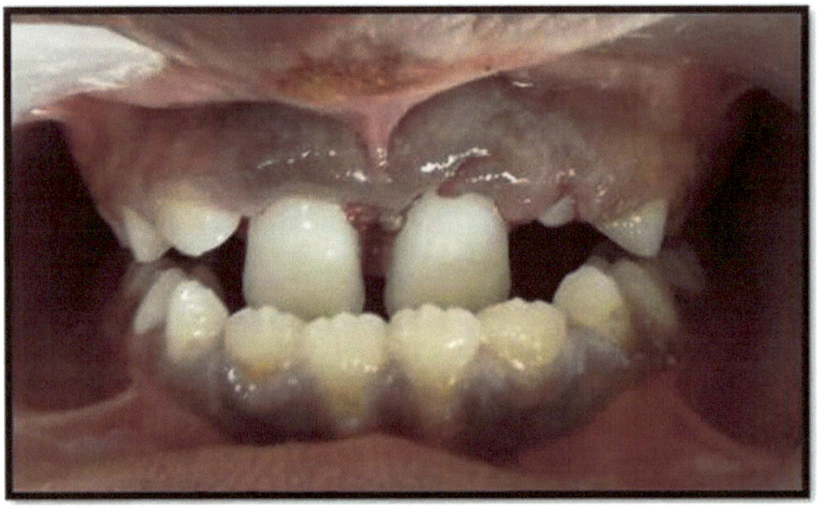

Fig (35). Ellis class VII, Luxation of #11 and #21.

Follow up

First follow up at 2 weeks for clinical and radiographic examination. Splint removal is done at 4 weeks and a follow up schedule of 6-8 weeks, 6 months and 1 year is given for clinical and radiographic examination. A regular follow up upto 5 years has been recommended. Pulp tests are also conducted to monitor pulpal status in the period.

Prognosis

Success of treatment in lateral luxation of permanent teeth depends on tooth remaining vital with radiographic signs of normal or healed periodontium. Injury, however, must always be regularly monitored for loss of vitality and/or external root resorption. Any sign of loss of vitality warrants stage appropriate endodontic therapy. The level of marginal bone must be compared from baseline in all radiographs to predict the future course.

Extrusive luxation **(peripheral dislocation, partial avulsion)-** Partial displacement of the tooth out of its socket.

Clinical Features (Fig. 36)

Patient presents with highly tender and excessively mobile tooth with slight displacement out of its socket. Gingival injury and bleeding may be observed. It is commonly associated with other TDIs, especially luxation injuries and maxillofacial trauma.

Investigations

Tooth appears to be out of its socket with radiolucent area apical to it on IOPA radiographs. Multiple angulations are required to rule out associated traumatic dental injuries and verify the extrusion from socket. Pulp sensibility testing usually gives negative results. This must be repeated periodically so that a definitive pulpal diagnosis can be made.

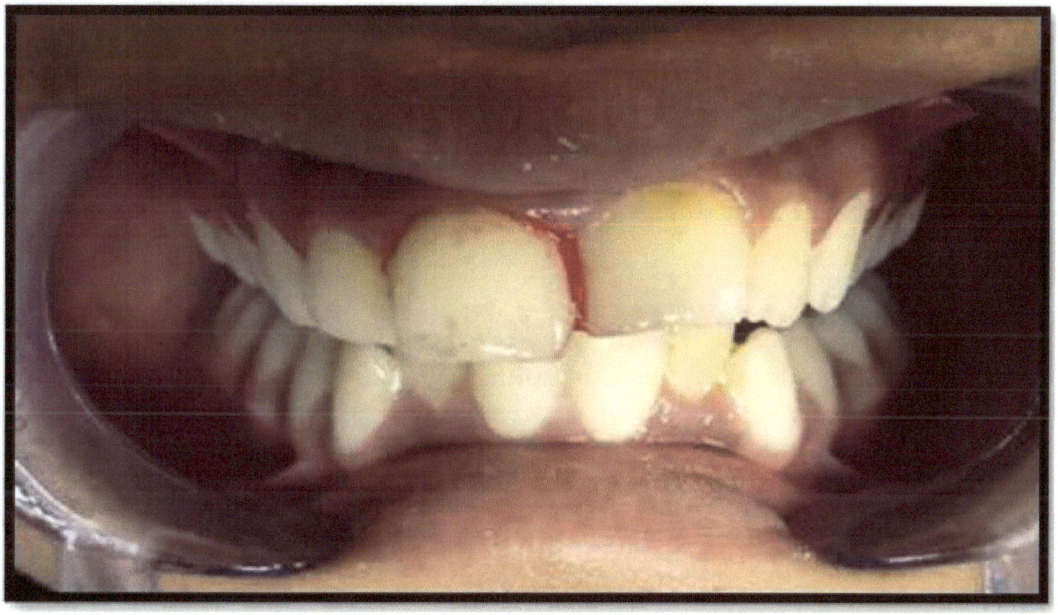

Fig (36). Ellis class VII, Extrusion of #11.

Treatment (Fig. 37)

Treatment depends on the degree of displacement, mobility, and root formation. All extruded teeth must be carefully repositioned in their socket, verified on radiographs, and stabilized for 2 weeks using flexible splint. The immature permanent teeth have been shown to re-establish their neurovascular supply while mature permanent teeth are expected to develop pulp necrosis, requiring root canal treatment. For splinted teeth, it is advisable to check and relieve any unusual occlusal contact along with pressure habits. Instructions for soft diet are helpful. Brushing with a soft brush and use of alcohol-free, 0.12%, chlorhexidine applied topically to the affected area with cotton swabs twice a day for one week has been recommended.

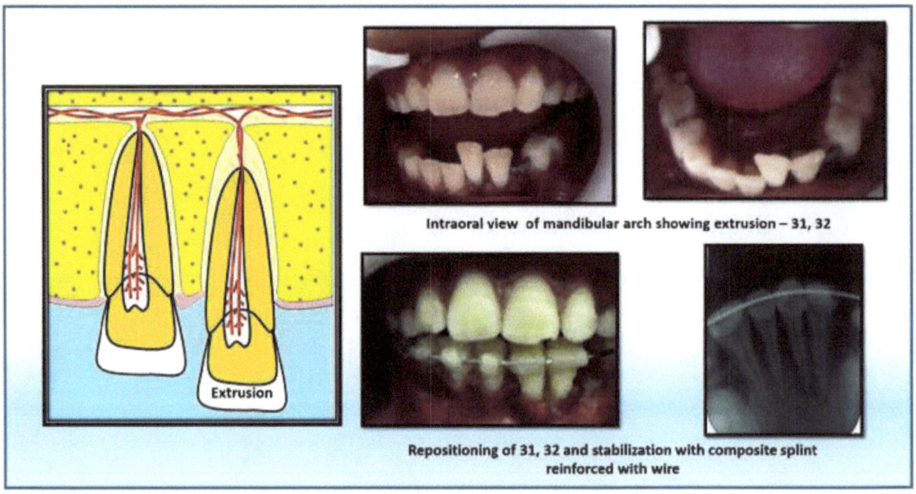

Fig (37). Treatment of Extrusion.

Follow up

First follow up at 2 weeks is for splint removal and clinical-radiographic examination. Further a schedule of 4 weeks, 6-8 weeks, 6 months and 1 year is given for clinical and radiographic examination. Status of the tooth must be observed for at least 5 years. Pulp tests are also conducted to monitor pulpal status in the period.

Prognosis

Extrusive luxation in immature permanent teeth has a good prognosis if repositioning and splinting is done in a short period of time. Tooth/teeth remain vital and continue with root development. Injury, however, must always be regularly monitored for loss of vitality and/or external root resorption. Any sign of loss of vitality, may be inevitable in mature permanent teeth and warrants stage appropriate endodontic therapy. The level of marginal bone must be compared from baseline in all radiographs to predict the future course.

Intrusive luxation **(central dislocation)** It is characterized by displacement of the tooth into the alveolar bone. This injury is accompanied by comminution or fracture of the alveolar socket.

Clinical Features (Fig. 38)

Patient presents with highly tender and immobile tooth with a displacement axially into the alveolar socket. On percussion, a high metallic (ankylotic) sound may be heard. Deviations in labial-palatal and mesio-distal direction can be present along with intrusion. It is usually associated with alveolar fracture and maxillofacial trauma.

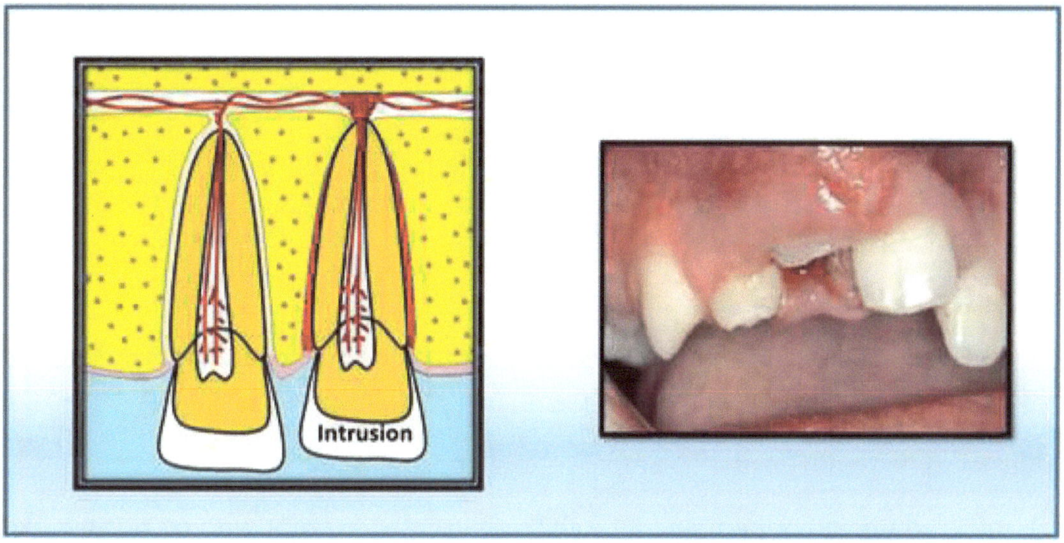

Fig (38). Intrusion.

Investigations

IOPA radiographs along with occlusal and other angulations are needed to confirm the position of intruded tooth. Periodontal ligament space may be absent from all or part of the root. The cemento-enamel junction of intruded tooth has been stated to be apical to adjacent tooth, sometimes even below the marginal bone. Pulp sensibility tests are likely to give negative results.

Treatment (Fig. 39)

Treatment depends on the degree of displacement, mobility, and root formation.
Immature permanent tooth.
All intruded teeth with incomplete root formation are allowed to erupt spontaneously. If there is no movement within a few weeks, orthodontic repositioning is initiated.
Mature permanent tooth.
If the displacement is more than 7 mm, the orthodontic or surgical repositioning must be initiated at the outset. The teeth which have been intruded less than 3 mm, have been recommended to re-erupt spontaneously. However, surgical, or orthodontic repositioning must be done if there is no movement in 2-4 weeks. This prevents ankylosis of the intruded tooth. If tooth is intruded by 3-7 mm, it can be repositioned surgically or orthodontically.

The immature permanent teeth have been shown to re-establish their neurovascular supply while mature permanent teeth are liable to develop pulp necrosis, requiring root canal treatment. Intermediate root canal filling by calcium hydroxide has been recommended for mature repositioned teeth. Endodontic treatment must be initiated in 2-3 weeks after repositioning.
A flexible splint for 4 weeks is used to stabilize the repositioned teeth. In these teeth, it is advisable to check and relieve any unusual occlusal contact along with pressure habits. Instructions for soft diet are helpful. Brushing with a soft brush and use of alcohol-free, 0.12%, chlorhexidine applied topically to the affected area with cotton swabs twice a day for one week has been recommended.

Follow up

For both spontaneous eruption and repositioned cases, a follow up schedule of clinical and radiographic examination at 2nd week, 4th week, 6th – 8th week, 6 months and 1 year has been recommended. This must be continued for 5 years. Splint must be removed at 4th week of follow up.

The intruded immature permanent tooth/teeth usually re-erupt with no or transient discoloration. The pulp vitality is also re-established in most cases as exhibited by continued root development. Locked teeth display an ankylotic tone on percussion which warrant the repositioning. Signs of loss of vitality, external resorption and discoloration require stage appropriate endodontic management.

- ***Sequelae of luxation injuries are*:**
  - Breakdown of attachment between periodontal ligament and tooth
  - External root resorption
  - Ankylosis
  - Obliteration of root canals
  - Pulp necrosis
  - Marginal bone loss

Ellis Class VIII Fracture (Fig. 40) [4]

A fracture of the crown en masse, must be treated by root canal treatment of the remaining root fragment followed by surgical or orthodontic extrusion of the fragment if possible and restoration with a post and core build up, and a suitable full coverage restoration later. However, if root apex is open, apexification must be initiated. This requires patience, meticulous follow up and regular appointments. After the apex has closed, the treatment can be carried out as detailed above.

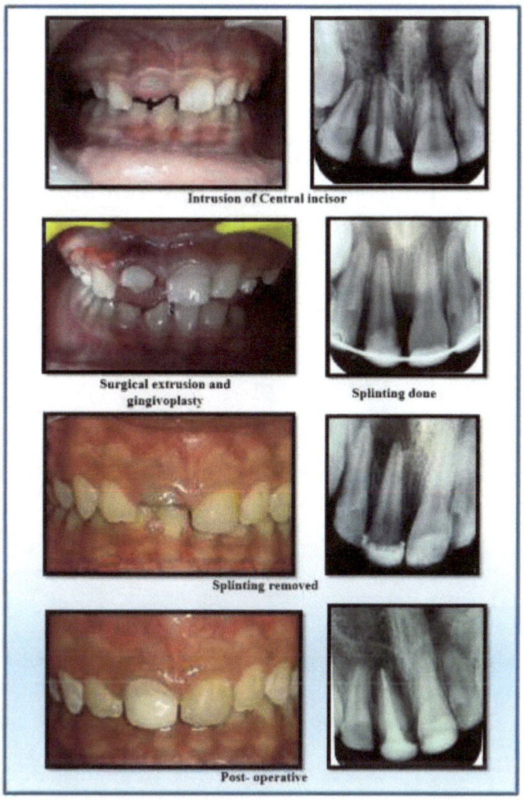

Fig (39). Treatment of Intrusion.

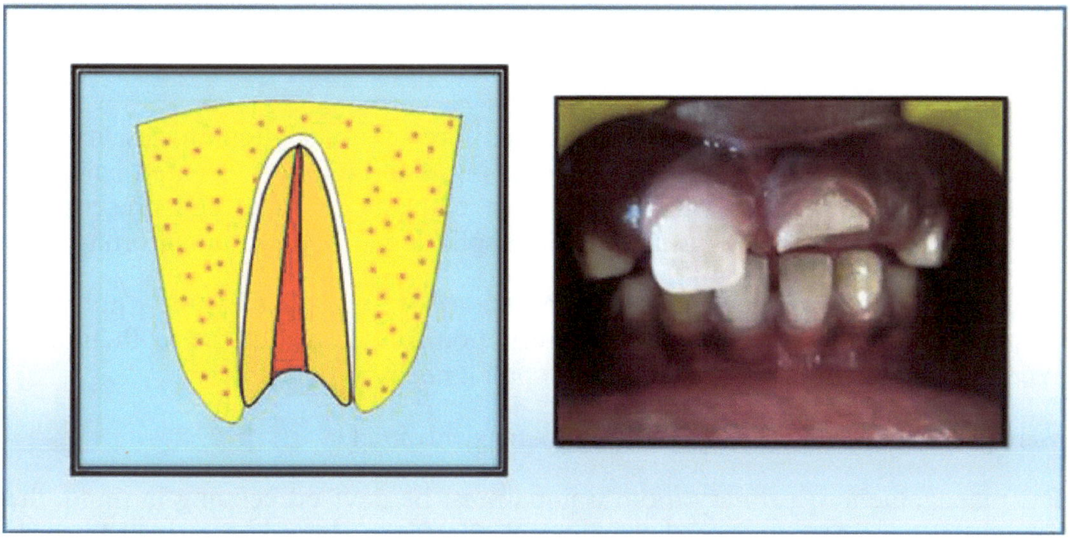

Fig (40). Ellis Class VIII fracture.

Ellis Class IX Fracture (Involving Primary Teeth) (Fig. 41) [18]

Treatment for enamel fractures, enamel-dentin fractures with and without pulp exposures remain same as for permanent teeth. However, if a tooth is near exfoliation, it better to extract. Teeth sustaining fractures of roots are often extracted, teeth sustaining concussion require no treatment. Subluxated teeth may require relieving of occlusion, splinting or extraction if subluxation is very severe.

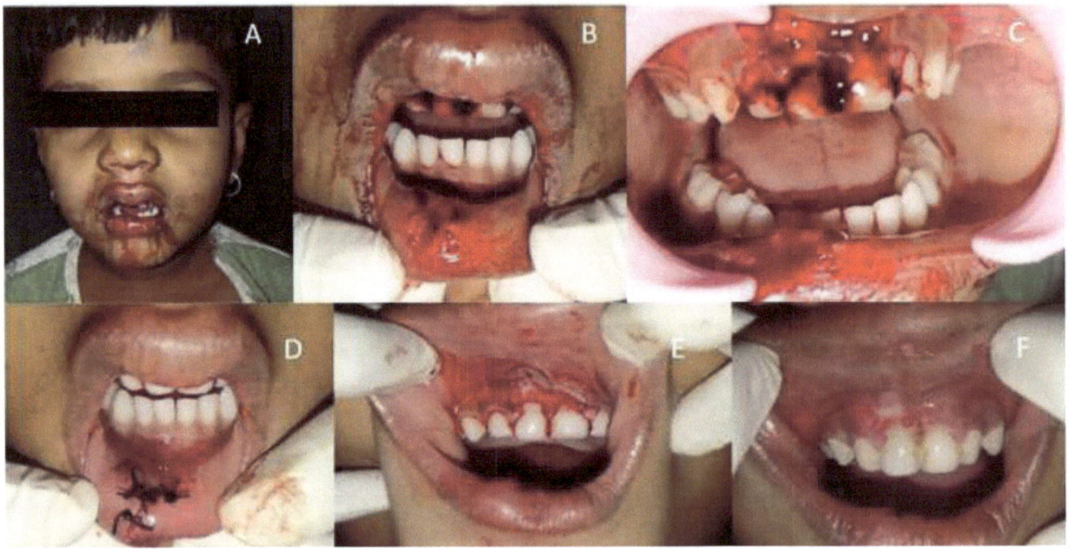

Fig (41). Ellis class IX fracture of a deciduous maxillary incisor. Trauma to primary teeth with soft tissue injury. A. Extra oral appearance eat time of trauma; B. Lower lip laceration; C. Luxation and gingival injury to maxillary anterior teeth no. 51, 61; D. Suturing of lip laceration; E. Debriding of maxillary injury; F. Healing at 7 days.

Due to pliability of the alveolar bone in children trauma often causes luxation rather than fractures of the root. Luxation injuries must be evaluated carefully regarding direction and severity of trauma, maturity of tooth and presence of alveolar bone fracture. They usually require splinting and careful monitoring

Intrusive injuries are kept under observation. A "wait and watch" policy is adopted, and teeth are monitored for re-eruption. If the apex of the tooth appears to be in contact with the permanent tooth bud it needs to be extracted.

Management of traumatic injuries to primary dentition [19 - 21]:

The management of primary tooth trauma must be devised keeping in mind, the behavioral considerations of the child and all efforts should be guided towards prevention of sequelae to the developing permanent teeth.

The management of traumatic injuries to primary teeth differs from that of permanent dentition. It is important to keep in mind that there is close relationship between the apex of the root of the injured primary tooth and the underlying permanent tooth germ. Some of the complications that can occur to permanent tooth, following injury to primary teeth are [22 - 24]:

-Malformation to tooth structure (Dilacerations)
-Hypomineralisation
-Hypoplasia to permanent succadenuous tooth
-Arrested development
-Impacted teeth
-Eruption disturbances

Treatment guidelines for management of primary tooth fractures are like their corresponding injuries in the permanent dentition, though the operator should take into consideration the time for natural exfoliation of the tooth based on chronological and dental age of the child, co-operation, status of root resorption, concurrent dental caries, and proximity of the fracture to the developing permanent tooth (Table **4**).

Table 4. Treatment guidelines for primary tooth fracture.

Clinical findings	Treatment
<u>Uncomplicated crown fracture</u> Enamel/ dentin and enamel fracture without pulp exposure 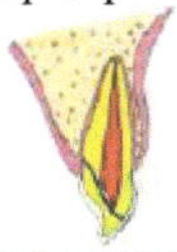	• Slight chipping - sharp edges smoothened. Restoration with tooth colored filling material.
<u>Complicated crown fracture</u> Enamel, dentin fracture with pulp exposure.	• In case of immature tooth with developing roots, pulp capping or partial pulpotomy is indicated to preserve pulp vitality. • In tooth with completely formed roots pulp capping/ partial pulpotomy or pulpectomy procedure can be done depending on the period of trauma occurrence, pulp health. • Both treatments should be considered, however in case of pulp necrosis, abscess formation, continuous pain, extraction is indicated. • Radiographic examination- pre-operatively (after trauma), post-operatively. Follow up radiographs 6-12 months (in case of endodontic intervention).

(Table 4) cont.....

Clinical findings	Treatment
Crown-root fracture Enamel, dentin and root fracture, with/without pulp exposure. 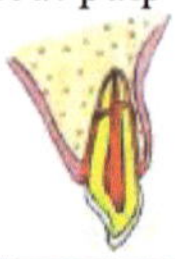	• Removal of any fragments followed by extraction of tooth carefully to avoid trauma to the subjacent tooth bud.
Root fracture Fracture of root (coronal 1/3rd, middle 1/3rd, apical 1/3rd) 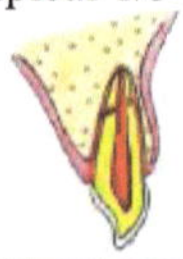	• Fracture segments immobile: Clinical & radiological follow up for 4 weeks. Parents warned of possible injury to permanent tooth germ. • Fracture segments mobile: Extraction of coronal segment, leave apical segment if not easily removable for physiological resorption.
Alveolar fracture Fracture of supporting alveolar bone with/without mobility of tooth-containing segment (displaced). Occlusal interference is often noted. 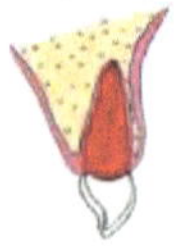	• Reposition any displaced segment under anesthesia and then splint. Monitor teeth in fracture line.

TREATMENT GUIDELINES FOR LUXATION INJURIES IN THE PRIMARY DENTITION (TABLE 5)

Luxation injuries are seen most in the upper incisors. It is one of the most dangerous injuries to the developing tooth germ and therefore the management of these injuries is aimed at saving/minimizing damage, by assessing displacement to the permanent tooth germ. The management of these cases include:

- Antibiotic therapy.
- Tetanus immunization (depending on the status of child).
- Radiographs (to know status of permanent tooth bud, post trauma).

Table 5. Treatment guidelines for luxation injuries in the primary dentition.

Clinical findings	Treatment
Concussion There is tenderness to palpation. Minimum increase in mobility, without bleeding from sulcular gingival. 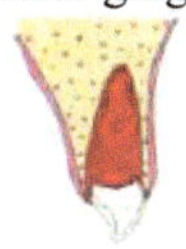	• Monitoring of the affected tooth for 6 months. Radiographic examination to check any damage to permanent tooth bud.
Subluxation There is tenderness to palpation, with comparatively increased mobility, without displacement and bleeding from gingival sulcus is seen. 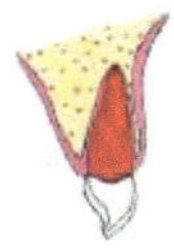	• Monitoring of the affected tooth for 6-12 months. Radiographic examination to check any damage to affected tooth and permanent tooth bud.
Extrusive luxation Increased mobility and tooth appear elongated compared to contra-lateral tooth and significant bleeding from gingival sulcus is seen. 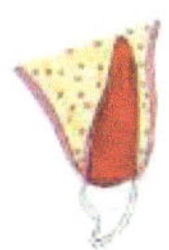	• Treatment decisions are based on the degree of displacement, mobility, root formation • For minor extrusion (<3 mm) in an immature developing tooth, careful repositioning or leaving the tooth for spontaneous alignment are acceptable treatment options. • Extraction is the treatment of choice for severe extrusion in a fully formed primary tooth.
Lateral luxation There is displacement of root tip towards palatal/lingual direction, with minimum amount of mobility. 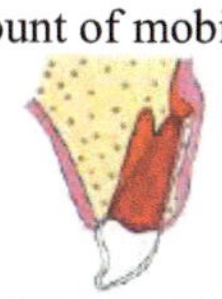	• In these displacement cases- with minimum of occlusal interference, the tooth is gently repositioned by combined labial and palatal pressure, under local anesthesia, otherwise without/minimal occlusal interference the tooth is allowed to reposition spontaneously/ selective grinding is indicated. • In case the crown is dislocated in a labial direction with severe displacement, extraction is the treatment of choice.
Intrusive luxation The root tip displaced towards buccal cortical plate or vertically and can be impinging upon the permanent tooth bud. 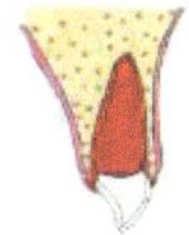	• If the apex is displaced toward or through the buccal cortical plate, allow 6 months for spontaneous re-eruption. Advise parents of potential damage to permanent tooth. • If the root tip is displaced into the developing tooth germ, extract. • On signs of swelling, spontaneous bleeding, abscess and fever, extract. • Radiograph: Ideally lateral film is taken to confirm intruded tooth has not displaced permanent tooth germ, if so, extraction recommended.

(Table 5) cont.....

Avulsion The tooth is displaced out of the socket 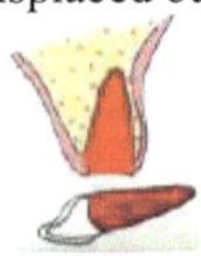	• Replantation not recommended, avoiding damage to succedaneous tooth bud. • Radiographic examination to check any damage to permanent tooth bud • Space loss may not occur if primary canines are present • Permanent tooth eruption may be delayed due to scar tissue formation/ bone remodeling

The common complications after TDI to primary and permanent tooth have been shown in Table **6**.

Table 6. Complication of traumatic injuries to teeth.

A) Primary teeth	**B) Permanent Teeth**
• Failure of eruption • Color changes • Infection • Space loss • Ankylosis • Injury to developing tooth bud • Abnormal exfoliation	• Color change • Infection • Loss of space • Ankylosis • Loss of alveolar bone support • Resorption of root • Abnormal root development • Difficulty in mastication • Poor esthetic • Difficulty in speech

Combination Traumas-(Fig. 42, 43) [4, 10]

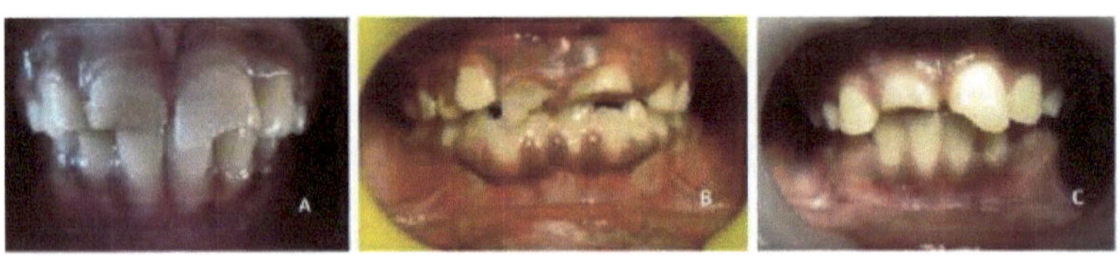

Fig (42). Complex presentations of fractured teeth A-#11Ellis class IV. #21Ellis class II;B-#11 Ellis class, #21Ellis class VIII;C-#11 Ellis class IV,#21 Ellis class II.

Traumatic episodes present with varied clinical situations which are a combination of different types of injuries. Management of these combination traumas is difficult and require effective clinical judgement for better prognosis. The basic objective of any management strategy must be preservation of tooth vitality and survival of the pulp with special considerations for chances of infections and damage to injured tooth, supporting structures and succedaneous tooth. Sequence of treatment should also follow the same guidelines. When more than one tooth shows signs of traumatic injury, triage should be done to decide which tooth requires more urgent attention than the other.

International Association of Dental Traumatology (IADT) & Dental Trauma Guide

The International Association of Dental Traumatology (IADT) is a professional organization whose mission is to promote optimal prevention and treatment service in the field of traumatic dental injuries through interaction with dental and medical colleagues, the public, and interested parties in education, sports, industry, and appropriate governmental agencies.

It is a global association which has researchers and clinicians from diverse dental and medical specialties having keen interest and expertise in Dental Trauma research. The journal of IADT- Dental Traumatology has been regarded as one of the best resources for scientific evidence and data regarding traumatic dental injuries and sports dentistry. IADT guidelines for management of TDI in primary and permanent dentition have been widely accepted and globally acclaimed.

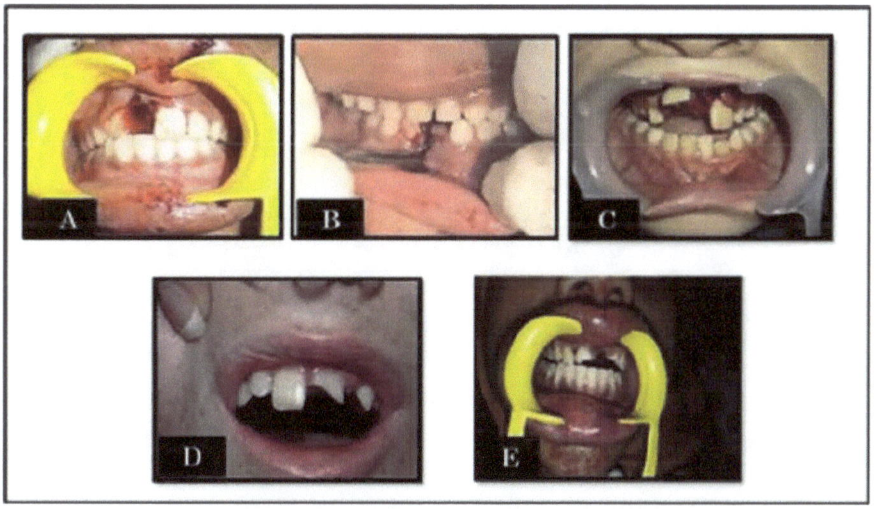

Fig (43). Complex presentation of traumatic dental injuries A- #11 Avulsion and #21 Ellis class II; B- Ellis class IX showing dent-alveolar fracture of mandible and luxation of #71, #81; C-#11 Ellis class VII with labial luxation, #32 intrusion; D- #11 palatal luxation #21 Ellis class II;E-#11 Ellis class II and #21 avulsion.

The assessment of traumatic injuries has been arranged as a dental trauma decision protocol to logically assess traumatic dental injuries (Fig. **44**) [25].

Trauma Prevention

Traumatic dental injuries are accidental in nature and their prevention has been ignored in past. An increased awareness of public, teachers, sports teachers, and students regarding etiology of TDI, risk profiling of individuals and steps for making environment safe has been stated as best practice for dental trauma prevention. Sports persons, athletes, coaches, and sports authorities must be educated regarding mouth guards and other protective gears.

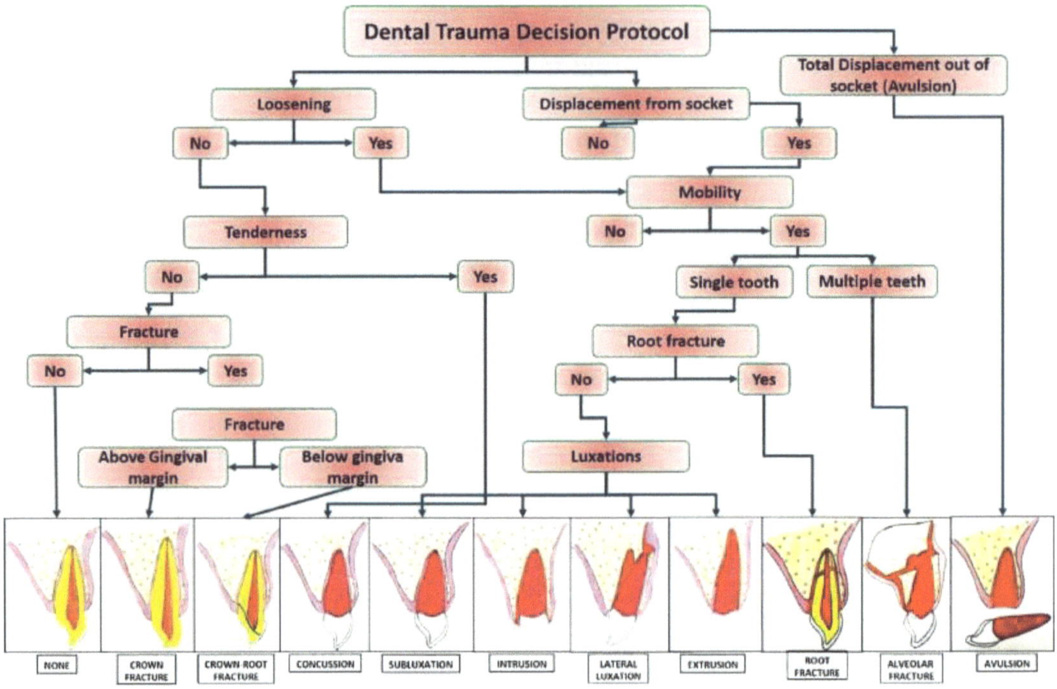

Fig (44). Dental trauma decision protocol.

Who Healthy Cities Program [26], defines a healthy city as one that continually creates and improves the physical and social environment and expands community resources for enabling the mutual support among populations/groups for living. It has been emphasized as major trauma prevention scheme for future. Another community program- The WHO Health Promoting Schools Program, includes TDI as a public health problem and devices measures to create awareness and prevention.

CONCLUSION

Traumatic injuries to anterior teeth in children are common and are on the rise. Management of such injuries is an arduous task requiring tact, a tender approach and considerable clinical acumen and skill. All predisposing factors should be addressed along with management of the acute dental injury to reduce likelihood of future episodes of trauma. Many times, the clinician needs to take a quick decision for management of TDI and the decision-making process is based on scientific evidence and often complex criteria that allow the best possible output in terms of patient benefit. The successful management of traumatic injuries to teeth gives a sense of immense satisfaction during dental practice and helps in practice building as well.

CONSENT FOR PUBLICATION

Not applicable.

CONFLICT OF INTEREST

The authors declare no conflict of interest, financial or otherwise.

ACKNOWLEDGEMENT

Declared none.

REFERENCES

[1] Guideline on management of acute dental trauma. Pediatr Dent 2008-2009-2009; 30(7) (Suppl.): 175-83.
[PMID: 19216418]

[2] McTigue DJ. Diagnosis and management of dental injuries in children. Pediatr Clin North Am 2000; 47(5): 1067-84.
[http://dx.doi.org/10.1016/S0031-3955(05)70258-3] [PMID: 11059350]

[3] Eyuboglu O, Yilmaz Y, Zehir C, Sahin H. A 6-year investigation into types of dental trauma treated in a paediatric dentistry clinic in Eastern Anatolia Region, Turkey. Dent Traumatol 2009; 25(1): 110-4.
[http://dx.doi.org/10.1111/j.1600-9657.2008.00668.x] [PMID: 18721195]

[4] Andreasen JO, Bakland LK, Flores MT, *et al.* Traumatic Dental Injuries A Manual. 3rd ed., Oxford, United Kingdom: Wiley-Blackwell 2011.

[5] DiAngelis AJ, Andreasen JO, Ebeleseder KA, *et al.* International Association of Dental Traumatology guidelines for the management of traumatic dental injuries: 1. Fractures and luxations of permanent teeth. Dent Traumatol 2012; 28(1): 2-12.
[http://dx.doi.org/10.1111/j.1600-9657.2011.01103.x] [PMID: 22230724]

[6] Das AN, Geetha K, Varghese Kurian A, Nair R, Nandakumar K. Interdisciplinary Approach to a Tooth with Open Apex and Persistent Sinus. Case Rep Dent 2015; 2015: 1-4.
[http://dx.doi.org/10.1155/2015/907324] [PMID: 26425373]

[7] Cvek M, Mejàre I, Andreasen JO. Conservative endodontic treatment of teeth fractured in the middle or apical part of the root. Dent Traumatol 2004; 20(5): 261-9.
[http://dx.doi.org/10.1111/j.1600-9657.2004.00272.x] [PMID: 15355385]

[8] Kenchappa M, Gupta S, Gupta P, Sharma P. Dentine in a capsule: Clinical case reports. J Indian Soc Pedod Prev Dent 2015; 33(3): 250-4.
[http://dx.doi.org/10.4103/0970-4388.160404] [PMID: 26156282]

[9] Garcia-Godoy F, Murray PE. Recommendations for using regenerative endodontic procedures in permanent immature traumatized teeth. Dent Traumatol 2012; 28(1): 33-41.
[http://dx.doi.org/10.1111/j.1600-9657.2011.01044.x] [PMID: 21794081]

[10] Andersson L, Andreasen JO, Day P, *et al.* International Association of Dental Traumatology guidelines for the management of traumatic dental injuries: 2. Avulsion of permanent teeth. Dent

Traumatol 2012; 28(2): 88-96.
[http://dx.doi.org/10.1111/j.1600-9657.2012.01125.x] [PMID: 22409417]

[11] Kargul B, Welbury R. An audit of the time to initial treatment in avulsion injuries. Dent Traumatol 2009; 25(1): 123-5.
[http://dx.doi.org/10.1111/j.1600-9657.2008.00732.x] [PMID: 19208024]

[12] Zhao Y, Gong Y. Knowledge of emergency management of avulsed teeth: a survey of dentists in Beijing, China. Dent Traumatol 2010; 26(3): 281-4.
[http://dx.doi.org/10.1111/j.1600-9657.2010.00877.x] [PMID: 20572844]

[13] Trivedy C, Kodate N, Ross A, *et al.* The attitudes and awareness of emergency department (ED) physicians towards the management of common dentofacial emergencies. Dent Traumatol 2012; 28(2): 121-6.
[http://dx.doi.org/10.1111/j.1600-9657.2011.01050.x] [PMID: 22107050]

[14] Arikan V, Sönmez H. Knowledge level of primary school teachers regarding traumatic dental injuries and their emergency management before and after receiving an informative leaflet. Dent Traumatol 2012; 28(2): 101-7.
[http://dx.doi.org/10.1111/j.1600-9657.2011.01042.x] [PMID: 21790991]

[15] Brown CL, Mackie IC. Splinting of traumatized teeth in children. Dent Update 2003; 30(2): 78-82.
[http://dx.doi.org/10.12968/denu.2003.30.2.78] [PMID: 12705028]

[16] Feierabend S, Jockel-Schneider Y, Klaiber B. Treatment of a crown-root fracture with concomitant root fracture. Quintessence Int 2011; 42(3): 239-42.
[PMID: 21465011]

[17] Tewari N, Pandey RK, Jindal G. Management of crown root fracture in primary 'double tooth': a case report. Dent Traumatol 2011; 27(1): 71-3.
[http://dx.doi.org/10.1111/j.1600-9657.2010.00948.x] [PMID: 21143391]

[18] Malmgren B, Andreasen JO, Flores MT, *et al.* International Association of Dental Traumatology guidelines for the management of traumatic dental injuries: 3. Injuries in the primary dentition. Dent Traumatol 2012; 28(3): 174-82.
[http://dx.doi.org/10.1111/j.1600-9657.2012.01146.x] [PMID: 22583659]

[19] Needleman HL. The art and science of managing traumatic injuries to primary teeth. Dent Traumatol 2011; 27(4): 295-9.
[http://dx.doi.org/10.1111/j.1600-9657.2011.01005.x] [PMID: 21535401]

[20] Kupietzky A, Holan G. Treatment of crown fractures with pulp exposure in primary incisors. Pediatr Dent 2003; 25(3): 241-7.
[PMID: 12889700]

[21] Padmanabhan M, Pandey R, Tewari N, Aparna R. Evaluating intrusive injuries in primary dentition from computed tomographic scans: A preliminary report. Indian J Dent Res 2014; 25(3): 311-5.
[http://dx.doi.org/10.4103/0970-9290.138322] [PMID: 25098986]

[22] Al-Khayatt AS, Davidson LE. Complications following replantation of a primary incisor: A cautionary tale. Br Dent J 2005; 198(11): 687-8.
[http://dx.doi.org/10.1038/sj.bdj.4812382] [PMID: 15951774]

[23] Tewari N, Pandey RK. Root hypoplasia: an unusual sequela to primary tooth trauma. Dent Traumatol 2010; 26(1): 115-7.
[http://dx.doi.org/10.1111/j.1600-9657.2009.00842.x] [PMID: 20089069]

[24] Tewari N, Pandey R. Multiple abnormalities in permanent maxillary incisors following trauma to the primary dentition. J Indian Soc Pedod Prev Dent 2011; 29(2): 161-4.
[http://dx.doi.org/10.4103/0970-4388.84691] [PMID: 21911957]

[25] Day PF, Barber SK. Review of the Dental Trauma Guide; an interactive guide to evidence-based trauma management. Evid Based Dent 2011; 12(4): 117-20. [http://dx.doi.org/10.1038/sj.ebd.6400830] [PMID: 22193658]

[26] https://www.who.int/healthpromotion/healthy-cities/en/

CHAPTER 11

Sports Related Dental Injuries

Rishika Choudhary[1,*], **Harsimran Kaur**[1] and **Ramakrishna Yeluri**[1]

[1] *Teerthanker Mahaveer Dental College and Research Centre, Moradabad. U.P India*

Abstract: Sports dentistry is an emerging section of dentistry. All sports-associated persons must have knowledge about injuries during all sports-related events. Since the very beginning, it has been known that participation in sports carries an extensive risk of sustaining dental injuries, with the increased popularity of sports like contact sports, semi-contact sports, and more support for children to participate at an early age. Dental injuries have become one of the most recurrent types of orofacial injuries that may occur during involvement in various sports activities and have a high rate of incidence between sports-related injuries normally during school physical education classes and club activities. The commonest orofacial injuries involve both soft tissue and hard tissue injury i.e.: facial bones, tooth intrusions, luxation, crown and root fractures, complete avulsions, and Dento-facial fractures. Prevention is of utmost importance to aesthetics for reducing the psychological and economic consequences of traumatic injuries. The most substantial feature in averting sports-related orofacial injuries is wearing protective devices like face masks, mouth guards, and helmets. The use of these protective devices by athletes has been shown to provide an effective safeguard against suffering.

Keywords : Mouthguard, Sports Dentistry, Sports Injuries.

INTRODUCTION

The face is the most exposed area of the body and is usually the least protected. Sports-related facial injuries account for 8% of all facial soft tissue injuries. Nearly 11-40% of all sports-related injuries involve the facial regions [1]. Sports dentistry is referred to as the branch of sports medicine that deals with the prevention and treatment of dental injuries and related oral diseases associated with sports and exercise (Table **1**). This branch of dentistry had its beginning in the 1980s and is related to the prevention and therapy of orofacial injuries occurring in athletes. In general, about 13% of trauma to the orofacial structures in children arises due to sports-related activities. Numerous dental injuries experienced throughout sports are avulsion, luxation injuries to the tooth,

* **Corresponding author Rishika Choudhary:** Teerthanker Mahaveer Dental College and Research Centre, Moradabad. U.P; India; E-mail: rishika.choudhary@gmail.com

Satyawan Damle, Ritesh Kalaskar & Dhanashree Sakhare (Eds.)

concussion, and fracture of the facial bones [2]. Dental trauma in sports is the major linking channel between sports and dentistry. The combined impact of violence, traffic accidents, and sporting activities has contributed to the establishment of traumatic dental injuries as a public dental health problem.

Table 1. Definitions.

Sports	**"A sport is an organized, competitive, entertaining, and skillful activity requiring commitment, strategy, and fair play, in which a winner and loser can be defined by objective means."**
Contact Sports	"Contact sports are defined as those sports in which players physically interact with each other, trying to prevent the opposing team or person from winning."
Semi-contact Sports	"Semi-contact sports are those sports in which body contact occurs sometimes as per the demands of a situation. For example, Football, Hockey. Limited contact sports, like volleyball, basketball, and fencing, have a high probability of occasional, inadvertent contact, mostly due to loss of balance or control."
Non-contact Sports	"Non-contact sports are sports where participants compete alternately, in lanes, or are physically separated such as to make nearly impossible for them to make contact during a game without committing an out-of-bounds offense, or more likely, disqualification. Examples include precision sports such as golf or curling, tennis, cricket, volleyball, swimming, sprinting, and gymnastics."
Sports Dentistry	"Is a branch of dentistry that is closely related to dental traumatology and includes prevention and treatment of sports-related dental/orofacial injuries, information collection, information dissemination, and promotion of research on the preventive procedures related to injuries of such a specific etiology."

Epidemiology of Sports-Related Dentistry (Table-2)

Today more children are getting involved in sports activities and their involvement is beginning at an earlier age. Sports account for 36% of injuries to children and youth. Injury rates are even higher for unorganized sports. Participation in organized and recreational sports poses a significant risk of dental injuries. Dental injuries are one of the most common types of injuries sustained by athletes. They are also one of the most preventable types of sports-related injuries. The table below depicts the causes and types of sports-related injuries.

SPORTS-RELATED INJURIES

Common Athletic Injuries

Soft Tissue Injuries

Soft tissue injuries to the face are common and this is the most exposed part of the human body to get injured. Certain common soft tissue injuries include Abrasions, contusions, and lacerations [3]. These soft tissue injuries (Fig. **1A**) are likely to happen most commonly on top of the bony prominence of the facial skeleton. Lacerations of the lip can also be seen as a regular injury.

Table 2. Epidemiology of sports-related injury.

Cause/ (%)	Type of injury (%)
Bicycle (9.3)	A crown fracture not involving pulp (42.7)
Swimming/diving 4.9	A crown fracture involving pulp (4.6)
Impact with person (15.9)	Root fracture (0.4)
Impact with object (15.3)	Luxation (3.5)
Hit by ball (3.7)	Avulsion (4.0)
Unspecified (13.2)	Concussion (1.0)

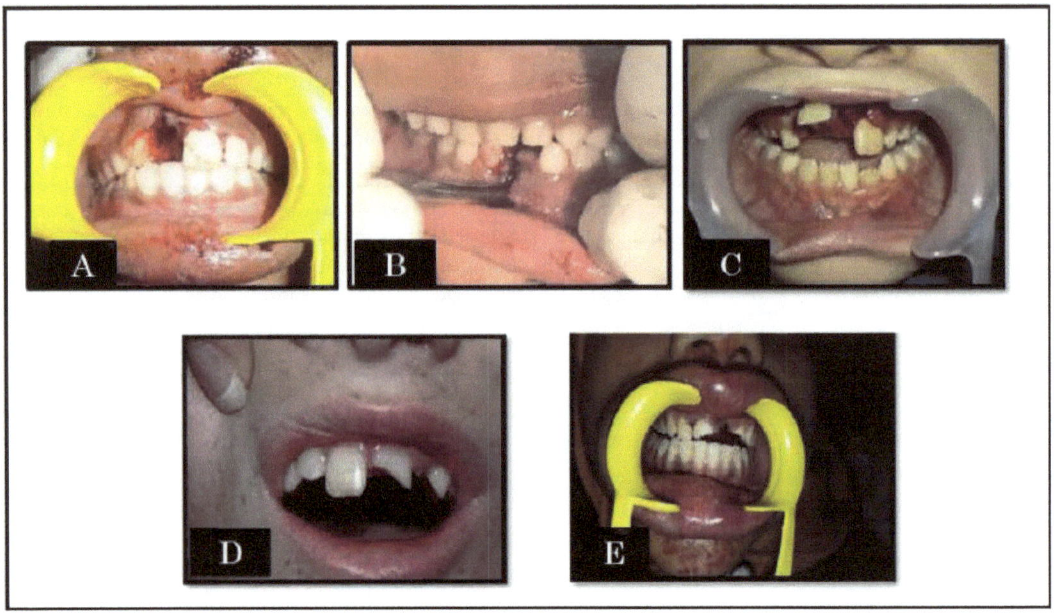

Fig (1). -Type of injury: A - Soft tissue injury, B - Fracture of mandible, C - Tooth intrusion, D - Crown fracture, E - Avulsed tooth

Fractures

The cheekbone (zygoma) is the most recurrent area of trauma in the facial bonAbout 10% of the maxillofacial fractures are seen in this region. A study was conducted by Linn and coworkers in which 319 patients were examined who were given treatment for sports-related injuries; the outcome proved that males were more prone to fractures of zygoma as compared to females and it is due to the strong physical contact in males during sports activities. The prominent shape of the zygoma makcs it morc pronc to trauma. 10% of the maxillofacial fractures from activities related to sports are seen in the mandible due to collision of an athlete with the other player, any armamentarium, or a solid surface (Fig. **1B).** Controlling airway is mandatory for instant protection in a fracture involving the mandible. The condyle is the most at-risk part of the mandible in children as well as adults. There is a high tendency for long-term facial deformity of the fractures involving this region.

TMJ Injuries

Most of the time any hit to the mandible does not result in the fracture of the mandible but the force generated from the hit will get transferred to the temporomandibular disc and its surrounding structures and this will cause injury to the same. In case of trauma, the movement of the condyle can occur that much posterior that the retrodiscal tissues get compressed. If the condyle is forced forwardly in case of any acute malocclusion, then it can cause edema and inflammation of the same. At times, this kind of trauma will result in intracapsular bleeding, and it often leads to ankylosis.

Tooth Intrusion

The forces directed axially usually drive the tooth into the alveolar process which leads to the intrusion of the tooth (Fig. **1C**). The intrusion of the tooth is a brutal form of displacement injury. Necrosis of the pulp falls out in approximately 96% of these cases and is seen mostly in mature teeth. In the case of an immature root, the tooth is likely to erupt faster as compared to the tooth with fully formed roots. The tooth with fully formed roots can be treated by orthodontic extrusion, tooth repositioning, and splinting.

Crown and Root Fractures

The commonest trauma to the succedaneous dentition is the crown fracture which can be represented in many ways. A crown infraction is the simplest type of crown fracture. In this enamel, cracking occurs, and the tooth structure is not compromised. This does not need any specialized therapy other than vitality testing to ensure the vitality of the pulp. If the tooth turns non-vital endodontics treatment should be conducted.

Fractures involving the dentin are normally reactive to the temperature and various additional impulses (Fig. **1C**). The most extreme fracture of the crown with a closed apex tooth results in the fully exposed pulp. A horizontal impact on the tooth may result in a root fracture causing mobility of the tooth. To ascertain the site and extremity of the fracture, radiographic assessment is required.

Avulsion

Complete avulsion of a tooth is a challenging dental injury related to sports (Fig. **1E**). Reimplantation of the avulsed tooth may be presented with various levels of success. Time of the avulsed tooth outside the socket plays a vital role in the success or failure of the treatment. There is a better possibility of an avulsed tooth retrieving its normal function when the fibers of the periodontium that are adhered to the root are hardly destroyed [2]. Andreasen and Andreasen have reported that approximately 90% of the achievement was noticed after reimplantation of the tooth within 20 minutes of the injury. Guyette noticed that the periodontal fibers that are adhered to the root of the reimplanted tooth undergo necrosis and the tooth undergoes resorption and is finally lost.

Risk Factors for Sports Injuries

These are extrinsic and intrinsic risk factors.

a). Extrinsic Factors

These are those prognosticators of injury that are individualistic. These are the injury predictors that are interconnected to the kind of task challenged by a specific sport.

b). Intrinsic Factors

- Age
- Gender
- Body size
- Central motor control
- Psychological and psychosocial factors
- General mental ability
- Other factors

Prevention of Sports-Related Injuries

Emergency Treatment (Table 3)

Most sports-related dental injuries occur in regions including the upper lip, upper jaw, and maxillary incisors with the primary cause of direct external force due to a fall, collision with sports equipment, or player-to-player contact. Several types of these injuries are not reversible and their likelihood of happening is persistent.

Various injuries related to sports are avertible. Furthermore, as the predictive risk factors related to such injurics arc morc distinctly recognized and explained, the pattern and evolution of new protective devices may grant positively to future athletic injury prevention [4].

Table 3. Dental emergency kit for sporting events.

Mouth mirror	2*2 4*4 Sterile Gauze
Pen Light	Sterile small wire cutter (for removal of broken Orthodontic Wire)
Scissors	Spare Commercial Mouthguard
Rope Wax	Emergency Tooth Preservation Solution Save – a –Tooth for the Avulsed tooth
Zinc Oxide Eugenol (*i.e.*, IRM)	Mixing Pad
Spatula	-

Shielding Devices in Sports Dentistry (Table 4)

The key to averting injuries related to sports is wearing devices like face masks, mouth guards, and helmets.

Table 4. Lists of sports activities.

Bandy	Handball	Skydiving
Acrobatics	Gymnastics	Skiing
Baseball	Ice hockey	Soccer
Boxing	Martial art	Surfing
Field events	Rugby	Volleyball
Field hockey	Skateboarding	Wrestling

Helmets

Helmets are essential in preventing or minimizing brain or head injuries in sports (Fig. 2). These helmets are fabricated precisely and examined strictly relative to the effect of individual sports. A helmet fabricated for a boxer might be unacceptable for a cricketer or cyclist. The fitting of the helmet should be proper to avert injury from wearing.

Face Shields

A depletion in facial injuries has been seen when the face shield was introduced especially in ice hockey. Benson *et al.* [5] differentiated the potency of half and full-face shields in the players of ice hockey. Of 319 athletes who wore full-face shields, 195 (61.6%) had at least one injury during the study season, whereas of 323 who wore half-face shields, 204 (63.2%) were injured. The risk of sustaining a facial laceration and dental injury was 2.31 and 9.90 times greater, respectively, for players wearing half vs. full face shields.

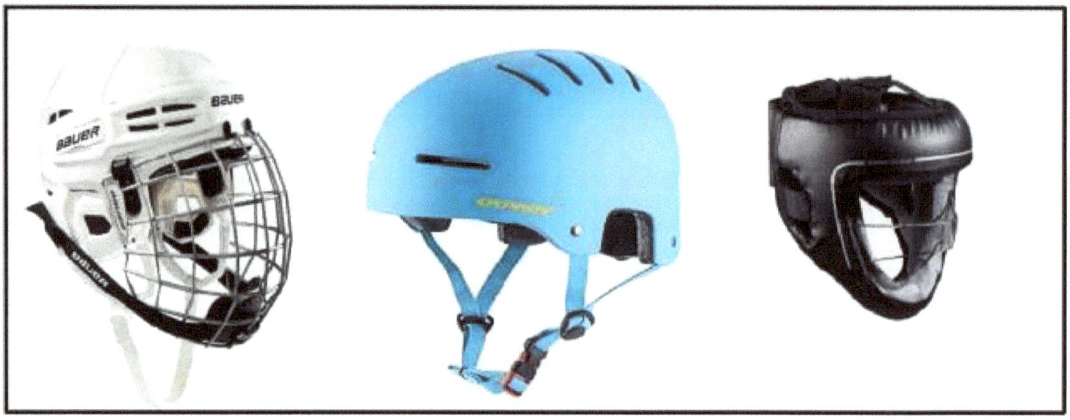

Fig (2). - Distinct types of Helmets.

Mouthguard

The mouthguard is a device worn over the teeth that protects them from blows to the face and head. Sports guards or mouth protectors are synonyms for mouth guards. These are important pieces of athletic equipment for anyone participating in a sport that involves falls, body contact, or flying equipment. This includes football, basketball, baseball, soccer, hockey, skateboarding, gymnastics, mountain biking, and any other sports-related activity that might result in an injury to the mouth [2]. The American Dental Association and Academy for Sports Dentistry (AAAD) [6] recommend properly fitted mouth guards for variety of sports (Fig. **3**) and recreational activities which predispose the participants to oral injuries. The list of such activities is given in the below-mentioned table.

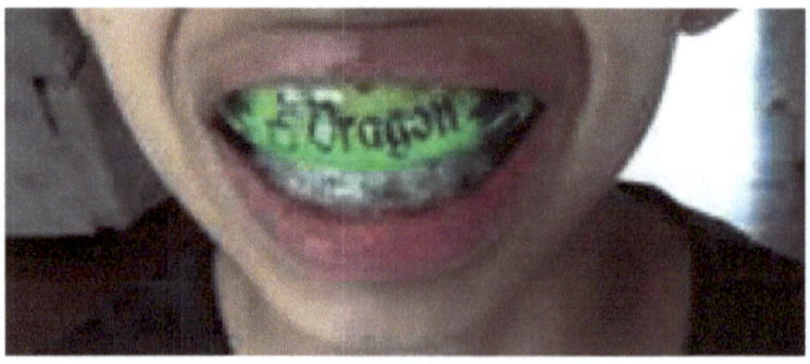

Fig (3). Mouth fitted with Mouthguard.

A well fabricated, custom-fitted mouthguard with an adequate fit lowers the incidence of concussion and any injuries to the dentofacial region. Mouthguards relieve the stress concentrated on the frontal teeth by disseminating and soaking up the shock energy and promptly ceasing the pulsing of the upper anterior. Approximately, 51.6% of national hockey league athletes wear a mouthguard during their sports activities. A professional athlete cannot be forced to wear a mouth guard, instead the owners or league administrative personnel must educate their athletes making mouthguard wearing compulsory. One of the major fears expressed by the athletes towards the use of mouthguards was their belief that these safety protectors may cause hindrance in breathing [2].

Functions of Mouthguards

Mouthguard prevents the athlete from sports-related traumatic injuries as:

1. It acts as a buffer between the soft and hard Dento-oral structures, thus

preventing any laceration and bruising during trauma.

2. It provides cushioning effect between teeth through undeviating frontal impact and redistributes the impact of a blow.

3. It protects the contrary dentition from seismic contact against each other.

4. It prevents the injury to mandibular angle during impact.

5. It behaves as a shock absorber between the maxilla and mandible and hence helps in decreasing neurologic trauma. Otherwise, it may be transferred from the condyles against the skull base with the outcome of concussion.

6. It provides a positive reinforcement against neck injuries.

7. It provides a psychological benefit to athletes as it offers confidence in terms of protection.

8. It fills empty spaces, thereby providing support to adjacent teeth. This benefit permits the athlete to take out his/her removable prosthesis during competition.

A routine, professional examination is necessary for the fit and function of the mouthguard. This depends on numerous factors such as the age of the athlete, the type of sport, and the athlete's compliance to care for the appliance. The number of appointments for such an appliance is decided by the dental professional, which further depends on the related athlete.

Selection of Material

Several materials have been suggested for mouth guards, such as [7]

i. Polyvinyl acetate-polyethylene or ethylene-vinyl acetate (EVA) copolymer,
ii. Polyvinylchloride
iii. Latex rubber
iv. Acrylic resin and
v. Polyurethane.

Three basic types of mouthguards are available:

1. Type I: Stock prefabricated mouth guard

2. Type II: Mouth-formed mouthguard

3. Type III: Custom-made (over a dental cast) mouthguard

TYPE I: Stock Mouth Guards (SMGs)

ADA has recommended that the stock mouth guards (Fig. **4**) may be bought from the sources like a pharmacy, departmental store, or sports goods store. SMGs are composed of rubber, polyvinyl acetate copolymer, or polyvinyl chloride. The advantage of SMGs is that it is cost-effective. The disadvantages include their availability only in limited sizes, improper fit, inhibition in speech and breathing, and the need of closing the jaws to hold the mouth guard in place. SMGs are the least preferred type, economical and potent. Few sizes are available in the market (Fig. **5**) thus needing modification for proper fit and function. SMGs provide comparatively less protection.

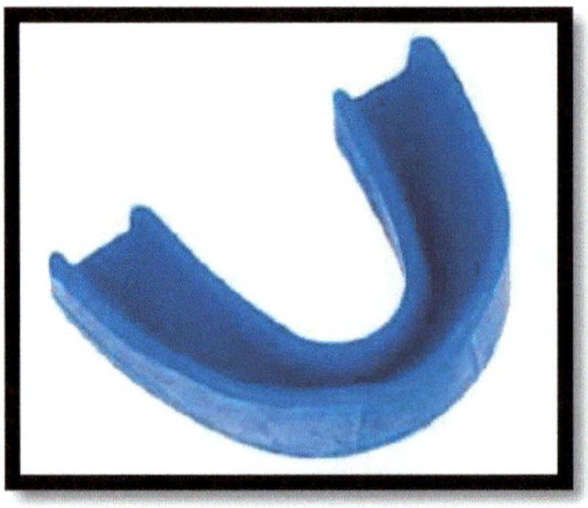

Fig. (4). Stock mouthguard.

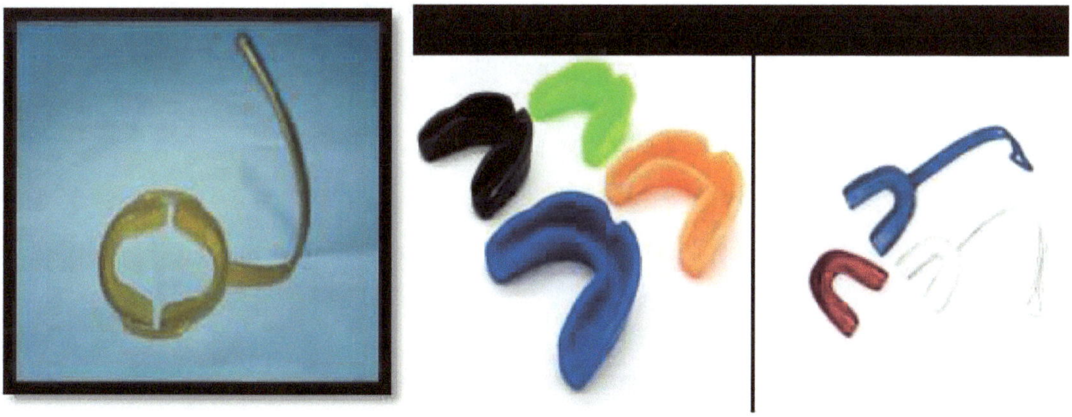

Fig. (5). Distinct types of stock mouthguards.

On condition that the person becomes insensible; the appliance might be lifted from its position causing airway obstruction. Due to improper fitting, mouth guards may develop discomfort and irritation while wearing by an athlete. However, orthodontic specialists recommend SMGs, as this appliance protects the soft tissues while allowing tooth movement. However, Academy for Sports Dentistry (ASD) does not recommend SMGs as an orofacial protective appliance due to their inadequate protection of teeth.

TYPE II: Mouth-formed Protectors (MFPs)

MFPs are available in two varieties:

i. The shell liner
ii. The thermoplastic mouthguards

The first type is made up of silicone rubber or a preformed shell with a liner of plastic acrylic. The liner is to be kept in the athlete's oral cavity and molded around the teeth and finally allowed to set. The second type *i.e.,* the preformed thermoplastic has a lining that is submerged in boiled water for approximately 10-45 sec, after which it is transmitted to the cold water and then adjusted to the teeth. This type of MFPs is also known as boil and bite guard. This type of mouthguard is the most popular of the available three types and is used by more than 90% of athletes (Fig. **6**).

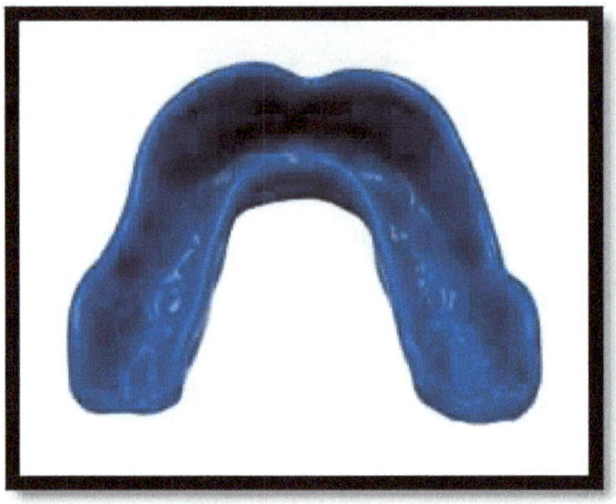

Fig (6). Mouth-formed mouthguard.

Fabrication of Mouth-Formed Protector's Mouthguard

The following steps (Fig. **7A** - **D**) are compulsory to attain a peculiar adjustment of mouth guards [8].

a. Primarily, the appropriate dimensions and the desired color of the mouthguards are chosen from commercially available materials.
b. It is then immersed in boiling water for 10-45 seconds to make it resilient and comfortably adjustable.
c. This is followed by the reduction in the temperature by keeping it in cold water, it is immediately transferred in the athlete's mouth, where it is formed, in the beginning with the use of pressure by the dentist's fingers, and pressure of the lips, tongue, cheeks and biting pressure by the athlete.
d. Then the mouth guard is ready for use.

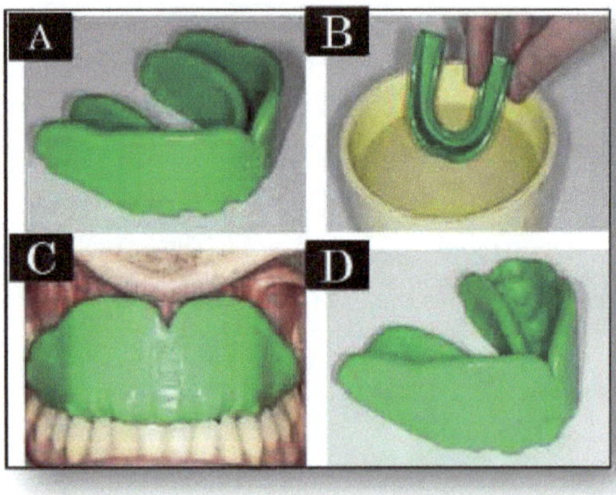

Fig (7). – Steps of fabrication of Mouth-formed protector's mouthguard: A - Available Mouthguard, B - Put in boiling water, C - Moulding to the patient's mouth, D - Customized to the patient's oral cavity.

TYPE III: Custom-Made Mouthguards (CMMs)

CMMs are the superior of the three types of mouthguards and the most expensive to the athlete. ADA has recommended this type of mouth guard for athletes to prevent sports-related injuries. CMM is composed of a thermoplastic polymer (Fig. **8**). It is fabricated by the dental professional likely to adjust accurately to the oral cavity of an athlete. Several benefits of CMMs include accurate fit, ease of speech, comfort, and retention. The best benefit of such a type of mouthguard is that it significantly reduces the incidence of a concussion due to the forward placement of the mandible.

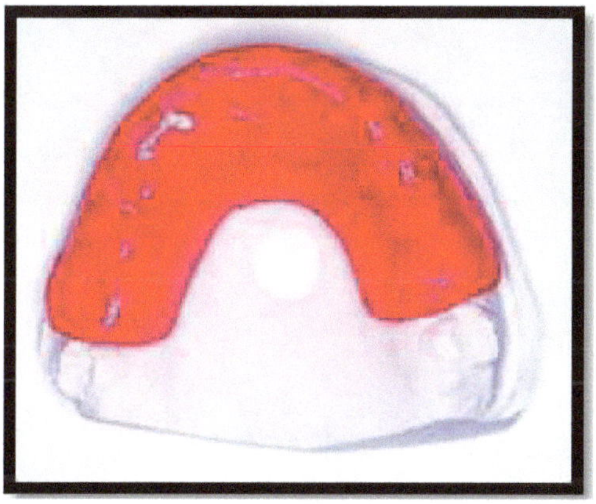

Fig (8). Custom-made mouthguard.

Fabrication of Type III Mouth Guards

The principal steps for making:

a. First and foremost, impressions are made of maxillary and mandibular arches.

Impressions made from alginate or hydrophilic material should be as precise as feasible and they should record all the areas properly. To give sufficient support to the impression material metal trays should be utilized. The minimum disinfection protocol must be followed before dispatching the impression to the laboratory.

a. Fabrication of the casts (Fig. **9A**) by pouring stone into the impression to duplicate the teeth.
b. Recording the interrelation of both the arches that the mouthguard will deliver.
c. This is followed by the construction of the mouth guard.

d. Then the mouth guard is trimmed and polished.
e. Finally placing the mouth guard into the oral cavity followed by an examination of occlusal equilibration. (Fig **9B**).

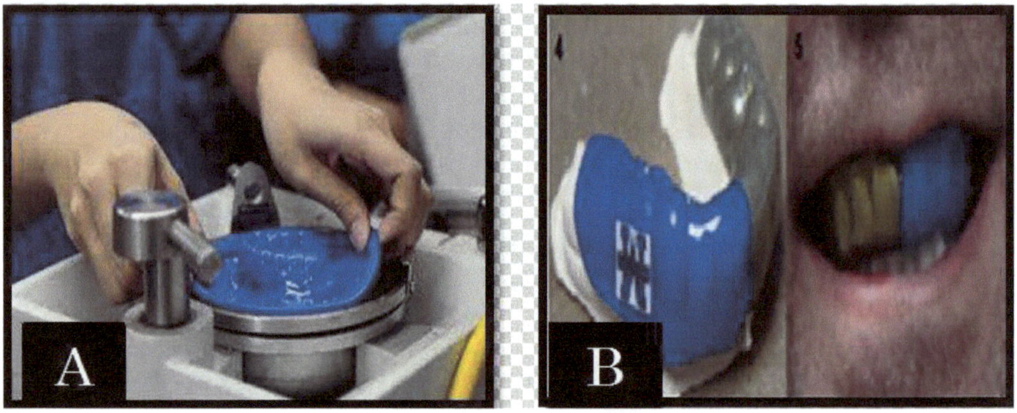

Fig (9). - Mouthguard: A - Fabrication of the mouthguard, B - Mouthguard fitted into the patient mouth.

CMMs can be divided into two types:

I. Custom vacuum-formed mouthguard (CVFMS)
II. Pressure-laminated mouthguards (PLMS).

CVFM is the most common and widely fabricated mouthguard by a dental professional (Fig **10A** - **H**). It provides adequate protection from sports-related traumatic dental injuries. It also offers the least amount of hindrance in breathing and speaking. These are prepared from a single sheet of EVA polyvinyl acetate-polyethylene copolymer that includes the heating of the sheet followed by its placement on the cast and finally, it is suctioned through a vacuum that acquires the shape of teeth and the associated oral structures. Such procedures decrease its thickness occlusally by 25% and buccolingually by more than 50%. These mouth guards cannot be used for a longer period as the change in shape occurs after wearing these for a few weeks only.

Pressure-laminated mouthguards (PLMs) are fabricated from multiple sheets of laminating ethylene- vinyl acetate (EVA) materials. These layers are fused together forming a thick and protective mouthguard. It is more retentive compared to other types of mouth guards.

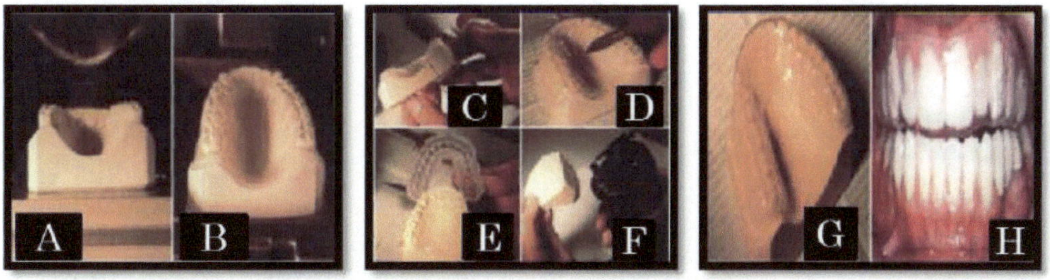

Fig (10). - Fabrication of Custom vacuum-formed mouthguard: A - A 5.5 – inch square sheet of polyvinyl acetate-polyethylene is positioned on the vacuum machine and heated until the sheet shows a 1–2-inch sag, B - The heated is switched off as the vacuum is switched on while the softened material is compressed over the dental model. The vacuum should be kept on for approximately 2 minutes, C - When the model is completely cool, excess material is trimmed with scissors and peeled away, D - The palatal region is cut out in a U shape with a utility knife, E - After soaking in water, the mouth guard is then carefully removed from the model, F - Final finishing of rough edges can be accomplished by using polishing stones or rubber wheels and then flamming the mouth guard lightly with an alcohol torch, G - The completed custom-fabricated mouthguard is now ready for delivery, H - Following placement in the mouth, the mouthguard is adjusted if necessary and then given to the athlete.

It shows very minor distortion when worn for an extended interval. These are typically fabricated by dental professionals or dental laboratories. It is mandatory to collaborate with the technician and notify her/him regarding the shape of the mouthguard, the kind of sports protection, layers of laminate, and the position of erupting teeth. The thickness of the custom-made mouthguard should be 3-4mm posteriorly and 5mm anteriorly. Covering of the teeth should be done till the first molar including all the surfaces properly and should extend palatally approximately 10mm beyond the gingival margin. It should protect the premaxillary region by extending labially (Fig **11A, B**). This design has been shown to be comfortable, functional, and adaptable.

The color of the mouthguard is an individual preference that can be accommodated with this system. When constructing mouth guards for patients playing certain sports like hockey, lacrosse, and ice hockey, the potential danger from a hard stick or ball/puck, means that more than two layers of laminate are required to increase the thickness, thus enhancing the appropriate level of protection. Bonding of various layers can be done together if a system is used that engages a machine like Drufomat. On the contrary, the thickness of the mouthguard should not be much as it can cause the stretching of the upper lip that increases the chances of splitting during sports. Several advantages of PLMs include effective communication, no interference with breathing, reduced wear in chewing, agreeable wear, and allows the uniform thickness of guard material.

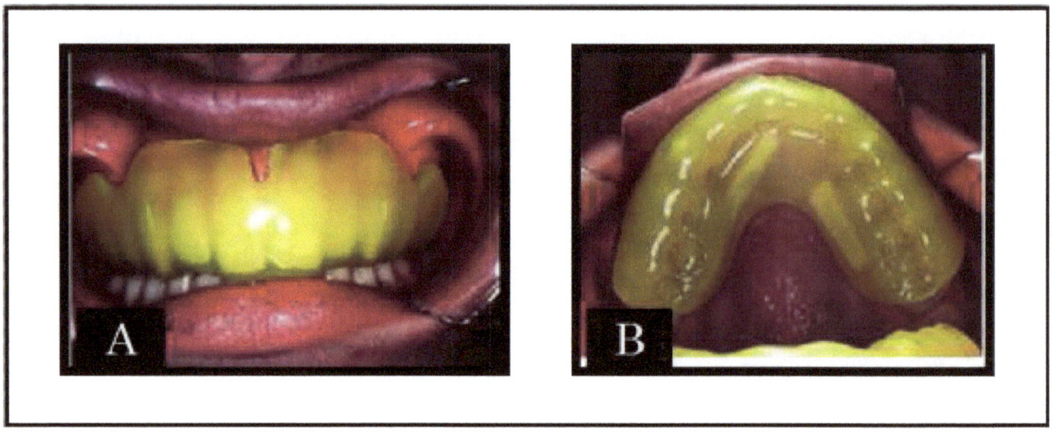

Fig (11). - Ideal shape of mouthguard, labial view: **A** - Labial view, **B** – Occlusal view.

Fabrication of Mouthguard using Digital Technology

Yanagi *et al.* [9] used high elastic rubber MG to manufacture mouthguards using a 3D printer. In their study, the same ready-made plaster model was used as the master model. They used a dental scanner to scan a plaster model and obtained a Standard Tessellation Language (STL) full form data of the plaster model. Then, software is used to design an MG which has 2.5 mm thickness onto the STL data, and fabricated high-elastic silicone rubber MGs (Digital-MGs) using a 3D printer (Fig. **12**).

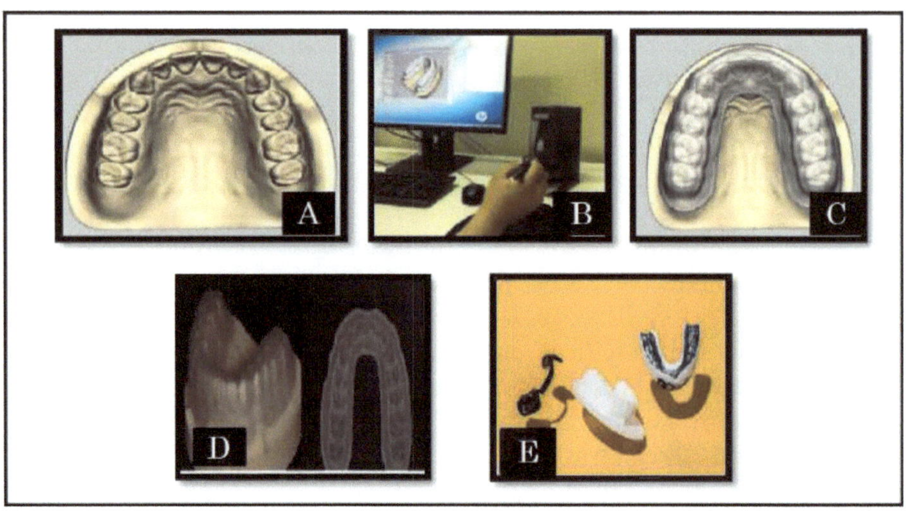

Fig (12). - Fabrication of mouthguard using digital technology: **A** - Standard Tessellation Language (STL) data of the plaster model, **B** - Design of MG with organic shape 3D modeling CAD software, **C** - Completed Digital designs, **D** - Fabricated Digital MG and inside, **E** - Completed Customized mouth guard (CMG) and inside caring for the mouthguard.

a. Cleansing it with mouth rinse or cold water prior to and following every usage. A toothbrush and dentifrice can also be used for cleaning purposes.
b. Storage and transportation of the mouthguard are to be done in a solid holder that must contain holes to permit the circulation of air.
c. Care must be taken not to expose the mouthguards to the increased temperatures as there are chances of shape distortion.
d. These should not be chewed on.
e. Should be examined routinely for any of the distortions.
f. Systematic dental follow-ups are required so that the dentist can examine the proper fit and condition of these guards.

Role of a Pediatric Dentist in Sports Dentistry

Because of the escalating number of children and adolescents participating in sports, many dentists are trained and provide their services to young athletes. In addition to the clinical aspects of sports dentistry, several other professional activities are available to dentists interested in enhancing their knowledge or expanding their involvement in this field.

These activities include volunteering for local mouth guard days, becoming a consultant to an athletic department, and serving as a sports team dentist. Some dentists may present seminars in their local communities on topics related to sports dentistry, provide information to governing agencies advocating the enactment of more stringent mouth guard regulations, or become involved in research projects studying various aspects of sports dentistry. An excellent way to become involved is to participate in the Special Olympics/Special Smiles program. Although various elements of sports dentistry, such as suturing techniques, restorations for the treatment of fractured incisors, and endodontic procedures, among others, already exist in the curriculum, few dental schools offer an interdisciplinary learning experience in sports dentistry. Such opportunities are strongly recommended in future curriculum planning, some of which are defined by the International Academy for Sports Dentistry in the dental school curriculum.

Since injuries sustained during mixed dentition or early permanent dentition have a long-term impact on the esthetic and functional status of an individual, it is essential for a pediatric dentist to have thorough knowledge about diagnosis, prevention, and management of such trauma. Also, Pediatric dentists can contribute to the education on the prevention and emergency management of sports-related injuries, by campaigning through school and community-based oral health programs.

CONCLUSION

Sports dentistry governs all the preventive and therapeutic measures of orofacial athletic injuries and related oral diseases and their manifestations. Pediatric Dentists as health professionals must have sound clinical experience and knowledge about sports related Dentofacial injuries and must work in collaboration with the teachers, coaches, trainers, parents, sports administrators, and other health care providers to provide deserved Dentofacial care. Last but not the least, sports dentistry should mandate the use of protective devices, especially mouth guards in all sports starting at the local and state levels, thus ensuring a safe future for prospects of the nation.

CONSENT FOR PUBLICATION

Not applicable.

CONFLICT OF INTEREST

The author declares no conflict of interest, financial or otherwise.

ACKNOWLEDGEMENTS

Declared none.

REFERENCES

[1] Saini R. Sports dentistry. Natl J Maxillofac Surg 2011; 2(2): 129-31. [http://dx.doi.org/10.4103/0975-5950.94465] [PMID: 22639498]

[2] Deogade SC, Dube G, Sumathi K, Dube P, Katare U, Katare D. Sports dentistry, and mouthguards. J Advan Med Res 2015; 11(6): 1-10.

[3] Guedes OA, Alencar AHG, Lopes LG, Pécora JD, Estrela C. A retrospective study of Traumatic Dental Injuries in a Brazilian dental urgency service. Braz Dent J 2010; 21(2): 153-7. [http://dx.doi.org/10.1590/S0103-64402010000200011] [PMID: 20640363]

[4] Ramagoni N, Rao SR, Singamaneni VK, Karthikeyan J. Sports dentistry: A review. J Int Soc Prev Community Dent 2014; 4(6): 139-49. [http://dx.doi.org/10.4103/2231-0762.149019] [PMID: 25374829]

[5] Benson BW, Mohtadi NG, Rose MS, Meeuwisse WH. Head and neck injuries among ice hockey players wearing full face shields vs half face shields. JAMA 1999; 282(24): 2328-32. [http://dx.doi.org/10.1001/jama.282.24.2328] [PMID: 10612320]

[6] Vastardis PD. Athletic mouthguards: indications, types, and benefits. Dent Today 2005; 24(12): 52-5. [PMID: 16396159]

[7] Maeda Y, Kumamoto D, Yagi K, Ikebe K. Effectiveness and fabrication of mouthguards. Dent Traumatol 2009; 25(6): 556-64. [http://dx.doi.org/10.1111/j.1600-9657.2009.00822.x] [PMID: 19788425]

[8] Tsaousoglou F, Topouzelis N. Fabrication processes of mouth guards. Balkan J Stomatol 2008; 12(1): 4-12.

[9] Yanagi T, Kakura K, Tsuzuki T, Isshi K, Taniguchi Y. Fabrication of mouthguard using digital technology. Dent 2019; 9(1): 1-5.

CHAPTER 12

Saliva and Oral Health

Vishwas Patil[1,*], **Vishwas Chaugule**[2] and **Heeral Shah**[2]

[1] *Department of Pediatric and Preventive Dentistry, D. Y. Patil Dental College & Hospital, Sant Tukaram Nagar, Pimpri, Pune, Maharashtra 411018, India*

[2] *Department of Pediatric and Preventive Dentistry, Sinhgad Dental College and Hospital, Sinhgad Rd, Pune, Maharashtra 411041, India*

Abstract: The mouth is a window to the body, and saliva plays an essential role in maintaining the integrity of oral structures. Saliva is that complex fluid that controls oral health through specific and nonspecific physical and chemical properties. The significance of saliva in our everyday activities and its medicinal properties are often taken for granted. However, when disruptions occur in the quality or quantity of saliva in an individual, he or she will likely experience detrimental effects on oral and systemic health. Often head and neck radiotherapy have serious and detrimental side effects on the oral cavity, including the loss of salivary gland function and a persistent complaint of a dry mouth (xerostomia). Thus, saliva has many beneficial functions that are essential to our well-being. Although saliva has been extensively investigated as a medium, few laboratories have further studied saliva's role in maintaining oral and general health and found saliva as a fascinating biological fluid that possesses the features of a perfect diagnostic tool. The presence of microbial, immunologic and molecular biomarkers in saliva offers these unique opportunities. These biomarkers aid in the early diagnosis and monitoring of oral diseases such as, dental caries, oral malignancies, infectious diseases and many more. Saliva has proved to be a good substrate for the early detection of oral diseases to evaluate therapeutic responses.

Keywords: Diagnostic Tool, Oral Health, Saliva, Salivary Gland, Salivary Immunoglobulins, Salivary Biomarkers, Sialorrhea, Xerostomia.

INTRODUCTION

Despite great improvements in the oral health of people in several countries, it is still a persistent global problem. Oral diseases such as dental caries, periodontal diseases, tooth loss, oral cancers, and oro-dental trauma have remained major public health problems. Poor oral health has a profound adverse effect on general health. Saliva is crucial for the health and proper functioning of the oral cavity.

* **Corresponding Author Vishwas Patil:** Department of Pediatric and Preventive Dentistry, D. Y. Patil Dental College & Hospital, Sant Tukaram Nagar, Pimpri, Pune, Maharashtra 411018, India; E-mail: docvishwaspatil@gmail.com

Satyawan Damle, Ritesh Kalaskar & Dhanashree Sakhare (Eds.)

Saliva is a biological fluid secreted by major and minor salivary glands. The major salivary glands arc parotid, submandibular, and sublingual glands. Minor salivary glands are widely disseminated in the entire oral cavity. Saliva provides lubrication; facilitates mastication, digestion, and taste; it has antimicrobial properties; and serves as a buffer for acidic food. Moreover, saliva inhibits the demineralization of enamel and protects from caries. The physiological secretion generates 0.75–1.5 L per day, with a decrease during the nighttime. Saliva contains 99% water and the remaining 1% (mucins, enzymes, immunoglobulins), electrolytes, lipids, and inorganic substances.

Dilution of quantity and quality of saliva is associated with complications which increases the suffering and leads to many diseases. However, the presence of a systemic disease impacts salivary microbiota. Thus, saliva, a diagnostic tool in predicting future disease risk would be a significant help in precision medicine. There are many advantages to utilizing saliva as a substrate for diagnostic analysis [1].

Physical Properties of Saliva

Saliva is the watery mixture of secretions from the salivary and oral mucosal glands that lubricate chewed food, moisten the oral walls, and contain ptyalin. Table (**1**) depicts the physical properties of saliva which are imparted by its constituent elements.

Table 1. Physical properties of saliva.

S. no	Physical property	-
1.	Daily secretion	500-1500ml/24 hours
2.	Flow rate	0.25-0.5ml/min
3.	Consistency	Cloudy, colourless, opalescent fluid
4.	pH	Whole saliva:6.35-6.85 Parotid gland saliva: 5.5-6.5 Submandibular and sublingual gland saliva: 7.0-7.5
5.	Specific gravity	1.002-1.012
6.	Freezing point	0.07˚C- 0.34˚C
7.	Viscosity	Parotid gland saliva: 1.5 Submandibular gland saliva: 3.4 Sublingual gland saliva: 13.4

Composition

Saliva is an exceptionally dilute fluid, composed of more than 99.5% water and 0.5% solids. The solids are further classified as organic, inorganic, cellular and gases (Fig. **1**).

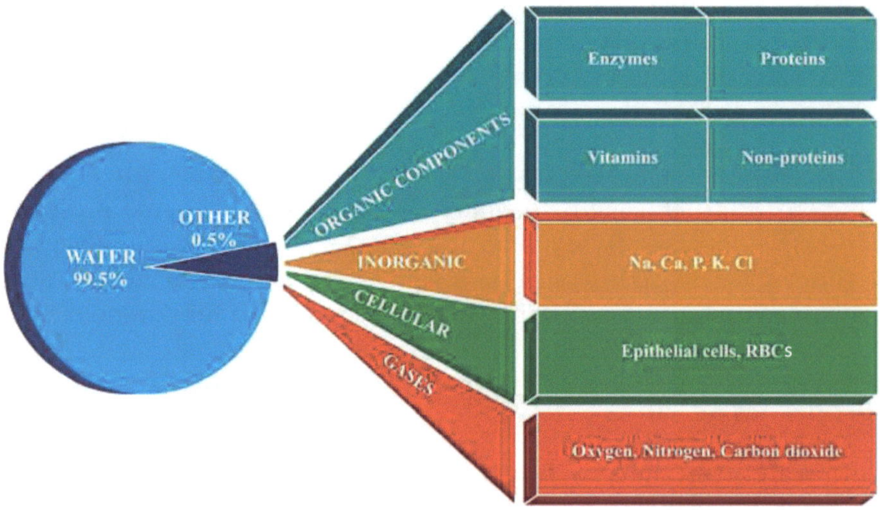

Fig (1). Composition of saliva.

- **Organic components-**
  a. **Enzymes:** amylase, lingual lipase, lysozyme, esterase, maltase, kallikrein
  b. **Proteins:** mucins, lactoferrin, albumin, immunoglobulins, blood group antigens, Interferon-gamma (IFN-g) levels
  c. **Non- proteins**: nitrogenous substances: urea, creatinine, sialin, statherins.
  d. Vitamin B-complex and vitamin C
- **Inorganic components -** Sodium, calcium, potassium chloride, bicarbonate, fluoride, phosphate, iodine, magnesium

Major salivary glands contribute most of the secretory volume and electrolyte content to saliva, whereas minor salivary glands contribute little secretion volume and most blood-group substances. Fig. (**1**) illustrates the composition of whole human saliva.

Factors Affecting the Salivary Secretion

Multiple factors influence the salivary flow and its composition. Hence, great variations are seen among individuals and the same individual under different circumstances. Following are the factors that affect the physical and/or chemical properties of saliva.

1. Age and gender
2. Salivary glands' size and body weight
3. Salivary flow index
4. Medications
5. Degree of hydration
6. Body posture and lighting
7. Physical exercise
8. Psychic stimuli
9. Circadian and circannual cycle
10. Systemic diseases and nutrition [1]

Functions of Saliva

The major functions of whole saliva [1] are enlisted in Fig (**2**).

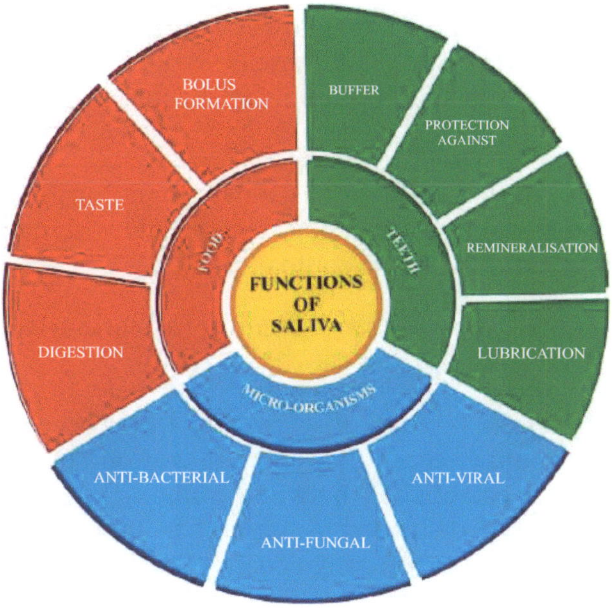

Fig (2). Functions of saliva.

Effect of Saliva on Oral Tissues

The homeostasis of the oral tissues is maintained by saliva which is often referred to as the "Gatekeeper of the oral cavity." Salivary secretions play a significant role in the maintaining of homeostasis, which when disturbed, causes various diseases like dental caries, periodontal diseases, and pathologies of the oral cavity.

Saliva and Dental Caries

Dental caries is a multifactorial disease with an interplay of four foremost factors-host (saliva and teeth), microflora, substrate (diet) and time. Saliva, also referred to as 'oral fluid,' serves as the main vehicle for solubilizing and transporting protective and potentially harmful substances to biofilm-covered tooth surfaces. Both salivary flow rate and composition (buffering agents, antimicrobial proteins) are key factors that modify the caries process. Hence, it is also termed the bloodstream of a tooth [2].

Salivary Clearance/Oral Clearance

It is how saliva dilutes and eliminates food substances such as sugars and acids from the oral cavity. The clearance rate is determined by the salivary flow rate, the volumes of saliva in the mouth before and after swallowing and the swallowing rate. It has been shown that lower residual volume of saliva, and higher salivary flow rates facilitate the increased rate of oral clearance. This promotes the removal of a substantial number of bacteria and thus balances the oral microbiome.

Persistent reduced salivary flow rates are associated with prolonged retention of food and microbes in the oral cavity. Hence, individuals with decreased salivary flow rates develop more carious lesions comparatively.

Inorganic Components of Saliva: Demineralization-Remineralization Concept

Dental caries is a dynamic process that results from net imbalance where demineralization of the tooth exceeds the remineralization ability. Under normal conditions, equilibrium is established between mineral loss and mineral gain. However, this balance can be disturbed by several factors like plaque fluid pH, presence/ absence of fluoride and buffering capacity of saliva.

Demineralization of the hydroxyapatite crystal occurs when calcium and phosphate concentrations in saliva surrounding the tooth are under-saturated in comparison to hydroxyapatite. Regaining the equilibrium in this case, calcium ions from the apatite are released until saturation is achieved or the pH rises. The critical pH for hydroxyapatite with respect to saliva is 5.5. Saliva acts as a remineralizing agent and as a delivery vehicle of ions, like fluoride, which can then get incorporated into the tissues and help in the remineralization of the tooth.

Therefore, saliva helps in reducing dental caries by controlling the ph. Stephan's curve (Fig. **3**) varies among individuals. It is determined by the buffering capacity of saliva where phosphates, bicarbonates and calcium protect the tooth from caries.

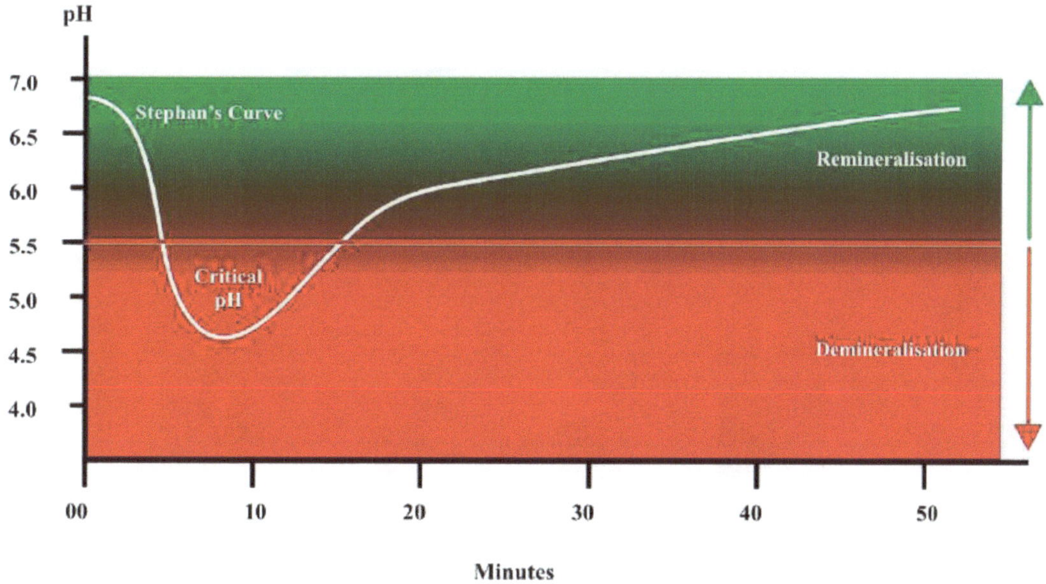

Fig (3). Stephan's curve.

Individuals with good buffering capacity neutralize the acids to a greater extent resulting in lesser dental caries. The amount of calcium and phosphorous in saliva also indicates a considerable variation depending on the flow rate. The calcium and phosphorous content of saliva are low in caries active persons.

The presence of fluoride or fluorapatite makes the tooth more resistant to demineralization. In these cases when the surface starts to demineralize, a much lower critical pH is required to demineralize the tooth surface. When the surface demineralizes, fluoride ions are released into the surrounding environment, which supersaturates the saliva faster aiding in the remineralization of the tooth. Fig. (**4**) depicts the dynamic process of demineralization and remineralization at the tooth-saliva interface.

Antimicrobial Properties of Saliva

Major antimicrobial proteins in human saliva are usually divided into non-immune (innate) and immune (acquired) factors, the latter representing antigen-stimulated immunoglobulins.

Non-immunoglobulin proteins

Table (**2a**) enlists the non-immunoglobulin salivary proteins which aid in the antimicrobial action of saliva.

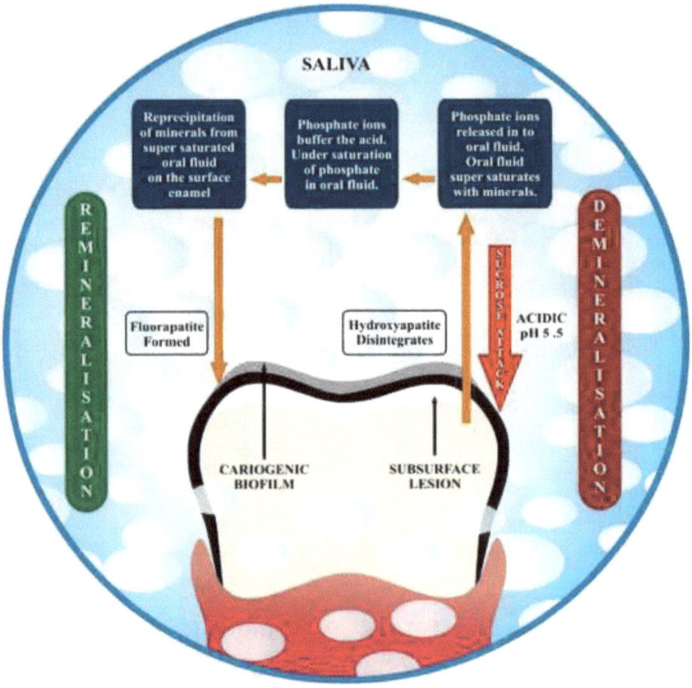

Fig (4). Demineralization-remineralization process at the tooth-plaque interface.

Table 2a. Functions of salivary non-immunoglobulin proteins.

Protein	Major target or function
1. **Lysozyme**	• Present in the saliva of newborn babies at levels equal to those of adults. • Lysozyme is a strongly cationic protein that activates bacterial autolysins that destroy the bacterial cell walls hence called – "suicide packages." • Gram-negative bacteria are more resistant to lysozyme because of their protective outer lipopolysaccharide layer. • Gram-positive bacteria, such as Mutans streptococci, are protected by cell-produced extracellular polysaccharides.
2. **Lactoferrin**	• Lactoferrin has bacteriostatic, bactericidal, fungicidal, antiviral and anti-inflammatory activity. • The biological activity of lactoferrin is due to its high affinity for iron (Fe^{3+}) and helps in scavenging the essential metal from pathogenic micro-organisms. This leads to a bacteriostatic effect.

(Table 2a) cont.....

Protein	Major target or function
3. **Peroxidases**	• There are two different peroxidase enzymes in the whole saliva: a) Salivary peroxidase (sometimes called sialo peroxidase) b) Myeloperoxidase. • Salivary peroxidase is secreted by the parotid and submandibular glands; the myeloperoxidase is a leukocyte-derived protein entering the mouth via gingival crevices. • Both enzymes catalyze the oxidation of salivary thiocyanate ions (SCN-) by H_2O_2 to the antimicrobial component, hypothiocyanite (OSCN-).
4. **Agglutinins**	Agglutination of microorganisms either results in their rapid removal from the oral cavity when the saliva is swallowed or, if the agglutinated microorganisms are more adherent, could promote their colonization of epithelial and dental surfaces.
5. **Amylase**	α-Amylase is the most abundant salivary enzyme, accounting for 40-50% of the total salivary gland-produced protein.
6. **Histatin**	Exhibits strong in vitro killing and growth inhibitory activities towards C. albicans, which is an opportunistic oral fungus
7. **Mucins**	The salivary mucin MUC5B prevents the attachment of Streptococcus mutans to the tooth surfaces by keeping the bacterium in the planktonic state and repelling bacteria from the tooth surface.

Immunoglobulins (Table 2b).

Table 2b. Functions of salivary immunoglobulin proteins.

Protein	Major target or function
1. **Secretory IgA**	• This is a predominant class of immunoglobulin in a modified form called as secretory immunoglobulin A or S-IgA • S-IgA differs from its serum counterpart in that it mostly exists as a dimer of IgA to which are attached two other molecules, one being termed a secretory component and another J chain. • S-IgA is particularly resistant to proteolytic enzymes, due to its association with secretory components. • It has the potential for producing a local response to an antigen.
2. **IgG, IgM**	Enhancement of phagocytosis

The result, "caries to be or not to be", is a complex phenomenon and is based on multiple factors. Saliva is an important biological and protective factor in the remineralization process.

Saliva and Periodontium

Dental plaque, in sufficient concentration, can disturb the host-parasite relationship and produces dental caries and periodontal disease. Dental calculus is the consequence of the mineralization of bacterial plaque which forms most abundantly on the tooth surfaces opposite the orifices of the main salivary glands [3]. It may be prevented by mineralization inhibitors present in saliva such as statherin and proline rich proteins.

Saliva and Oral Health- Applied Aspects

Salivary Gland Hypofunction

There is an unfound belief that children cannot suffer from salivary hypofunction and that infants drool and young children always have an excess of watery saliva. The subjective sensation of dry mouth, xerostomia is a well-recognized problem in adults, however, less attention has been paid to this issue in children [4].

Classification of Xerostomia

- Profound - Saliva flow absent/ reduced
- Severe- 250mg/day
- Moderate - 250-500 mg/day
- Normal- 500 -1500 mg/day

Etiologic Factors

The following factors contribute to the etiopathogenesis of xerostomia-

1. Excessive fluids loss- exertional sports activities, GIT fluid loss from diarrhoea or vomiting.
2. Medications- Antidepressants like methylphenidate and amphetamines; antihistamines; diuretics; bronchodilators and inhaler medications contribute to salivary dysfunction.
3. Diabetes mellitus- fluid loss due to polyuria.
4. Thyroid gland disorders- coexistence with Sjogren's syndrome is common.
5. Psychogenic causes- mood changes affect the autonomic nervous system
6. Chemotherapy and Radiotherapy- damage acinar cells and affect the blood flow of glands.
7. Graft vs Host diseases- damage the skin, oral mucosa and salivary glands
8. HIV Infections- affect salivary glands and reduce the salivary parameters dramatically.
9. Ectodermal dysplasia (ED)- salivary glands are ectodermal in origin and hence may be affected.
10. Down syndrome- salivary flow rate found to be 36% lower in these cases
11. Salivary gland agenesis- may be partial or complete. Non-drooling infants, caries on lower incisors on the lingual aspect are classical signs.

12. Autism spectrum disorder (ASD)- Rothia species is more prevalent and hence, modification of oral microbiomc is necessary [5, 6].

Changes in Salivary Composition due to Hyposalivation

Hyposalivation results in changes in the quality of the whole saliva. They are-

1. It favours multiplication of acidogenic bacteria and yeast.
2. Increased concentration of IgA and IgG, lactoferrin, lysozyme, β_2 microglobulin.
3. Increased salivary amylase activity
4. The concentrations of acidic and basic proline-rich proteins like cystatins, histatins and statherins appear to be reduced in irradiated patients [4].

Management

It should be tailored to the individual patient. It is used as a multidisciplinary model. Patient education should include counselling on daily oral hygiene and regular dental visits. Topical fluoride and other restorative interventions must be used. Emphasis on frequent dental visits is essential.

1. **Management of Systemic Conditions and Medications.**

2. **Home care programs**- in children with ongoing salivary gland dysfunction, life-long, therapy utilising salivary substitutes CPP-ACP, fluoride applications, intermittent chlorhexidine therapy and diet counselling is essential to prevent early loss of teeth.
3. **Candidiasis prevention and control-** topical therapy with Nystatin / Clotrimazole may provide an effective treatment. Lozenges and pastilles in such patients are usually not recommended as it becomes difficult to dissolve them and irritation to the oral mucosa is likely to happen.
4. **Pharmacotherapy with salivary stimulants:**
   - Currently, pilocarpine and cevimeline are two sialogogues that are approved by US Food and Drug Administration for treating dry mouth. The recommended dosage for pilocarpine is 5 mg four times a day and cevimeline is 30 mg three times a day.
   - Chewing gum
   - Paraffin wax (1-1.5mg) 3-5 times daily
   - Lemon mucilage citric acid
5. **Saliva substitutes**–make the patient feel more comfortable. Available in different forms of solutions (Hypromellose, V.A. Oralube), sprays (Saliva orthana, Glandosane) and lozenges (Polyox) [5, 7].

Drooling/ Hypersalivation/ Ptyalism

Drooling (also known as ptyalism, sialorrhea, or slobbering) is when saliva flows outside the mouth, defined as "saliva beyond the margin of the lip." It is normal in infants but usually stops by 15-18months of age. Sialorrhea after the age of four is considered as pathologic. Anterior drooling is defined as saliva spilled from the mouth that is visible. Posterior drooling occurs when saliva spills through the oropharynx and into the hypopharynx. The primary factors which may cause drooling are enlisted below.

Causes of Drooling

1. **Systemic causes** –
   - Neuromuscular/sensory dysfunction- cerebral palsy, Parkinson's disease, mental retardation, motor neuron disease, pseudobulbar/bulbar palsy, stroke
   - Medication side effects- antipsychotics (clozapine), tranquillizers, anticonvulsants, anticholinesterases, lithium
   - Infections – rabies
   - Gastric- gastroesophageal reflux
2. **Local causes -**
   - Oral- Inflammation, teething
   - Infection- dental caries, oral cavity infection, tonsillitis, peritonsillar abscess
   - Anatomic- macroglossia, nasal blockage, oral incompetence, dental malocclusion, orthodontic problems, head and neck surgical defects.
3. **Physiological Causes-**
   - Pregnancy [8]

Effect of Untreated Drooling of Saliva

1. **Physical effects:** Perioral chapping (skin cracking), maceration with secondary infection, dehydration, foul odor, aspiration/ pneumonia, speech disturbance, interference with feeding.
2. **Psychological effects:** Isolation, barriers to education (damage to books or electronic devices), increased dependency and level/intensity of care, decreased self-esteem, and difficult social interaction.

Management

Treatment of sialorrhea is best accomplished with a multidisciplinary team approach. The goal of the treatment of drooling is a reduction in excessive salivary flow while maintaining a moist and healthy oral cavity. Primarily, reversible causes of drooling should be treated. Less invasive and reversible methods are preferred before surgery is undertaken.

1. Non-invasive modalities: include oral motor therapy, orofacial regulation therapy using functional appliancces, spcech thcrapy, biofeedback, positive and negative reinforcement, oral prosthetic devices, and pharmacological therapy (anticholinergic drugs).
2. Minimally invasive modalities: use of botulinum toxin, photocoagulation of salivary ducts and tongue acupuncture are minimally invasive procedures.
3. Invasive modalities including surgery and radiotherapy: Neurectomy and salivary gland duct and gland surgeries have been mentioned as invasive modalities for the treatment of sialorrhea surgically [9].

Saliva- A Diagnostic tool

It is surprising for most people to learn that saliva has been used in diagnostics for more than two thousand years. Ancient doctors of Chinese medicine have concluded that saliva and blood are "brothers." Body fluids provide a wide perspective regarding the biological processes and health of different organs. The human body is composed of a variety of fluids such as blood, urine, and saliva with a high quantity of proteins that can be associated with several systemic and oral diseases. Human saliva has been one of the most appealing diagnostic tools for an early diagnosis, a better treatment and an improved prognosis. Proteomic studies of saliva help in the identification of new proteins and peptides that can help quantify the biological activity in pathological states. The most assayed salivary biomarkers are cortisol, testosterone, progesterone, aldosterone and hydroxyprogesterone. Saliva is characterized by four major types of salivary proteins. They are PRPs, cysteine, statherin and histatins. Saliva proteome knowledge base is the first database that contains all the proteomic data being accessible to the public. Plasma-derived biomarkers in saliva facilitate the continuous monitoring of the oral and general health status [10].

Clinical Applications of the Salivary Diagnosis in the Era of "Omics"

For the salivary diagnosis to become a routine in clinical practice, it is necessary to know specific salivary biomarkers of both healthy and diseased states. The genomic, transcriptomic, proteomic and metabolomic approaches are currently being used to characterize these diagnostic biomarkers in saliva. Thus, the use of saliva as a diagnostic fluid will be increasingly accepted, allowing for enhanced systemic and oral health [11].

Advantages Offered by Saliva as a Diagnostic Tool

1. High sensitivity
2. Cost-effectiveness
3. Real-time diagnostic value

4. Multiple samples can be obtained in a non-invasive way
5. Provides new and non-invasive perspective in obtaining a diagnosis

Salivary Biomarkers for Oral and Systemic Diseases

Following oral and systemic diseases can be diagnosed using the salivary biomarkers-

Periodontal Diseases

Various salivary biomarkers have been studied for the diagnosis and prognosis of periodontal diseases, which are characterized by three phases in which specific biomarkers are seen to increase.

a. Inflammation- E_2, IL-1, IL-6 and TNF-α
b. Connective tissue disintegration-E_2, IL-1, IL-6, TNF-α and MMP8
c. Bone turn-over- NF-α and IL-1

Other salivary biomarkers associated with periodontal diseases are- Salivary soluble toll-like receptor two, IL-4, Dipeptidyl peptidase, increased levels of Aspartate aminotransferase (AST) and alkaline phosphatase (ALP), lower uric acid levels and albumin.

Sjogren's Syndrome (SS)

Severe alterations in the levels of IL-4, IL-5 and cytokine clusters are noticed. It is accompanied by significant changes in the proteome and transcriptome. The sialo chemistry (analysis of saliva's chemical components) offers a great value for the diagnosis of Sjogren's syndrome. Increased immunoglobulin levels, inflammatory mediators, albumin, sodium and chloride and decreased phosphate level are indicative of Sjogren's syndrome.

Cardiovascular Disease (CVD)

Levels of IL-1β, IL-6 and TNFα and prostaglandin E_2 are raised whereas levels of α-2- Hs glycoprotein in saliva seem to decrease in patients with CVD. α amylase salivary activity could be used as a good marker of catecholamines during the evaluation of patients in different stressful situations.

Viral Infections

The existing tests for viral infections are based on salivary biomarkers like viral DNA/ RNA, antigens and antibodies. Current tests available are based on the proteomic analysis and existing antibodies for hepatitis A, B, C, HIV 1, rubella and mumps.

Dental Caries

In the last few decades, there has been an increasing interest in the utilization of saliva for bacteriological tests that indicate caries risk. These tests are based on the identification of Lactobacillus species and Mutans streptococci and their quantification in saliva.

Saliva's buffer capacity varies with glandular activity. The bicarbonate raises the pH of saliva and its buffering capacity during stimulation. Thus, the levels of bicarbonate showing abnormalities suggest a predisposition to dental caries.

Infectious Diseases

Saliva contains viruses and/or bacteria responsible for systemic diseases that can be identified by PCR. Another way to diagnose infectious disease by the salivary examination is through monitoring the presence of antibodies to microorganisms. In recent years, researchers have shown that salivary tests for detection of antibodies to HIV, represent a non-invasive alternative to monitor the effectiveness of antiretroviral therapy and progression of AIDS.

Psychological and Genetic Disorders

Salivary cortisol levels represent an important biological marker of stress. Levels of phosphate, potassium and chloride are increased in individuals with intense activity of the sympathetic nervous system, which is commonly seen in situations of emotional stress.

Salivary α amylase activity is regulated by the sympathetic autonomic nervous system and has importance in the psychology of stress. These levels increase under various conditions of physical and psychological stress before any other clinical signs are perceived. Therefore, salivary α amylase acts as an effective biomarker in saliva to evaluate psychological and metabolic stress.

Malignancy

Level of soluble CD44 in saliva has been evaluated as a potential molecular marker for head and neck cancer at all stages. The role of biomarkers has been expanded to cover all aspects of patient care from early cancer detection to more accurate tumour staging to post-treatment tumour surveillance. Saliva is the fluid that drains the lesions and there is increased RNA and proteins of oral cancer on it [11].

FUTURE PERSPECTIVE OF SALIVA AS A BIOLOGICAL FLUID FOR SARS-COV-2

The potential use of saliva for SARS-COV-2 detection is scientifically well-founded. Being a noninvasive specimen type, saliva is well suited for serial viral load monitoring. The SARS-COV-2 RNA load in the saliva is reported to be the highest after the first week of symptom onset, followed by a gradual decline. This underlines that saliva is a viable candidate for SARS-COV-2 detection in the early disease phase. In the light of these promising results, the search for salivary biomarkers associated with the development and progression of COVID 19 could allow a better distinction between asymptomatic, mild, moderate or advanced diseases [12].

CONCLUSION

Saliva is the most easily available and non-invasive body fluid of the human body that permanently bathes the oral cavity and is trying to cope with an ever-changing milieu. Saliva includes a large number of organic and inorganic compounds which function as a "mirror" of the body's health. In addition to other functions, it constitutes the first line of defense against oxidative stress. As a diagnostic fluid, saliva offers multiple advantages over serum. It provides a cost-effective approach for the screening of large populations. Saliva as a diagnostic tool for oral and systemic diseases has numerous advantages over other body fluids and based on specific biomarkers, can provide an accurate diagnosis. Thus, the use of saliva as a diagnostic fluid will be increasingly accepted allowing for enhanced systemic and oral health as we explore saliva as a potential alternative to blood and tissue-based diagnostics. With the advent of novel and more sensitive techniques with standard reference values, salivary diagnostics will become the technique of choice in the future.

CONSENT FOR PUBLICATION

Not applicable.

CONFLICT OF INTEREST

The authors declare no conflict of interest, financial or otherwise.

ACKNOWLEDGEMENT

Declared none.

REFERENCES

[1] Edgar M, Dawes C, Mullane D, Eds. Saliva and oral health. 135-50.

[2] Nikiforuk G. 9 Saliva and Dental Caries. Understanding dental caries. Karger Publishers 1985; Vol. 1: pp. 236-60.

[3] McDonald RE, Avery DR, Weddell JA. Gingivitis and periodontal disease. Dentistry for the child and adolescent, ed. 2010; 8;9: 366-402.

[4] Pedersen AM, Bardow A, Jensen SB, Nauntofte B. Saliva and gastrointestinal functions of taste, mastication, swallowing and digestion. Oral Dis 2002; 8(3): 117-29. [http://dx.doi.org/10.1034/j.1601-0825.2002.02851.x] [PMID: 12108756]

[5] Walsh LJ. Dry mouth: a clinical problem for children and young adults. Int Dent SA 2007; 9(5): 48-58.

[6] Tschoppe P, Wolgin M, Pischon N, Kielbassa AM. Etiologic factors of hyposalivation and consequences for oral health. Quintessence Int 2010; 41(4): 321-33. [PMID: 20305867]

[7] American Dental Association. Managing xerostomia and salivary gland hypofunction. A Report of the ADA Council on Scientific Affairs. 2015.

[8] Güvenç IA. Güvenç IA. Sialorrhea: a guide to etiology, assessment, and management. Salivary Glands–New Approaches in Diagnostics and Treatment. 2018.

[9] Meningaud JP, Pitak-Arnnop P, Chikhani L, Bertrand JC. Drooling of saliva: A review of the etiology and management options. Oral Surg Oral Med Oral Pathol Oral Radiol Endod 2006; 101(1): 48-57. [http://dx.doi.org/10.1016/j.tripleo.2005.08.018] [PMID: 16360607]

[10] Tiwari M. Science behind human saliva. J Nat Sci Biol Med 2011; 2(1): 53-8. [http://dx.doi.org/10.4103/0976-9668.82322] [PMID: 22470235]

[11] da Silva AC, da Silva DR, de Macedo Ferreira SA, de Sousa Rodrigues AD, Albuquerque AD, Marinho SA. Salivary diagnostics, current reality and future prospects in emerging trends in oral health sciences and dentistry Mar 11. Intechopen 2015.

[12] Ceron J, Lamy E, Martinez-Subiela S, *et al.* Use of saliva for diagnosis and monitoring the SARS-CoV-2: a general perspective. J Clin Med 2020; 9(5): 1491. [http://dx.doi.org/10.3390/jcm9051491] [PMID: 32429101]

CHAPTER 13

Systemic Fluorides and Dental Health

Joby Peter[1,*], **H. Sharath Chandra**[2] and **Dhanashree Sakhare**[3]

[1] *Department of Pediatric and Preventive Dentistry, Annoor Dental College and Hospital, Muvattupuzha, Kerala, India*

[2] *Department of Pediatric and Preventive Dentistry, SJM Dental College, Chitradurga, Karnataka, India*

[3] *Lavanika Dental Academy, Melbourne, Australia*

Abstract: Dental caries remains a significantly prevalent public health problem globally for both developing countries and deprived inhabitants in developed countries. The WHO Oral Health Programme persists in emphasizing the importance of public health methods for the effective use of fluorides in the prevention of dental caries. Early research and development were concerned with waterborne fluorides, both naturally occurring and their controlled addition, with emphasis on the effects of fluoridation on the prevalence and incidence of dental caries. More recently, systematic reviews summarizing these extensive databases have indicated that water fluoridation and fluoride toothpaste both substantially reduced dental caries. Fluoride must be present in the right place, namely in saliva and dental plaque at the right time to interfere with the tooth decay process. This process is a swing and balance affair between acid dissolution and remineralization of the tooth surfaces. In addition, in conditions where the incidence and prevalence of dental caries in the community are high to moderate, or when there are firm indications that the incidence of caries is increasing, a supplementary source of fluoride should be contemplated.

Keywords: Community Oral Health, Dental Caries Prevention, Fluorides, Systemic Fluorides.

INTRODUCTION

Once in a millennium, we come across significant discoveries, the ramifications of which span an entire century. One such discovery was the inverse correlation between the prevalence of dental caries and fluoride concentration which is a great forward stride in the field of public health. The fact that the presence of fluoride in drinking water drastically decreased the prevalence of dental caries was established in the 1940s, although the mechanism of action was not known, it

* **Corresponding author Joby Peter:** Department of Pediatric and Preventive Dentistry, Annoor Dental College and Hospital, Muvattupuzha, Kerala, India; E-mail: jobspeter77@gmail.com

Satyawan Damle, Ritesh Kalaskar & Dhanashree Sakhare (Eds.)

was thought to be primarily systemic. Since then, various preventive measures and programs using fluoride were implemented in controlling dental caries. A substantial decline in the caries prevalence has been observed in different parts of the world during the last 15-20 years, both in countries using water fluoridation as a caries preventive measure and in countries without water fluoridation. It is remarkable that caries reduction has occurred at the same time and with similar magnitude in regions which are far apart like the Nordic region (North Europe and North Atlantic countries) on one hand and Oceania region (Australia and New Zealand) on the other.

Many countries have used fluoride in different forms for caries prevention like community water fluoridation programs, salt fluoridation and fluoride tablets, but more emphasis has been given to topical fluorides by most countries. However, one aspect which remained common for the prevention of dental caries at the community level is fluoride which endured the test of time and various trials. Fluorides now have become an integral part of every oral health program and WHO had passed a resolution at World Health Assembly in 2007, that universal access to fluoride for caries prevention was to be part of the basic right to human health (Fig. **1**).

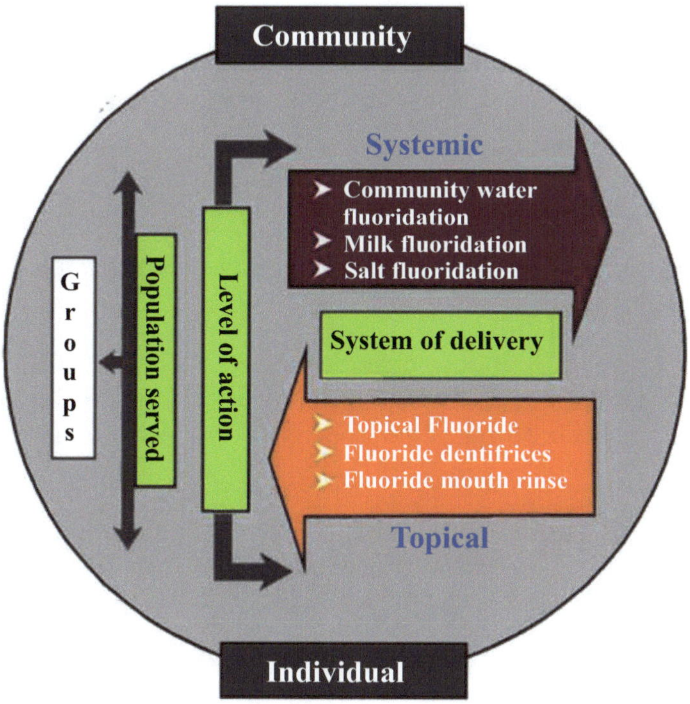

Fig (1). Fluoridation program for prevention of Dental caries.

Historical Evolution of Fluorides

In 1901, Dr Fredrick McKay in Colorado Springs, Colorado, USA, started detecting a permanent stain on his patient's teeth, particularly those who had lived in that area all their lives, and the locals called it **'Colorado Stain'.** McKay was not able to find any reference to them in any of the available scientific literature. He described the stain by calling it 'mottled enamel' as: A minute white flecks, or brown or yellow spots or areas, which are scattered irregularly or streaked over the surface of a tooth, or it may be a condition where the entire tooth surface is of a dead paper-white like the colour of a China dish.

Important Milestones in the History of Fluorides

1901: Dr Fredrick McKay of Colorado (USA) discovered permanent stains on the teeth of his patients, which were referred to as **'Colorado stains'** and he named it **'Mottled Enamel'.**

1908: McKay at the annual meeting of the State Dental Association in Boulder said that this condition was not only confined to Colorado but extended to other towns as well.

1912: McKay came across an article written by Dr I.M. Eager (1902), a U.S. Marine hospital surgeon stationed in Italy who reported that a high proportion of Italian residents in Naples had ugly brown stains on their teeth known as **"Denti di chiaie".**

1916: In a major study by McKay and G V. Black, who examined 6,873 individuals and reported that mottled enamel develops due to the presence of an unknown factor in the domestic water that the people ingested during the period of enamel calcification.

1930: Another interesting finding observed by Kemp and McKay is that there was no mottling of enamel occurred in people who grew up in Bauxite before 1909, the year in which Bauxite had changed its supply from shallow wells to deep drilled wells.

1931: Churchill H.V., the chief chemist of an aluminum company in New Kensington, Pennsylvania, after thorough spectrographic analysis of the rare elements, noted that Fluoride was present in Bauxite water at a level of 13.7 ppm.

1931: **Shoe leather survey**- Trendley. H. Dean was assigned the job to continue McKay's work and to find out the extent of the geographical distribution of mottled enamel in the U.S. by the U.S. Public Health Service. About 5,824 children from 22 cities in 10 states were screened for fluorosis and found that mottling was present in those areas where the water concentration was 3 ppm or more. This survey confirmed that the concentration of fluoride in drinking water was directly correlated with the severity of fluorosis in the enamel (Fig. **2**).

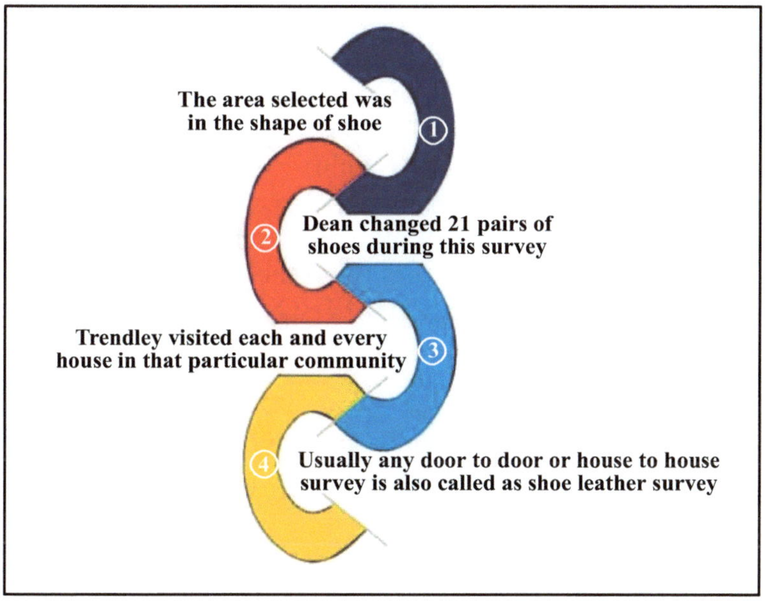

Fig (2). Shoe leather survey.

1934: Trendley H. Dean introduced the mottling index, which is popularly known as Dean's Index for fluorosis.

1942: The important milestone discovery was made by Dean et al. that at 1 ppm F in drinking water, a 60% reduction in caries experience was observed.

1945:The world's first artificial fluoridation plant at Grand Rapids, U.S.A.

1946: Klein examined children of Japanese ancestry who had been transferred from a community containing 0.1 ppm fluoride or less to Arizona where water contained 3 ppm of fluoride. It was observed that: teeth in the process of eruption received maximum benefits from fluoride. Teeth exposed to fluorides shortly after eruption were also protected, although to a lesser degree [1].

Thus, from all the above-mentioned studies and findings, fluoride was identified as an essential element for reducing dental caries, and this led to the introduction of various methods of application of fluorides for individuals and water fluoridation projects for communities.

According to Dean's study data, at a natural fluoride concentration of around 1 mg/litre, the increased resistance to dental caries was of substantial public health importance whereas the prevalence, severity, and cosmetic impact of dental fluorosis were not significant. This paved the way for studies to check the hypothesis that artificially raising the fluoride level of public drinking water would have the same effects. The first intervention study was undertaken under the direction of USPHS in Grand Rapids in 1945, results of which were published in 1953 after 6 years of fluoridation. Additional studies were started in 1945 and 1946 in New York State, Illinois, and Ontario, Canada. Further intervention studies were carried out in the Netherlands (1953), New Zealand (1954), the UK (1955-56), and East Germany (1959). All these interventional studies demonstrated a clinically important reduction in the incidence of dental caries. In 1994, the World Health Organisation (WHO) recommended the optimal concentration of fluoride in the range of 0.5mg-1.0mg/litre, varying according to climatic conditions.

The word fluorine is derived from the Latin term **'fluore'** meaning **'to flow'**. 'Fluorine' is a yellowish-green diatomaceous gas, which is never obtained in its free elemental form because it is a highly electronegative and reactive anion. The highest fluoride value has been recorded in the Nakuru Rift Valley of Kenya (2800mg/kg - 5600 mg/kg in soil) [2].

Fluoride as an Element

Properties of fluoride are given in Fig. (**3**).

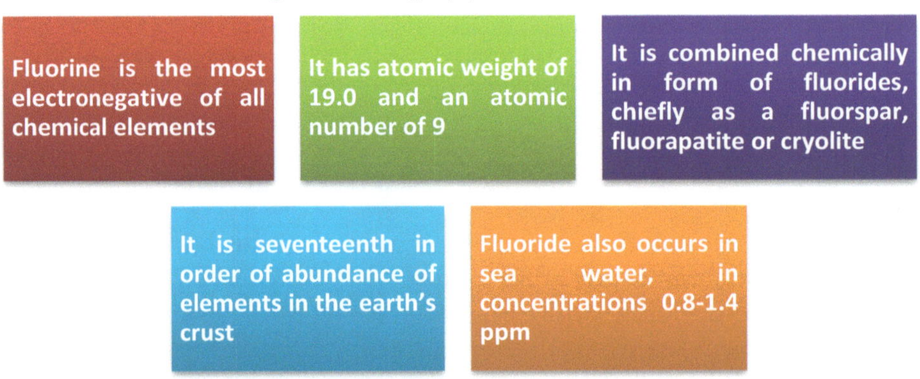

Fig (3). Various properties of fluorides.

Passage of Fluorides in the Environment

Fluoride derived from volcanic eruptions or mining industries is present in the atmosphere and enters the soil by deposition as dust, snow, fog, or rain. Fluoride leaches from the soil into groundwater and is taken up by vegetation. Plants take up fluoride by absorption from the air, soil, and deposition from dust. It enters the food chain and ultimately returns to the soil as waste. The average daily intake of fluoride by adults from dry food substances is in the range of 0.2 to 1.8 mg, and the average daily intake from water containing 1 ppm fluoride is about 1.5 mg. The total fluid intake in children between 1-12 years of age ranges from 700-1300 ml/day, which at a level of 1 ppm fluoride would result in ingestion of about 0.7 mg/day and for the younger bottle-fed group of children to about 1.3 mg fluoride/day [3].

Fluorides prevent dental caries not only by systemic incorporation into developing enamel, but also by topical action post-eruption of the tooth. The caries inhibiting effect tends to persist if fluoride exposure is continued but tends to be gradually lost after fluoride exposure is discontinued. The periodic or continuous renewal of fluoride content of tooth enamel is required to maintain maximum caries inhibiting effect.

Pharmacokinetics of Fluoride

The majority of the fluorides are absorbed and transported in the body and subsequent excretion occurs in the form of fluoride ions. The absorption is passive in nature and no active transport mechanism is found to be involved. Peak plasma concentrations of fluoride usually occur within 30-60 minutes since half-time for absorption is approximately 30 minutes. Absorption from the stomach occurs freely and is inversely proportional to the pH of gastric contents. Dietary calcium and other cations in high concentrations form insoluble complexes with fluoride which reduces fluoride absorption from the gastrointestinal tract. About 10% of the daily fluoride intake is not absorbed from the gastrointestinal tract and elimination of absorbed fluoride occurs almost exclusively via the kidneys. Approximately 99% of fluoride in the body is associated with calcified tissues. Approximately 55% of the ingested fluoride is retained in the body in children and it is 36% in adults [4].

Systemic Fluorides

Systemic fluoride is a method of providing regular, low-level exposure to fluorides that are ingested into the body and become incorporated into forming tooth structures during tooth development stages. The actual mechanism of action of systemic fluorides is different from the topical fluoride with the former method being superior by making fluoride available widely in a cost-effective way. Systemic fluorides play an important role in reducing the susceptibility to caries.

Definition- Systemic fluoride is defined as the fluoride that is ingested by the mouth usually through a community's drinking water or supplements.

A relationship between natural fluoride, regulated levels of fluoride in drinking water and decline in the prevalence of dental caries, at the beginning of the 20th century, led to worldwide research into the action of fluoride. Systemic fluorides have both systemic effects on the tooth and also topical effects on the surface of the tooth.

Mechanism of Action of Fluoride

Conversion of Hydroxyapatite to Fluoridated Hydroxyapatite:

Dental enamel is a crystalline structure made of hydroxyapatite crystals. The hydroxyl ion in the hydroxyapatite crystal is liable to isomorphous substitution by fluoride ion due to:

- Similar charge (OH^-, F^-)
- The higher affinity of F^- for calcium
- Smaller size (OH^-=0.33A^0, F^-= 0.29A^0)

This hydroxyl ion replacement with fluoride ion renders the hydroxyapatite crystal more stable and more resistant to dissolution by acid. Hydroxyapatite crystals of enamel have inherent voids due to missing hydroxyl groups, ingested fluorides fill these voids, thus crystals attain stability with the formation of more and stronger hydrogen bonds. This leads to lower solubility of enamel crystals, hence greater resistance to dissolution in acids (Fig. **4**) [5].

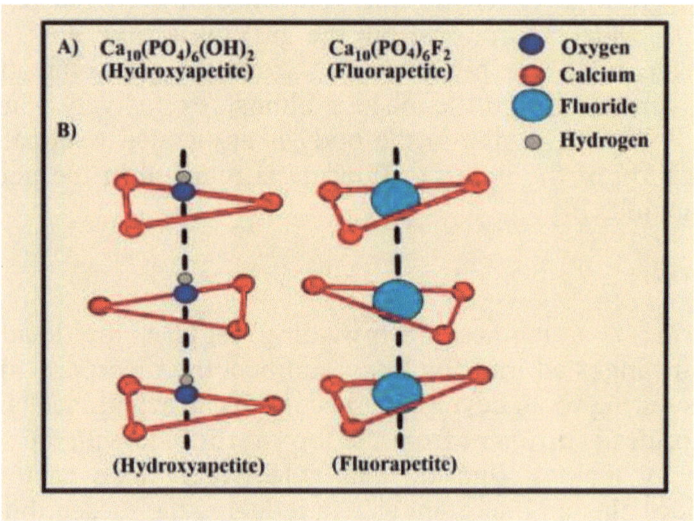

Fig (4). Crystalline structure of Hydroxyapatite and Fluorapatite crystals.

In the crystal, the orientation of OH^- is reversed at various places with some OH^- pointing upwards and some downwards. When this reversal occurs, two adjacent OH^- cannot point in the opposite direction because H atoms will be too close and would not fit in the lattice. A vacancy or void occurs which introduces instability into the crystal and increases its solubility. As the dimensions of F^- and OH^- are similar, F fills the vacancy and gets attached to OH^- by hydrogen bonds (Fig. **5a**, **b**). This has been proved by several studies in which fluoridated hydroxyapatite is less soluble in-vitro as compared to hydroxyapatite alone. Hence teeth that acquire a high level of fluoride during development are supposed to have greater resistance to caries (Fig. **6**).

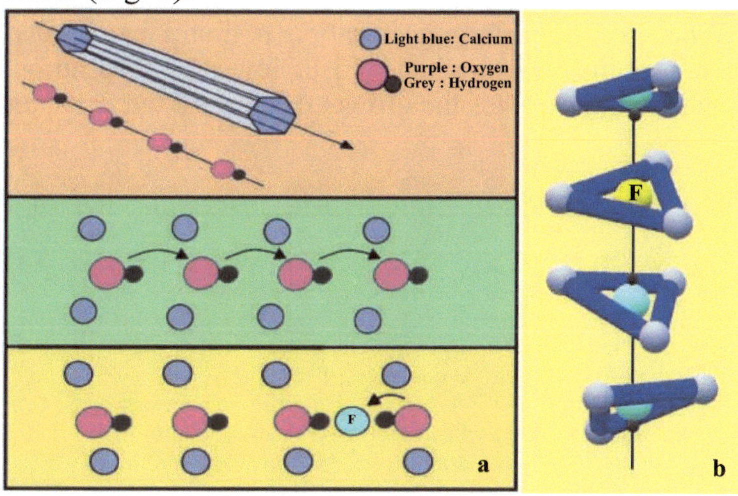

Fig (5). **a-** Conversion of Hydroxyapatite to Fluor hydroxyapatite crystals, **b-** 3D view of fluor hydroxyapatite crystals.

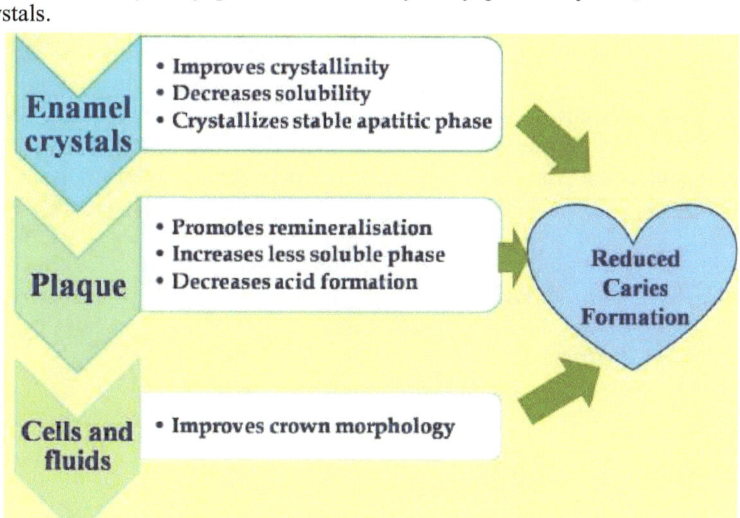

Fig (6). Mechanism of action of fluorides.

Increased Rate of Post-Eruptive Maturation

When a tooth erupts in the oral cavity, there are certain areas of the tooth which are yet to be completely developed. Fluoride when present increases the deposition of minerals in these areas. Hence newly erupted tooth becomes more resistant to acid attack by deposition of both organic material and inorganic mineral ions on the enamel surface.

Interference with Microbial Activity

Fluoride or hydrofluoric acid is capable of interfering with bacterial metabolism and growth. When the fluoride concentration within a bacterial cell reaches a certain level, it becomes bactericidal and at lower concentrations, fluoride is bacteriostatic which only reduces the growth of bacteria but does not kill them [5] (Table **1**).

Different ways of Interference of Fluoride with Microbial Activity

Table 1. Interference with microbial activity.

- The action of fluoride is mainly on inhibition of bacterial enzymes, enolase. It is a metalloenzyme of glycolysis that converts 2-phosphoglycerate (2PGA) to P-enolpyruvate (PEP) and requires Mg^{++} ion for its activity. F^- forms complex with Mg^{++} thereby inhibiting the enzyme and is increased when the environment is acidic. Fluoride diffuses into the bacterial cell in the form of hydrofluoric acid (HF) in acidic conditions which is more lethal.
- PEP (P-enolpyruvate) is required for the transportation of glucose in microbes like *S. Salivarius*.

  $$Glucose + PEP \rightarrow Glu - 6 - P + Pyruvate.$$

  The addition of F^- inhibits the production of PEP by inhibiting the enolase dependent step in glycolysis, thus indirectly inhibiting the transportation of glucose.
- Inhibits the transport of glucose through proton motive force (PMF). Bacterial cells are capable of pumping protons (H^+) out of the cytoplasm into the external medium. This creates an electrochemical proton gradient (Δ pH) between the cytoplasm and the external environment.
- Inhibits H^+ - ATPases which is a membrane bound enzyme necessary to extrude protons from the cell thereby maintaining the electrochemical gradient across the cell.
- Inhibits the other bacterial phosphatases which utilize Mg^{++} as the co-enzyme.
- Reduces the cellular content of both K^+ and inorganic phosphate. This results in a reduction in aciduance of streptococcal growth and metabolism.

Alteration of Tooth Morphology

Teeth that have developed under the influence of fluoride have been reported to possess shallow fissures, less steep cuspal inclines and rounder cusps. Systemic fluorides are effective if present during the time of tooth formation and development. After tooth eruption, topical fluorides play a vital role in increasing the resistance of the tooth to decay (Fig. **6**). Fluoridated drinking water is considered to have an additional beneficial effect because of prolonged contact with the tooth surface and consequently a topical mode of action along with systemic action [5].

Prevents Demineralization and Enhances Remineralization

The solubility of enamel increases dramatically with a decreased pH. A high concentration of fluoride in oral fluids leads to absorption and/or ion exchange at the crystal surface lowering enamel dissolution (Fig. **7**) [6].

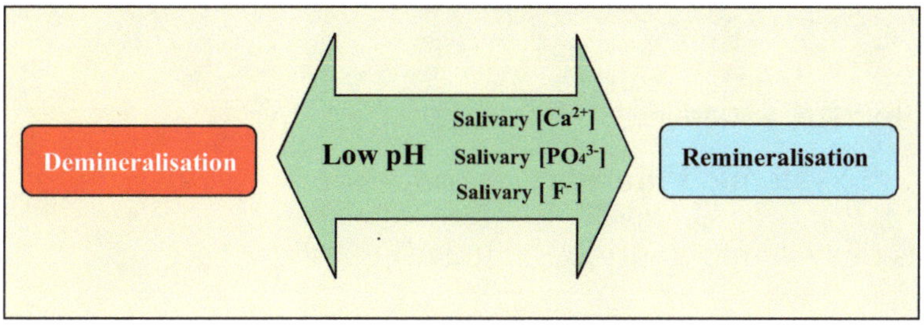

Fig (7). Demineralisation and Remineralisation process.

The formation of fluor hydroxyapatite (FHAP or FAP) results in a mineral with an even greater level of acid resistance. Thus, remineralization of the incipient carious lesion may result in the repair of the existing lesion with less soluble minerals and render that portion of the tooth less susceptible to future episodes of demineralization (Figs. **8** & **9**).

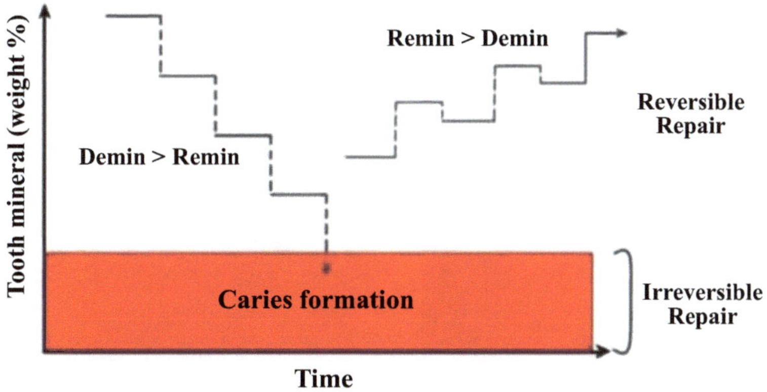

Fig (8). Demineralisation and Remineralisation cycle leading to reversible and irreversible repair.

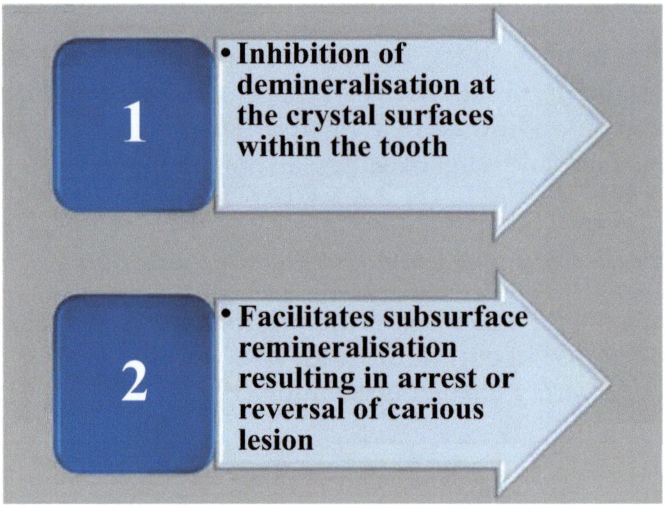

Fig (9). Effect of fluoride on demineralization and remineralization of tooth.

Classification of Systemic Fluorides

Various modes of systemic fluorides include (Fig **10**).

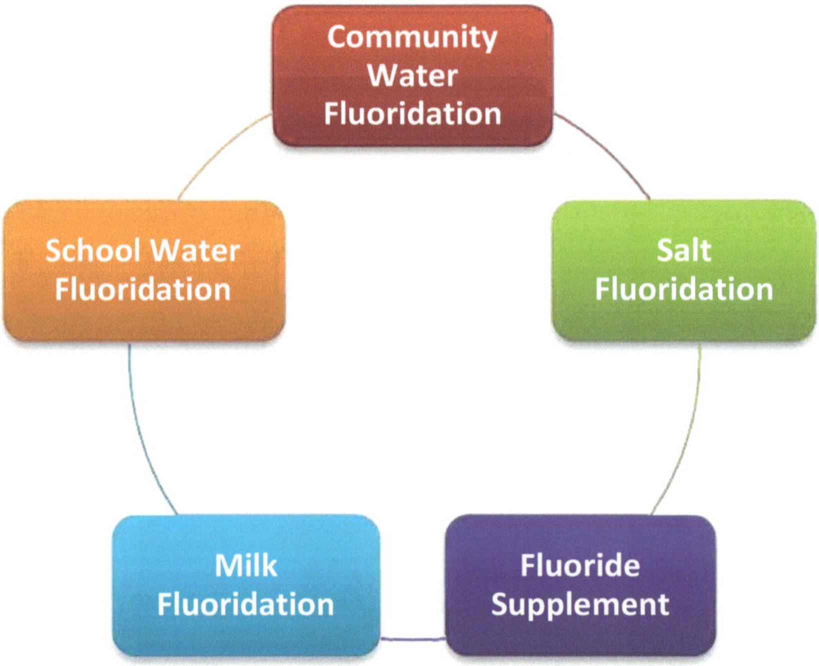

Fig (10). Classification of Systemic Fluorides.

COMMUNITY WATER FLUORIDATION

Definition

- It is defined as the controlled adjustment of the concentration of fluoride in a communal water supply to achieve maximum caries reduction and a clinically insignificant level of fluorosis.
- It is also defined as the upward adjustment of the concentration of fluoride ions in the public water supply in such a way that the concentration of fluoride ions in the water may be consistently maintained at 1 ppm.

Community water fluoridation is one of the most common methods of delivering fluorides which is a cost-effective and wide range of reach. In addition to systemic effects fluoridated water also has topical effects, thus maintaining continuous maintenance of low levels of fluoride in the mouth for cariostatic effect [2, 7].

History of Water Fluoridation

The relationship between the natural fluoride content of drinking-water with reduced caries prevalence was first shown in the 1930s. The practice of adjusting the natural concentration of fluoride in drinking water to improve dental health began in 1945 in the city of Grand Rapids in the USA.

Some of the Landmark Studies

Grand Rapid- Muskegon Study

On January 25th, 1945, sodium fluoride was added to the Grand Rapids water supply and Muskegon town was kept as a control. After 6 ½ years in 1951, Arnold et al. observed that the caries experience of 6–15-year-old children who are residents of Grand Rapids was half that of Muskegon (Fig. **11**).

Newburgh –Kingston Study

On the 2nd May 1945, sodium fluoride was added to the drinking water of Newburgh on the Hudson River and Kingston town was kept as a control. After 10 years of fluoridation Ast et al. in 1956 reported that the DMF rate decreased from 23.5% to 13.9%, establishing the fact of caries inhibitory property at 1 ppm fluoride in drinking water.

Evanston- Oak Park Study

It is one of the most detailed fluoridation studies, lasting for 14 years. In January

1946, a fluoridation experiment began in Evanston, Illinois and as the control town, the nearby community of Oak Park was selected. There was a reduction of 49% in DMF values after 14 years of fluoridation in Evanston.

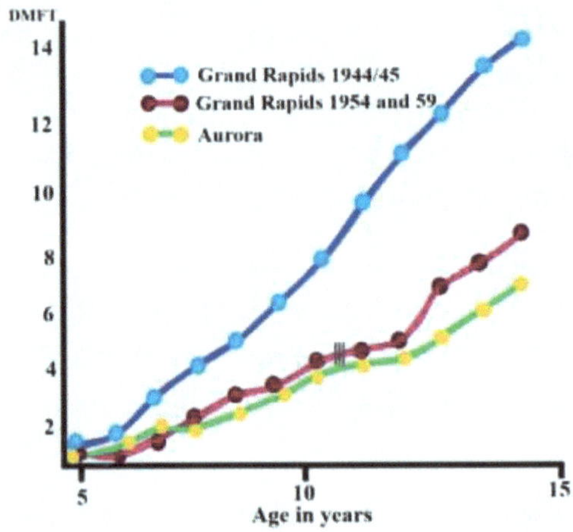

Fig (11). Comparison of DMFT index (Decayed, Missing, Filled Teeth) of Grand Rapids before fluoridation (1944/45) and 10-15 years after fluoridation (1954-59) and Aurora (a town in Illinois, USA which has naturally fluoridated water).

The Brantford- Sarnia-Stratford Fluoridation Caries Study

In June 1945, fluoride was added to the water supply of Brantford, Ontario, Canada, and the community of Sarnia acted as the control town. As an auxiliary control the community of Stratford, where fluoride was naturally present in drinking water at a level of 1.3 ppm was used. After 17 years of fluoridation in Brantford, Et Al in 1951, Brown and Poplove in 1965 reported that caries experience was similar to that of Stratford which is a natural fluoride area and it was 55% lower than Sarnia, the control town.

Tiel – Culemborg Study

In March 1953, community drinking water in Tiel was fluoridated to a level of 1.1 ppm and Culemborg acted as control which has a water fluoride level of 0.1 ppm. After 13 years of fluoridation, the number of anatomical sites of teeth affected by dental caries was 58% lower in Tiel than in Culemborg.

Requirements for Community water fluoridation

- Dental caries prevalence is high or moderate in the community, or caries levels are increasing.

- Countries that have attained a moderate level of technological and economic progress.
- Availability of municipal water supplies reaching many homes.
- Evidence that people drink water from the municipal supply rather than from wells or tanks.
- Availability of the requisite equipment needed in a treatment plant.
- Availability of a reliable supply of fluoride chemicals of acceptable quality.
- Availability of trained workers in the water treatment plant who can maintain the system.
- Availability of sufficient financial resources for the initial installation and running costs. (Fig. **12**) [2].

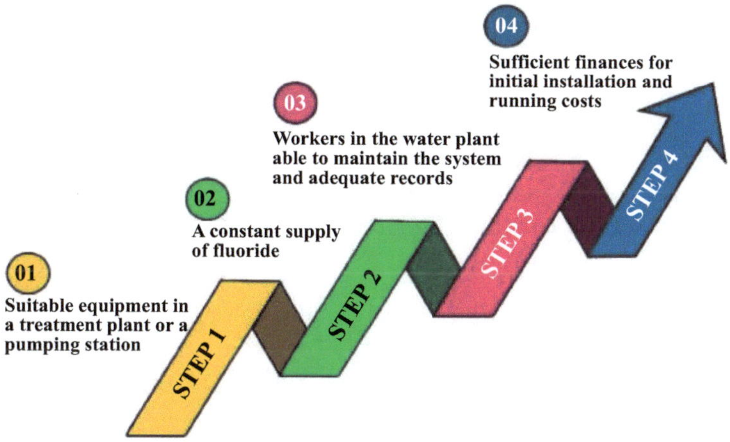

Fig (12). Requirements for Community Water Fluoridation.

Different forms of Fluoride used in Water Fluoridation

- Fluorspar
- Sodium fluoride
- Silicofluoride
- Sodium silicofluoride
- Hydrofluorosilicic acid
- Ammonium Silicofluoride

The 3 types of fluoridation equipment commonly used for fluoridation of water supplies are: (Fig. **13**).

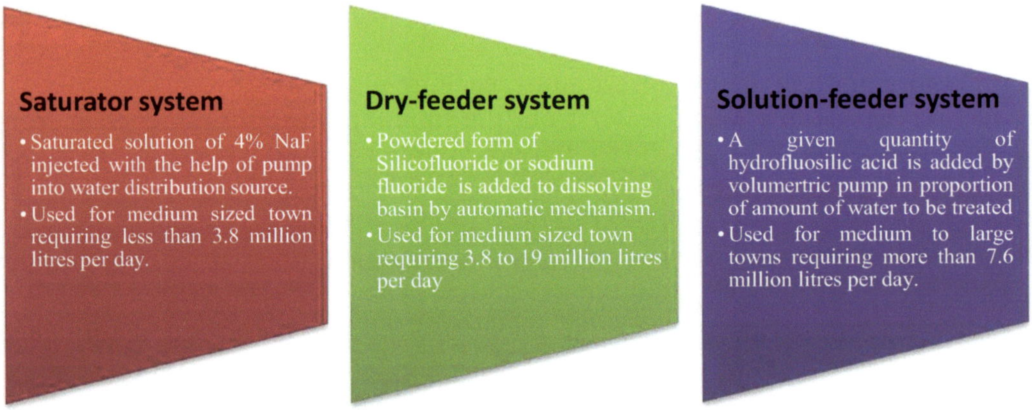

Fig (13). Different fluoridation systems for Community Water Fluoridation.

Estimation of Fluoride Concentration in Drinking Water

500ml of water to be evaluated is collected from its source in a clean dry polystyrene container. 2cc of 6N HCI is added to inhibit microbial growth or enzymatic changes & stored at 40^0C for analysis which is utilized within 2-3 months.

Estimation of Fluoride Concentration in the Water can be Done By

I. Fluoride electrode coupled with standard pH meter- Two pH meters, namely the Orion 901 microprocessor ion analyzer and Orion 407 are used. A specific ion meter has an inbuilt facility for converting the electrode potential into a concentration of fluoride in ppm. The unknown concentration of fluoride in a sample can be calculated by one of the following:

a. Typical Calibration Curve
b. By applying the electrode potential difference equation (Nernst equation)
c. Direct ppm reading.

2. Scot - Sanchis method : In this method, the reaction between the fluoride and the red zirconium lake of alizarine reagent is observed. The fluoride forms a colourless complex ion (ZrF6) and liberates free alizarine sulphuric acid, which is yellow in acid solution. When the amount of fluoride increases, the colour produced varies from yellow to red. The fluoride level in the sample is determined by comparing the colour during the reaction.

Recommended or most appropriate concentration of fluoride varies from 0.7 to 1.2 mg/L based on regional temperature. Regions with warmer climates tend to have a lesser level of fluoride recommendations as water consumption is more in those climates. The most appropriate concentration of fluoride meant the concentration at which maximum cariostatic effect is seen and minimum chances of enamel fluorosis.

Galagan and Vermillion (1957) gave an empirical formula for determining the optimal level of fluoride in drinking water-based daily fluid intake, body weight and climatic conditions. The optimal level of fluoride ppm F =0.34/E

E = -0.038+0.0062 t

E – Daily water intake in oz/lb. of body wt.

t – Maximum daily temperature of the region in degrees Fahrenheit

Richards et al made certain recommendations for water fluoridation based on the temperature of the region (Table **2**).

Table 2. Recommendations for water fluoridation based on temperature.

Temperature in °C	Recommended ppm
< 18.3	1.1 – 1.3
18.9 – 26.6	0.8-1.0
>26.7	0.5-0.7

Costs of Water Fluoridation

In the U.S.A, fluoridation was assessed in 1981 by the U.S. Public Health Service as costing an average of US $0.35 per person per year. In India, the approximate per capita cost is about Rs 0.25 per individual per year and the caries reduction of 50%. If there is a caries increment of 1 DMFS per year and the cost of restoring that tooth surface is Rs. 40/, the cost vs benefit ratio is 1: 160 inferring that for every Rs. 0.25 spent on water fluoridation, each individual would save Rs.40/.

Advantages and Disadvantages of Water Fluoridation

Water Defluorination

Defluoridation is defined as the downward adjustment of the level of fluoride in drinking water to the optimal level to the one that can arrest the prevalence of dental caries from causing an insignificant amount of fluorosis. There are five approved methods of defluoridation which are based on two principles (Table **3**) [8, 9].

i. An ion exchange process or adsorption and
ii. Addition of chemicals to water during treatment.

Five methods include

a. Bone charcoal
b. Contact precipitation
c. Nalgonda technique
d. Activated alumina
e. Clay

Table 3. Advantages and disadvantages of Community Water Fluoridation.

Advantages	Disadvantages
•Large number of people are benefited. •Consumption is regular •Fluoridated drinking water acts systemically during tooth formation to make dental enamel more resistant to dental decay, as well as has topical effect through the release in saliva after ingestion. •It is the least expensive way to provide fluoride to a large group of people. •Deprived communities where implementation of other health policies are less feasible.	•Interfere with human rights and ethical concerns. •Other modes are not considered •Centralized water supply is absent in most cities and rural areas.

Certain other advanced options like Electrodialysis, Distillation and Reverse osmosis are also available [2].

National Environmental Engineering Research Institute (NEERI) based in Nagpur in the year 1961 started the first work on defluoridation in India.

a. **Bone charcoal:** In contact with water, it absorbs most of the pollutants and fluoride. Drawback includes a foul taste of water treated by this method, hence careful planning is required and conflicts with the religious beliefs of certain communities.
b. **Contact precipitate:** In this method removal of fluoride is done by adding calcium and phosphate compounds and water is brought in contact with the already saturated bone charcoal medium.
c. **Nalgonda technique:** It was developed by National Environmental Engineering Research Institute (NEERI), Nagpur, India in the year 1974. The

process comprises the addition of aluminium sulphate and lime. This process involves the removal of fluoride by aluminium hydroxide micro-flocculation, sedimentation of micro-flocs in larger quantities and filtration of the flocs. During this flocculation process, small particles and negatively charged ions like fluoride are removed by attachment to the flocs by an electrostatic mechanism.

d. **Activated alumina:** When water passes through activated alumina, the aluminum grains adsorb pollutants and other remaining components like fluoride in the water.
e. **Clay:** It is an age-old method used in ancient Egyptian times. Clay is sedimentary earthy material that contains fine particles of hydrous aluminum silicates, minerals, and impurities. It can remove pollutants and fluoride.

SCHOOL WATER FLUORIDATION

It was first started at St. Thomas V. S Virgin Islands by US public health service division in 1954.

School water fluoridation is a suitable alternative to community water fluoridation because school-age children during school days would consume it, thus making it one of several effective alternatives for the prevention of dental caries in children. The concentration of the fluoride in the school water system must be adjusted upward to compensate for the reduced water intake since part of the day and year is spent at the school, and water consumption is less than in communities with fluoridated water supplies. The currently recommended level is 4.5 - 6.3 ppm of fluoride in the school water supply [3].

Advantages and Disadvantages

Venturi fluoride saturator is the most suitable for school fluoridation as they are simple fluoridators and effective in small instalments for small or medium-sized schools which requires almost no maintenance (Table **4**).

SALT FLUORIDATION

Fluoridated salt for the reduction of dental caries was first introduced in Switzerland in 1955 and later it expanded to many countries. It was only during 1980-82, table salt containing fluoride was authorized for human consumption. Salt containing fluoride reaches an individual in several ways like domestic salt, in bread, in large kitchens, and in meals at school exerting both systemic and topical effects [2].

Table 4. Advantages and disadvantages of School Water Fluoridation.

Advantages	Disadvantages
•Good results in reducing caries. • Minimal equipment. • Not expensive.	•Children do not receive the benefit until they go to school. •Not all children go to the school in poor countries and towns and villages. • Amount of water drunk cannot be regulated.

Salt fluoridation was cleared as a community preventive measure for dental caries only after clearing the following hurdles:

a. Successful clinical trials.
b. Recommendation of WHO, FDI and World Dental Federation.
c. European approval on including sodium and potassium fluoride as a food additive.
d. Local cultural, technological, and political adaptations.

WHO in 2007 approved the use of salt fluoridation as an alternative to water fluoridation in regions where it is not possible for certain reasons?

Fluoride concentration

Salt fluoridation is done by the addition of potassium fluoride and sodium fluoride to common salt to attain a concentration of 250-300 mg fluoride/kg salt. The community effectiveness of this concentration is like that of water fluoridation. The concentration of fluoride in the salt should appear on all commercially sold packages.

Requirements for Application of Fluoridated Salt

- Economic constraints for water fluoridation because of multiple sources of water.

- Regions with low fluoride drinking water.
- Political and community reluctance for water fluoridation.
- Centralized production of salt who expertise in adding and monitoring fluoride.
- Coordination between various sectors like health agencies, salt producers, communities, marketers, and distributors is mandatory [2].

Advantages and Disadvantages (Table 5)

Table 5. Advantages and disadvantages of salt fluoridation.

Advantages	Disdvantages
• No need for a community water supply as in the case of water fluoridation. • Cost is minimal compared to water fluoridation. • Individuals have choice to accept or reject it. • Non-fluoridated salt, like non-iodized salt, are available to the population.	• Fluoridated salt consumption is lowest when the need for fluorides is greatest - in the early years of life. • Risk of hypertension due to high salt consumption.

MILK FLUORIDATION

In early life, milk continues to be an essential food and it continues to give benefits from childhood and adolescence through old age. The concept of milk as a vehicle for fluoride started simultaneously in the US, Japan, and Switzerland in the 1950s. In 1988 first milk fluoridation scheme was developed in Bulgaria later it was expanded to other European countries.

Successful implementation of the milk fluoridation program depends on wider collaboration between health professionals, milk diaries, schools, and national and local governments [2, 3].

Fluoridated milk may be available in different forms like regular pasteurized milk, powdered milk, and milk cereal to children as daily needs at home and in schools including kindergarten.

Compounds used for milk fluoridation:

- Sodium fluoride
- Calcium fluoride
- Disodium Mono fluorophosphate

• Disodium silicofluoride.

The amount of fluoride required varies from 0.5mg to 0.85mg per child considering the child should drink 200ml of fluoridated milk per day for about 200 days a year.

Protection and reduction of the prevalence of caries in primary teeth it is recommended to consume fluoridated milk at early ages preferably before age of 4 years and at the eruption stage of a first permanent molar [2, 7].

Erickson stated that the bioavailability of fluoride from milk fluoridation is the same as that of availability of fluoride from water fluoridation 4hrs after consumption.

Fluoride level in the whole saliva increases within 20 to 60 minutes of ingestion of fluoridated milk. This is due to the re-secretion of absorbed fluoride through the salivary gland and retention of fluoride in the oral cavity after ingestion of fluoridated milk. Fluoridated milk also increases the plaque fluoride levels thus helping in remineralization.

Advantages and Disadvantages (Fig. 14)

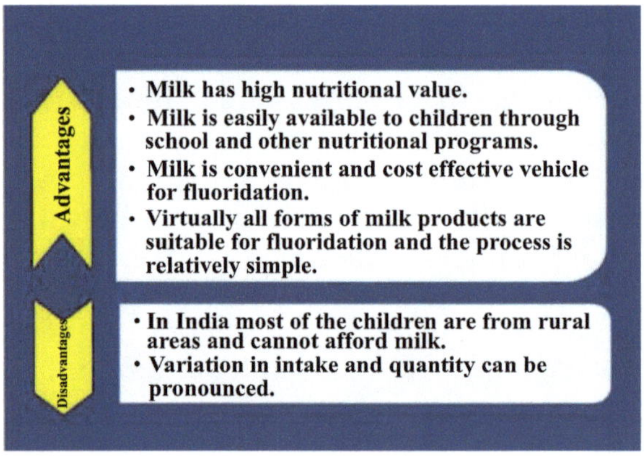

Fig (14). Advantages and disadvantages of Milk Fluoridation.

DIETARY FLUORIDE SUPPLEMENTS

Fluoride supplements were first introduced in the late 1940s and were intended as a substitute for fluoridated water for children in non-fluoridated areas. The most common method of systemic or dietary supplements includes [2]:

1. Fluoride drops with/ without vitamins.

2. Fluoride tablets with/ without vitamins

3. Lozenges intended to be sucked slowly or permitted to dissolve slowly in the mouth.

The most used Fluoride compounds are Sodium fluoride (NaF) and Acidulated phosphate fluoride (APF).

Fluoride tablets: They are available in 0.25mg, 0.5mg and 1mg of fluoride and in combination with vitamins they are available in 0.5mg and 1mg. Children should be motivated to chew and swish the fluoride tablet or allowed to dissolve in the mouth before swallowing. This facilitates both systemic and topical effects as fluoride comes in contact with the tooth surface [10].

Fluoride lozenges: Available in the same doses as tablets, lozenges should be sucked for topical and systemic effects.

Fluoride drops: It consists of a solution of sodium fluoride added to a child's drinking water or fruit juice by dropper. Mainly advised for children who have difficulty in chewing or swallowing tablets. Available in dose of 0.5mg/ml and with vitamins they are available in dose of 0.25mg/ml and 0.5mg/ml. The chances of inappropriate dose tendency are more as the volume of drops from the droppers may vary.

Indications for Use

- In areas where there are no central water supplies, where the fluoride concentrations of well-waters are low and where parental motivation is extremely high.
- As an interim measure in these communities with a central water system that has not yet implemented community water fluoridation.
- In areas where water fluoridation or salt fluoridation schemes cannot be implemented.
- An occupationally related situation where the parents need to shift the residence due to frequent change or workplace.

The Council on Dental Therapeutics of the American Dental Association recommends the dosage schedule for dietary fluoride supplements (Table **6**).

The dosage of fluoride dietary supplements is calculated on the following factors:

Target Population-Supplements are recommended for children residing in areas with inadequate water fluoridation. Supplements should be prescribed for daily use by infants and children up to 13 years of age. They may be prescribed for patients up to 16 years of age for added benefits to third molars (Fig **15**).

Table 6. Dosage of dietary fluorides according to the American dental association.

Age	Fluoride ion level in drinking water (ppm*)		
	Less than 0.3	**0.3 to 0.6**	**Greater than 0.6**
Birth to 6 months	none	none	none
6 months to 3 years	0.25mg/day**	none	none
3 years to 6 years	0.50mg/day	0.25mg/day	none
6 years to 16 years	1.0 mg/day	0.50mg/day	none
***1.0 part per million (ppm) = 1 milligram per litre (mg/L) **2.2 mg sodium fluoride contains 1 mg fluoride ion**			

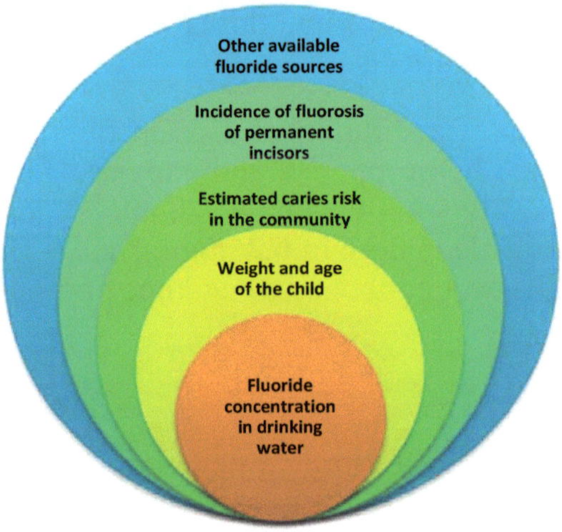

Fig (15). Factors influencing dosage of dietary fluoride supplements.

Benefits- Excellent caries reductions of 60 to 65% if used regularly from birth to 16 years. Fluoride supplements have the added advantages that provide both systemic and topical benefits for primary and permanent teeth.

Precautions- One of the major concerns with fluoride supplements is accidental ingestion which can cause stomach upset. They should be dispensed in a childproof container with a quantity of sodium fluoride from all the tablets in any container should not exceed 120mg. The risk of dental fluorosis reduces if the proper regimen is followed. Each day an individual should not consume more than 1 milligram of fluoride from all the available systemic sources.

Advantages and Disadvantages (Table 7)

Table 7. Advantages and disadvantages of dietary fluoride supplements.

Advantages	Disadvantages
• Gives additional fluoride exposure to tooth in regions where caries incidence is more and need for maximizing anticariogenic property.	• Limited application in community health care measure • Since fluoride absorption from supplements occurs once daily it might result in enamel fluorosis.

Toxicity of Fluoride

Fluoride is considered a double-edged sword; inadequate ingestion is related to increased caries prevalence and excessive intake leads to toxicity. It can be acute or chronic (Fig. **16** and Table **8**).

Table 8. Chronic fluoride toxicity.

Effect	Dosage	Duration
Dental fluorosis	Greater than 2 times optimal	Until 5 years of age
Skeletal fluorosis	10 to 25 mg/day	10 to 20 years of age
Renal failure	5 to 10 mg/kg	6 to 12 months

Acute Toxicity of Fluorides

The quantity of fluoride ingested, and the age and the weight of the individual determine the severity of the acute toxic effect. Hydrofluoric acid is formed by the combination of fluoride with hydrogen in gastric juices. HF acid is a stomach irritant and causes nausea and vomiting, diarrhoea, increased salivation, dehydration, and thirst. After two to four hours fatality is possible if first aid is not administered. Certainly, a Lethal Dose (CLD) is equal to 32 to 64 mg of fluoride per kg of body/ weight and 8-16mg F/kg is considered a Safely Tolerated Dose (STD). Management of accidental ingestion of fluoride includes (Table **9**) [11].

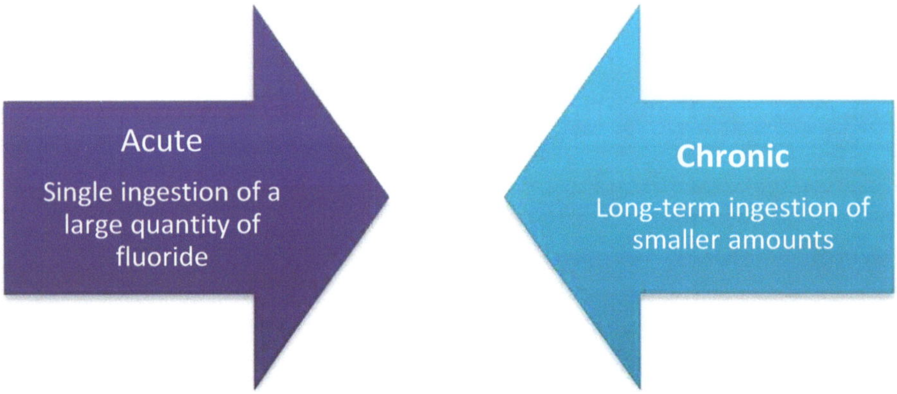

Fig (16). Types of fluoride toxicity.

Table 9. Management of acute fluoride toxicity by accidental ingestion of fluoride.

Milligram fluoride ion per kilogram body weight*	Treatment
Less than 5.0 mg/kg	• Calcium (milk) is given orally, to relieve GI symptoms. Observe for a few hours. • Inducing vomiting is not necessary
More than 5.0mg/ kg	• Inducing vomiting to an empty stomach with an emetic. • For children with Down's syndrome or severe mental retardation and with depressed gag reflex (age less than 6 months old) induced vomiting is contraindicated and endotracheal intubation should be performed before gastric lavage. • Soluble calcium in liquid form (*e.g.,* Milk, 5% calcium gluconate or calcium lactate solution) should be given. • Admit to hospital and observe for a few hours.
More than 15 mg / kg	• Admit to the hospital immediately and induce vomiting. • Cardiac monitoring should be done for arrhythmia. Observe for the peak in T-waves and prolonged Q-T intervals. • 10 ml of 10% calcium gluconate solution should be slowly administered intravenously. Additional doses may be given if clinical signs of tetany or Q-T interval prolongation develop. • Electrolytes, especially calcium and potassium should be monitored. Adequate urine output should be maintained using diuretics if necessary. • General supportive measures for shock

* Average weight/age, 1-2 years = 10 kg; 2-4years = 15 kg; 4-6 years =20 kg; 6-8 years = 23 kg.

Chronic Fluoride Toxicity

It occurs due to the ingestion of small amounts of fluoride over a long period. The effect of chronic fluoride toxicity on enamel causes dental fluorosis and on bones causes skeletal fluorosis (Table **9**) [11].

Safety of Fluoride Supplements

It is recommended that a child consume no more than 1 mg of fluoride per day from fluoride supplements and drinking water. Fluoride supplements should be prescribed in communities for which the level of fluoride in the drinking water is 0.7 ppm or less.

Frequent use of Small Amounts of Fluoride

Daily and regular exposure to low levels of fluoride will drastically reduce the risk of tooth decay for all age groups. This recommendation strongly supports using drinking water with optimal levels of fluoride which is followed by self-care practices such as brushing teeth twice a day with fluoridated toothpaste.

***a. Use supplements and high concentration fluoride products judiciously*:** For children with high risk for decay and who live in communities that have low fluoride concentration in their drinking water, fluoride supplements and professionally applied gels, foams and varnishes which has high fluoride concentration is recommended.

b. Parents should monitor the fluoride intake of children younger than 6 years old: For tooth development, the first, six years of life are an important period and any overuse of fluoride during this period can result in enamel fluorosis which is a developmental condition of tooth enamel appearing as white lines or spots. During the process of preventing early tooth decay, monitoring fluoride sources by parents is mandatory to reduce the occurrence of white spots. Children under the age of 6 years should use only a pea-sized amount of fluoride toothpaste and rice grain size for children less than 2 years of age.

c. Label bottled water with fluoride concentration: Consumers can make informed decisions on their fluoride intake if the labelling of bottled waters regarding fluoride concentration is voluntary.

d. Educating health professionals and the public: Collaborative efforts by professional organizations, public agencies and suppliers of oral care products are needed to encourage behaviour change to facilitate improved, coordinated use of fluoride products and regimens currently available.

CONCLUSION

Fluoride is a naturally occurring element that has many advantageous implications on the health of human beings if used appropriately. Fluoride is used worldwide as a preventive agent to decrease the incidence of caries and remains a standard recommendation. Understanding the mechanism of action of fluoride and its adverse effects if used inappropriately is imperative to obtain effective and efficient use of fluoride. They have both systemic effects on the tooth before the eruption and topical effects after the eruption of the tooth which makes the tooth caries resistant. The cost of any fluoridation method would be significantly less than the cost of treating the carious process of the tooth. Hence fluorides are highly recommended for public health prevention of dental caries.

CONSENT FOR PUBLICATION

Not applicable.

CONFLICT OF INTEREST

The authors declare no conflict of interest, financial or otherwise.

ACKNOWLEDGEMENT

Declared none.

REFERENCES

[1] Kanduti D, Sterbenk P, Artnik . Fluoride: A review of use and effects on health. Mater Sociomed 2016; 28(2): 133-7.
[http://dx.doi.org/10.5455/msm.2016.28.133-137] [PMID: 27147921]

[2] O'Mullane DM, Baez RJ, Jones S, *et al.* Fluoride and Oral Health. Community Dent Health 2016; 33(2): 69-99.
[PMID: 27352462]

[3] Buzalaf MAR. Review of fluoride intake and appropriateness of current guidelines. Adv Dent Res 2018; 29(2): 157-66.
[http://dx.doi.org/10.1177/0022034517750850] [PMID: 29461104]

[4] Mahmood M, Azevedo LB, Maguire A, Buzalaf M, Zohoori FV. Pharmacokinetics of fluoride in human adults: The effect of exercise. Chemosphere 2021; 262: 127796.
[http://dx.doi.org/10.1016/j.chemosphere.2020.127796] [PMID: 32755695]

[5] Rošin-Grget K, Peroš K, Sutej I, Bašić K. The cariostatic mechanisms of fluoride. Acta Med Acad 2013; 42(2): 179-88.
[http://dx.doi.org/10.5644/ama2006-124.85] [PMID: 24308397]

[6] Slayton RL, Urquhart O, Araujo MWB, *et al.* Evidence-based clinical practice guideline on nonrestorative treatments for carious lesions. J Am Dent Assoc 2018; 149(10): 837-849.e19.
[http://dx.doi.org/10.1016/j.adaj.2018.07.002] [PMID: 30261951]

[7] Aoun A, Darwiche F, Hayek SA, Doumit J. The fluoride debate: The Pros and Cons of fluoridation. Prev Nutr Food Sci 2018; 23(3): 171-80.

[http://dx.doi.org/10.3746/pnf.2018.23.3.171] [PMID: 30386744]

[8] Mobeen N, Kumar P. Defluoridtaion techniques- A critical review. Asian J Pharm Clin Res 2017; 10(6): 64-71.
[http://dx.doi.org/10.22159/ajpcr.2017.v10i6.13942]

[9] Biradar SV. Defluoridation – A review. Asian Technology and Innovation 2018; 6(27): 1-8.

[10] Goldberg M. Goldberg M. Fluorides in dental tissues: Caries Prevention and Fluorosis. JSM dent. 2020; 8(1): 1123.

[11] Martínez-Mier EA. Fluoride. J Evid Based Complementary Altern Med 2012; 17(1): 28-32.
[http://dx.doi.org/10.1177/2156587211428076]

CHAPTER 14

Topical Application of Fluorides

Mousumi Goswami[1,*] and **Palak Jain**[1]

[1] *Department of Pediatric and Preventive Dentistry, I.T.S. College of Dental Sciences and Research Center, Noida, Uttar Pradesh, India*

Abstract: Fluoride is present in natural water sources and occurs as an ionic form of fluorine trace element. It is a safe and effective agent used primarily to prevent dental caries, especially in children. Fluoride can remineralize calcium hydroxyapatite crystals in enamel by forming acid-resistant calcium fluorapatite crystals. It can be administered topically as well as systemically. Topical fluorides form a vital part of preventive oral health programs and help promote enamel remineralization, inhibit bacterial metabolism, and reduce the growth of bacteria in plaque. Various methods for delivering topical fluorides include self-applied toothpaste, gels, mouthwashes, professionally applied varnishes, and other gel forms. This chapter provides an overview of the different topically applied fluoride agents, their mechanism of action and the recommendations for their use in children.

Keywords: Dental Caries, Fluorides, Prevention.

INTRODUCTION

Fluoride has been the most critical caries preventive agent that has decreased the incidence of dental caries in recent decades. The Food and Drug Administration (FDA), United States and the World Health Organization (WHO) recognize fluoride as an essential nutrient and a vital trace element for normal growth and development. It can be administered systemically and topically and is a routine procedure performed in pediatric dentistry. The basic fluoride regimen recommended for preventive dental purposes is fluoridated toothpaste twice daily.

In 1969, WHO advocated using one ppm fluoride in community water and the introduction of topical fluorides for individual needs [1]. In communities with access to water fluoridation, topical fluoride application is limited to individuals at moderate to high risk for developing caries. Regular topical application may be considered for children in areas lacking systemic fluoridation facilities, having

* **Corresponding author Mousumi Goswami:** Department of Pediatric and Preventive Dentistry, I.T.S. College of Dental Sciences and Research Center, Noida, Uttar Pradesh, India; E-mail: mousumi_leo@yahoo.co.in

Satyawan Damle, Ritesh Kalaskar & Dhanashree Sakhare (Eds.)

suboptimal fluoride in drinking water and minimal usage of fluoride dentifrice duc to a lack of knowlcdgc [1].

Topical fluorides are fluoride-containing agents applied to the tooth surfaces at regular intervals to prevent caries. They exhibit anti-caries action by increasing the fluoride concentration in the outermost enamel surface [2].

Topical fluorides in the form of gels, foams, toothpaste and varnishes are considered the standard cornerstone in caries prevention for children and adolescents. Levels of fluoride in the saliva are crucial to assess the effectiveness of any topical fluoride agent. Salivary fluoride levels as low as 0.03–0.5 mg/L are considered effective and adequate to limit the demineralization process and promote enamel remineralization [3].

The protective ability of fluoride against dental caries is mainly due to its topical action and renders maximum protection to the smooth enamel surfaces. Consistent low fluoride levels in the oral environment prevent caries more effectively than high fluoride concentration with a prolonged time interval between subsequent exposures.

General Mechanism of Action of Topical Fluorides [4]

- Increased resistance to demineralization of the tooth structure.
- Enhancing remineralization of the demineralized tooth structure.
- Inhibition of the bacterial metabolic enzymes (enolase) necessary for acid formation.
- Inhibition of the adhesion of the plaque/ biofilm to the tooth structure.

Topical Fluoride Delivery Methods

Topical fluorides can be self-applied and professionally applied (Fig. **1**).

Self-Applied Fluorides

Individual patients may use self-applied fluoride agents independently but only at a dental professional's recommendation. They contain fluoride in low concentrations ranging from 200-1000 ppm or 0.2-1.0 mg F/ml. Various types of self-applied fluorides used are:

1) Fluoride Dentifrices

Fluoride dentifrices are comprised primarily of abrasive or polishing agents, detergents, binders, and flavouring agents. Sodium fluoride is the first active agent added to conventional dentifrices with dicalcium phosphate abrasives. It was followed by stannous fluoride incorporation, which was recognized and approved by the FDA (Food and Drug Administration) and ADA (American Dental Association).

Individuals brushing their teeth twice daily or more using dentifrices containing 1000 ppm or 1500 ppm or 2500 ppm of fluoride have been seen to significantly reduce the prevalence of caries [5].

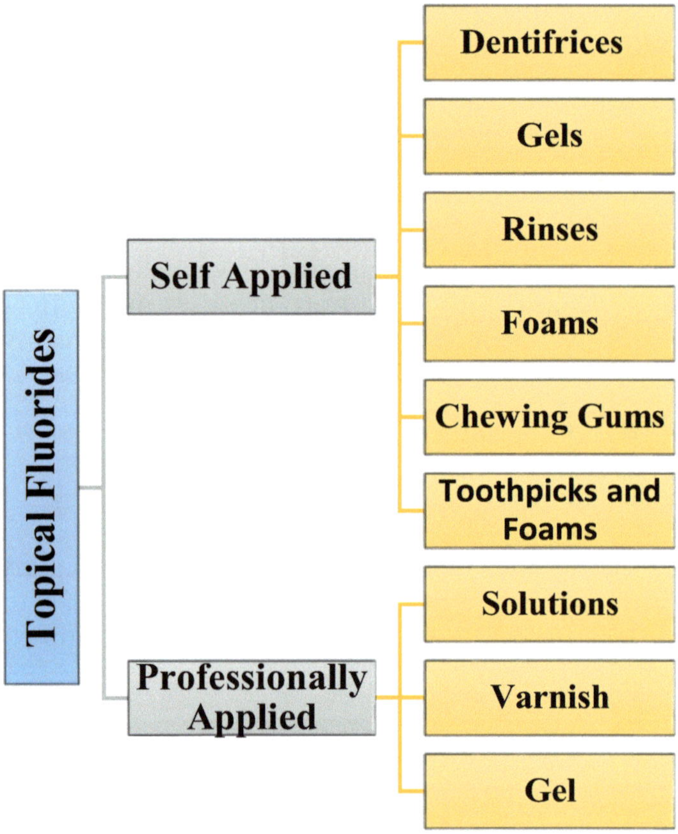

Fig (1). Illustrative diagram showing types of topical fluorides.

Fluoride Compounds in Dentifrices

- Sodium Fluoride
- Stannous Fluoride
- Monofluorophosphate
- Amine Fluoride
- Sodium hexametaphosphate

Fluoride Mouth Rinses

The use of fluoride mouth rinses was first stated in 1946 by Bibby et al. The Council of Dental Therapeutics of American Dental Association in 1979 recognized mouth rinses of neutral sodium fluoride and acidulated phosphate fluoride as effective agents for caries reduction.

Sodium Fluoride Mouth Rinse

These formulations are recommended as 0.2% (900ppm F) for weekly use or 0.05% (225 ppm F) for daily use. Before expectoration, a forceful swishing of 10ml of the mouth rinse around the mouth for 60 seconds is advised [6].

Preparation: At-home preparation for daily use involves the dissolution of 200mg NaF tablet (10mg NaF& lactose as filler) in 5 teaspoons of freshwater (approx. 25 ml). For the weekly regime, 2gm of NaF powder is dissolved in 1000ml of water. Preparation of 0.2% rinsing solution for schools may be done by dissolving 2 grams sodium fluoride powder in 100 ml of water [7].

Fluoride Gels

Gel-based fluoride agents include neutral sodium fluoride and acidulated phosphate fluoride (APF) with 5000 ppm fluoride concentration and stannous fluoride with 1000 ppm Fluoride. They are indicated in patients with moderate to severe caries activity. Fluoride in gel forms can be applied using foam-lined trays and allowed to contact teeth for 4 minutes.

Fluoride Foams

These have been developed to maintain an efficacious topical treatment and reduce the risk of fluoride toxicity.

Advantages

- They are lighter than conventional gel forms and require fewer amounts for topical application.
- The cleansing action by reducing surface tension allows the foam to enter the interproximal surfaces.
- These can be recommended for home use since they do not require suctioning.

Fluoridated Toothpicks and Dental Floss

Floss can aid in delivering topical fluoride in the proximal areas. Fluoridated toothpicks contain 0.1-0.2 mg F/ pick, whereas flosses are fluoridated with 0.3 mg

F/meter. It has also been seen that NaF impregnated toothpick promotes quick release of fluoride [8].

Fluoridated Chewing Gums

They contain fluoride in the range of 0.2-0.3 mgF/gm and are recommended in individuals with xerostomia as they aid in stimulating salivary secretions [9].

Professionally Applied Fluoride

It includes fluoride solutions, gels and varnishes (Tables **1-5**).

Solutions

Table 1. Table showing 2% NaF details.

Amount Of ppm	pH	Application Technique	No. of applications/ year
9,040 ppm	7	Knutson & Feldman technique (1948)	Four (at weekly intervals) At3, 7, 11 and 13 years of age.

Knutson and Feldman technique: The teeth are cleaned and isolated using sterilized cotton rolls and suctioning, and a 2% sodium fluoride solution is applied. Contact time of solution with teeth is approximately 3-4 minutes. The patient is then instructed to avoid eating, drinking or rinsing for the next 30 minutes.

Choking off phenomenon: NaF solution, when applied to the tooth surface, reacts with hydroxyapatite crystals resulting in the rapid formation of a large quantity of $CaF_{2,}$ which acts as a fluoride reservoir. An abrupt and significant cessation follows this in the rate of formation of CaF_2 that inhibits the subsequent uptake and diffusion of fluoride from the topical solution.

Advantages

- Chemically stable
- Acceptable taste owing to neutral pH of the solution.
- No gingival irritation or discoloration of teeth.
- Economical and cost-effective.

Disadvantages

- More follow up visits within a short period.

Table 2. Showing 8% SnF_2 solution details.

Amount of ppm	pH	Application Technique	No. of Applications/Year
19,360 ppm	2.4-2.8	Muhler technique (1957)	Single application annually.

Muhler technique (1957): Each tooth surface is cleaned and polished using pumice followed by isolation with cotton rolls and saliva ejectors and drying teeth with compressed air. One quadrant can be treated at one time. A freshly prepared 8% SnF_2 solution is continuously applied using a cotton applicator over the teeth, and the teeth are kept moist with the solution for 4 minutes. The solution is reapplied every 15-30 sec.

Advantages

- Tin and fluoride rapidly penetrate within 30 seconds.
- Acid-resistant tin fluorophosphate ($Sn_3F_3PO_4$) complex forms on the enamel surface.

Disadvantages

- Highly unstable in aqueous solution form and fresh preparation required each time.
- Unpleasant metallic taste.
- Gingival irritation may occur.
- Tooth discoloration may occur, especially in hypo calcified areas.
- Staining of tooth restoration margins may occur.

Table 3. Table showing 1.23% APF (Brudevold solution) details.

Amount of ppm	pH	Application Technique	No. of Applications/Year
12,300 ppm	3	Brudevold technique (1963)	Semi-annual/ Quarterly

Brudevold technique (1963): Prophylaxis of teeth is followed by isolation with cotton rolls on both lingual and buccal sides. APF solution is continuously and repeatedly applied using cotton applicators, and the teeth are kept moist for 4 minutes. Floss may be drawn through inter-proximal sites to ensure the application of the solution to these areas. The patient is then instructed to avoid drinking or rinsing the mouth for half an hour post-treatment.

Advantages

- Higher fluoride uptake and 50% more effective as compared to NaF.
- Easy preparation and longer shelf life.

- Cost-effective

Disadvantages

- 4 minute contact time of solution with teeth is essential.
- Unpleasant acidic and bitter taste mandates the use of suction.

Gels

Table 4. Table showing 1.23% APF gel details.

Amount of ppm	pH	Application Technique	No. of Applications/Year
12,300 ppm	4-5	Brudevold technique (1963) (Fig **2**)	Semi-annual/ Quarterly

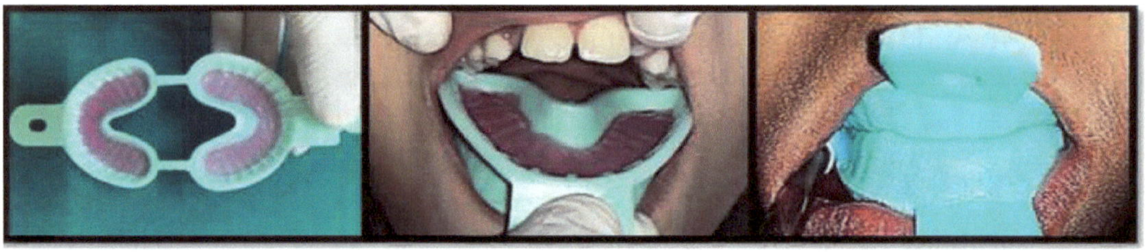

Fig (2). Application of Fluoride Gel: Loading the trays with APF gel, one-third of the trays are loaded, followed by Insertion of the loaded trays into the patient's mouth.

Brudevold technique (1963): APF gel is applied in the same manner with the exact mechanism of action as a topical solution. Various self-reusable/disposable trays in different sizes with sponge-like tray liners are available for its application.

Advantages

- Caries reduction efficacy is higher than APF solution.
- Thixotropic solution with an acceptable flavoured taste.
- It can be applied at home.
- Re-application is not required.

Disadvantages

- Gingival irritation may occur.
- Sensitivity in open carious lesions may be experienced, and therefore, restoration of teeth must be done before its application.

Varnishes

Table 5. Table showing varnish details.

Technique of Application	**Paint on technique (Fig. 3)**
Advantages	**Form a watertight protective seal that insulates against thermal and chemical challenges. With proper application and maintenance of oral hygiene, varnish can remain over the teeth surfaces for a prolonged period.**
Disadvantages	Patient compliance is required.
No. of Applications per year	Semi-annual

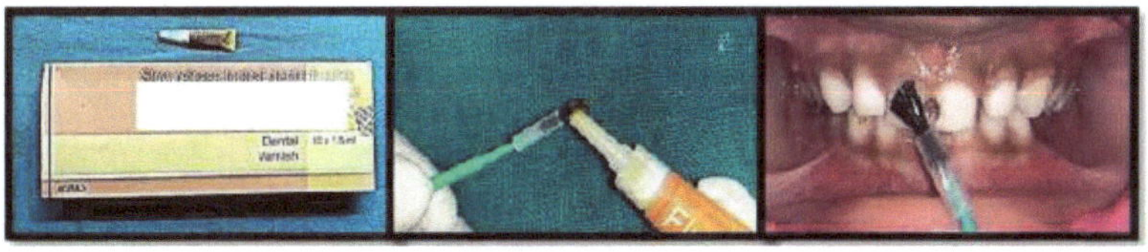

Fig (3). Fluoride Varnish application- Varnish is dropped onto a brush and painted onto the teeth surfaces.

Paint on technique: The patient is instructed to rinse the mouth, and teeth are isolated using cotton rolls. Additionally, saliva absorbers and ejectors can be used. It is followed by drying the teeth with compressed air. A cotton applicator is used to apply the varnish by swabbing or painting the tooth surfaces thoroughly. Reloading of fluoride varnish may be done continually for practical application.

Factors Affecting Uptake of Topical Fluorides

Certain factors are directly related, and some are indirectly related to the uptake of fluorides (Fig. **4**).

AAPD Recommendations [6] and European Directive for the Use of Fluorides [10]

Professional topical fluoride therapy in the form of 5% NaF varnish or 1.23% F gel is efficacious in reducing dental caries in children at caries risk. Home use of Prescription-strength 0.5 per cent fluoride gels and pastes and 0.09percent fluoride mouth rinse are an effective therapy for reducing chances of dental caries.

Tooth brushing frequency of twice a day using Fluoride toothpaste must be introduced as soon as the first tooth erupts. The toothpaste should be dispensed in the concentration and quantity recommended by the EAPD (Table **6**). Parents must assist or supervise children while brushing at least up to 7 years of age.

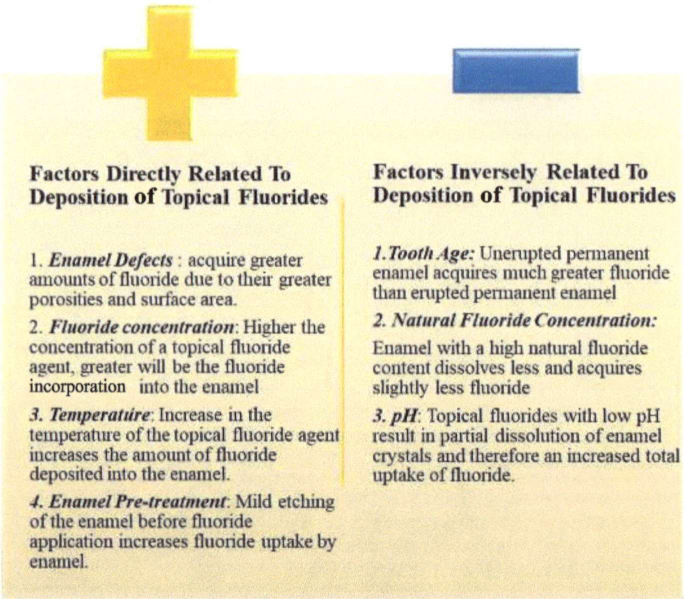

Fig (4). This figure showing factors affecting fluoride uptake.

Table 6. Recommended use of fluoride toothpaste for children by European Academy of Paediatric Dentistry (EAPD).

Age	Fluoride Concentration	Daily Use	Daily Amount
Six months-2 years	1000 ppm	Two times	Smear / Rice grain size
2-6 years	1000 ppm	Two times	Pea size
Six years and over	1450 ppm	Two times	1-2 cm

Recent Advances in Topical Fluoride Application

a) Silver diamine fluoride: Silver Diamine Fluoride (SDF) is a topical medication that can be used in varying concentrations; however, 38% is the most accepted for treating and preventing dental caries. It is a colourless, odourless liquid containing silver, ammonium and fluoride ions at a pH of 10.4 [11].

b) Slow-release fluoride devices: These devices release a predetermined quantity of fluoride inside the oral cavity over a long period when adhered to the tooth surfaces. They can release 0.02-0.2 ppm of fluoride for about 3-4months. Hydroxyapatite-Eudragit RS100. Diffusion Controlled Fluoride System is one of the latest slow-release F devices containing 18 mg of NaF and can release 0.15 mg F/day. Its use can significantly increase the salivary and urinary fluoride concentration for at least one month [12].

c) Elastomeric rings: To overcome the development of enamel white spot lesions during orthodontic treatment, F^- releasing biocompatible polyethene co-vinyl acetate rings have been fabricated that contain sodium fluoride in various percentages embedded into polyethene co-vinyl acetate polymer (PEVA) that aids in a well-controlled and efficient release of fluoride [13].

d) Fluoride containing restorative materials and prophylactic pastes: Fluoride releasing glass ionomer cement, composites, and prophylactic pastes may provide an additional benefit in preventive dentistry [14].

CONCLUSION

With the advances in dentistry, there has been a paradigm shift towards focusing on preventive aspects of controlling dental caries and enhancing oral health. Twice daily brushing with fluoridated toothpaste is considered the most effective regime in preventing caries. Professionally applied varnish, gel, and solution deliver more significant fluoride concentrations and promote remineralization and anti-caries effect. Dental professionals must counsel children and their parents/caregivers regarding the benefits of topical fluoride therapy and introduce regular fluoride application programs for those at a high risk of developing caries.

CONSENT FOR PUBLICATION

Not applicable.

CONFLICT OF INTEREST

The authors declare no conflict of interest, financial or otherwise.

ACKNOWLEDGEMENT

Declared none.

REFERENCES

[1] Whelton HP, Spencer AJ, Do LG, Rugg-Gunn AJ. Fluoride revolution and dental caries: evolution of policies for global use. J Dent Res 2019; 98(8): 837-46. [http://dx.doi.org/10.1177/0022034519843495] [PMID: 31282846]

[2] Harbi TAA, Meligy OAESE, Harbi SDA, Malik MA. Effectiveness of Topical Fluoride on Dental Caries: ALiterature Review. EC Microbiol 2020; 16(3): 1-9.

[3] Talwar M, Tewari A, Chawla HS, Sachdev V, Sharma S. Fluoride concentration in saliva following professional topical application of 2% sodium fluoride solution. Contemp Clin Dent 2019; 10(3): 423-7. [PMID: 32308314]

[4] ten Cate JM, Buzalaf MAR. Fluoride Mode of Action: Once There Was an Observant Dentist. J Dent Res 2019; 98(7): 725-30.

[http://dx.doi.org/10.1177/0022034519831604] [PMID: 31219410]

[5] Walsh T, Worthington HV, Glenny AM, Marinho VCC, Jeroncic A. Fluoride toothpastes of different concentrations for preventing dental caries. Cochrane Libr 2019; 3(3): CD007868. [http://dx.doi.org/10.1002/14651858.CD007868.pub3] [PMID: 30829399]

[6] American academy of pediatric dentistry fluoride therapy. The reference manual of pediatric dentistry. 2020; 288-91.

[7] Peter S. Essentials Of Public Health Dentistry. 6Ed, (Community Dentistry). ARYA, 2017.

[8] Särner B, Birkhed D, Huysmans MCDNJM, Ruben JL, Fidler V, Lingström P. Effect of fluoridated toothpicks and dental flosses on enamel and dentine and on plaque composition in situ. Caries Res 2005; 39(1): 52-9. [http://dx.doi.org/10.1159/000081657] [PMID: 15591735]

[9] Hassan TA, Aldik HBM, AL-Kadumi A. Release of Fluoride in Saliva the Use Chewing Gums with Different Fluoride Compounds NaMFP, SnF2 and Naf. Indian J Public Health Res Dev 2019; 10(10): 2019-23. [http://dx.doi.org/10.5958/0976-5506.2019.03145.0]

[10] Toumba KJ, Twetman S, Splieth C, Parnell C, van Loveren C, Lygidakis NA. Guidelines on the use of fluoride for caries prevention in children: an updated EAPD policy document. Eur Arch Paediatr Dent 2019; 20(6): 507-16. [http://dx.doi.org/10.1007/s40368-019-00464-2] [PMID: 31631242]

[11] Seifo N, Cassie H, Radford JR, Innes NPT. Silver diamine fluoride for managing carious lesions: an umbrella review. BMC Oral Health 2019; 19(1): 145. [http://dx.doi.org/10.1186/s12903-019-0830-5] [PMID: 31299955]

[12] Kachuie M, Khoroushi M. Prevention and treatment of white spot lesions in orthodontic patients. Contemp Clin Dent 2017; 8(1): 11-9. [http://dx.doi.org/10.4103/ccd.ccd_216_17] [PMID: 28566845]

[13] Ullah R, Zafar MS. Oral and dental delivery of fluoride: A review. Fluoride 2015; 48(3): 195.

[14] Bansal A, Ingle N, Kaur N, Ingle E. Recent advancements in fluoride: A systematic review. J Int Soc Prev Community Dent 2015; 5(5): 341-6. [http://dx.doi.org/10.4103/2231-0762.165927] [PMID: 26539383]

CHAPTER 15

Silver Diamine Fluoride and its Role in Prevention

Mousumi Goswami[1,*] and **Anam Mushtaq**[1]

[1] *Department of Pediatric and Preventive Dentistry, I.T.S. College of Dental Sciences and Research Center, Noida, Uttar Pradesh, India*

Abstract: Silver diamine fluoride (SDF) is a colourless and odourless combination of silver and fluoride solution with caries arresting properties. Clinical and in-vitro trials have proven its preventive efficacy for caries in high-risk individuals, which is considered a minimally invasive approach for arresting caries progression in cavitated teeth. This chapter gives an overview of the rationale of caries management by SDF, the mechanism of action, and the current evidence for its effectiveness as an anti-caries agent. The safety of SDF use in humans and its various limitations are also explained in the chapter.

Keywords: Anti-Caries Agent, Remineralization, Silver Diamine Fluoride.

INTRODUCTION

Silver diamine fluoride is a colourless liquid composed of silver, fluoride, and ammonia. It is available in various concentrations, of which 38% is considered the most effective. It is alkaline with a pH of 10. It forms a complex with ammonia; the silver particles have antimicrobial properties and act along with fluoride to prevent and arrest caries. SDF can arrest the progression of caries and prevent the development of new carious lesions. Its applicability as a preventive or therapeutic approach can help prevent or delay the requirement of extensive dental treatment until a child acquires a cooperative stage. SDF provides a much more easy-to-use and effective non-surgical alternative treatment for young patients with early childhood caries compared to traditional restorative options [1, 2].

Paradigm Shift

The bactericidal activity of silver ions has been known since ancient times. The first dental use of silver nitrate was in 1846 to treat erosion. Japan was the first country to approve SDF as a therapeutic agent in the 1960s. Since then, SDF has

* **Corresponding author Mousumi Goswami:** Department of Pediatric and Preventive Dentistry, I.T.S. College of Dental Sciences and Research Center, Noida, Uttar Pradesh, India; E-mail: mousumi_leo@yahoo.co.in

Satyawan Damle, Ritesh Kalaskar & Dhanashree Sakhare (Eds.)

been in the international market for over 40 years now, and in 2014, the United States Food and Drug Administration (FDA) cleared the use of SDF in the form of a commercially available 38% SDF solution [3].

Mechanism of Action [4-6]

Silver Diamine Fluoride Acts in the Following ways to Prevent and Halt the Caries Process (Fig. **1**).

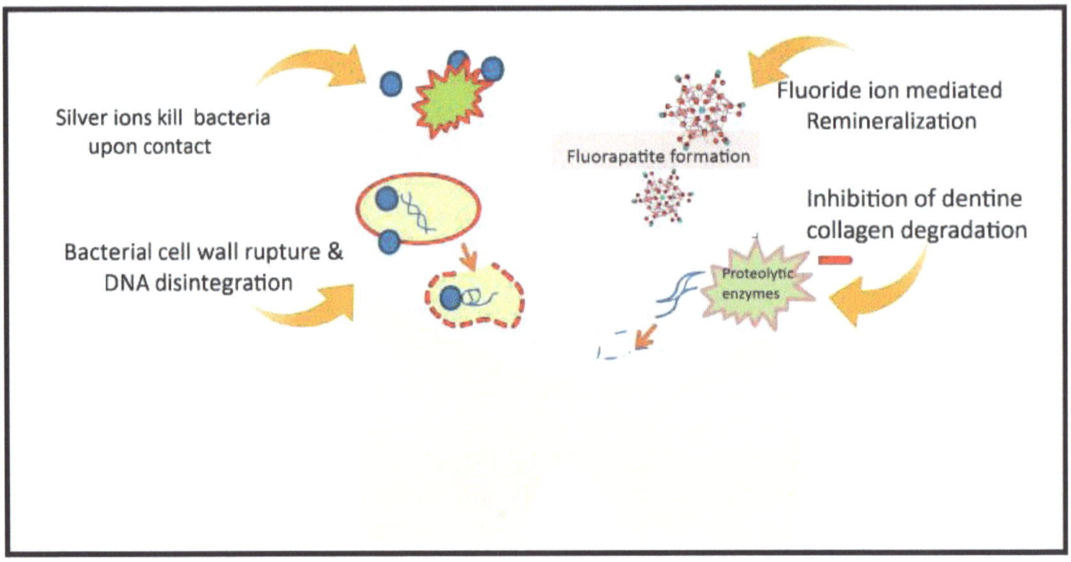

Fig. (1). Action of SDF on cariogenic bacteria.

- **Remineralization:** This is mediated by the fluoride ions (44,800 ppm) present in SDF that causes the formation of fluorapatite, silver phosphate and calcium fluoride compounds which enable remineralization and inhibit the demineralization process by rendering the treated surface more resistant to bacterial acids.
- **Bactericidal Activity:** The silver ion can penetrate up to 2 mm into a deep carious lesion to exhibit bactericidal effects. It interferes with bacterial metabolic processes by inhibiting DNA replication and cell wall synthesis leading to its rupture. The ionic silver may diminish the bacterial motility, or the organisms may be killed entirely. This inhibition occurs by the 'zombie effect' in which the active bacteria are killed upon contact with the silver-affected bacteria, ultimately causing plaque biofilm disintegration.
- **Inhibition of Collagen Degradation:** The progression of caries involves the destruction of the organic components of the tooth as well, which is comprised mainly of type 1 collagen. SDF can inhibit collagen degradation by inactivating

proteolytic enzymes like matrix metalloproteinase (MMP-2, MMP-8, MMP-9) and cathcpsins in dcntinc that arc a part of thc carics proccss.

The Overall Reaction can be Summarized as:

$$Ca_{10}(PO_4)_6(OH)_2 + Ag\ (NH_3)_2F = CaF_2 + Ag_3PO_4 + NH_4OH$$

The silver diamine solution reacts with the tooth minerals composed of the hydroxyapatite crystals forming a fluoride reservoir for remineralization. The silver compounds produced are responsible for the darkening of the lesion due to silver ion precipitation.

Indications and Contraindications of SDF (Fig. 2 and 3)

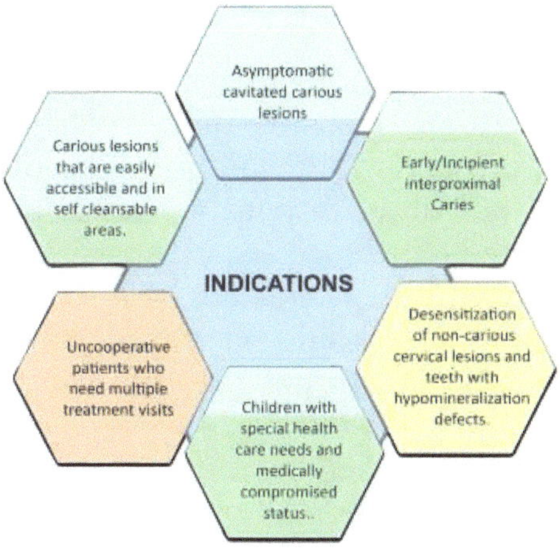

Fig. (2). Indications.

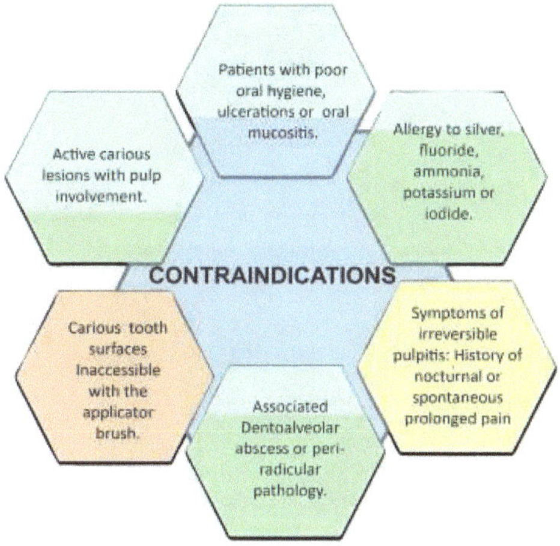

Fig. (3). Contraindications.

The technique of SDF application (Fig. **4**):

- Removes gross debris from cavities to allow adequate contact of SDF solution with carious dentin.
- Caries excavation before SDF application is not mandatory. It may be considered in aesthetic regions considering that it may reduce the areas of discoloration in carious dentin.
- A protective coating like petroleum jelly or cocoa butter is applied to the lips and skin to prevent tattooing with a brownish-black Henna-like appearance if the soft tissues contact the SDF solution.
- Isolation of areas to be treated must be done adequately using cotton rolls or other alternative isolation methods. Care must be taken not to accidentally coat the tooth surface in question, which may cause the ineffective application of SDF solution over it.
- A gentle flow of compressed air is used to dry the lesion area.
- Dispense a drop of SDF in a dispensing rubber/plastic cup. Bend the tip of a microsponge brush and dip it into the solution. Remove any excess liquid by dabbing the brush on the side of the dispensing container before application.
- Apply SDF onto the affected tooth surface and remove any excess solution using a gauze or cotton pellet to reduce any chances of systemic absorption.
- The contact time of the solution should be at least one minute. The application time is likely to be lesser in young patients and patients who are difficult to manage based on their cooperative ability.
- A gentle compressed airflow is used until the solution-treated region becomes dry. The area is kept isolated appropriately for as long as three minutes.

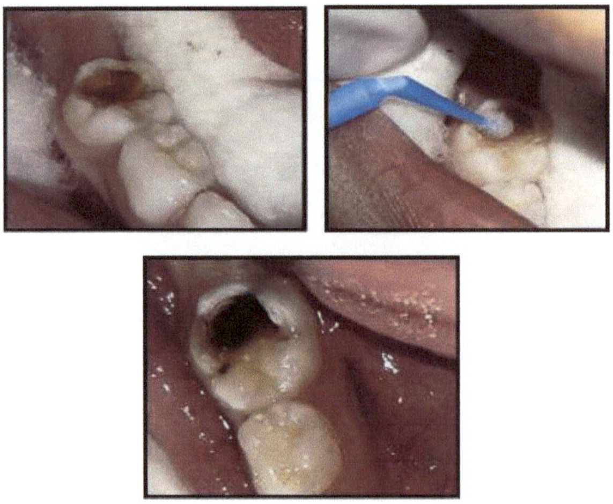

Fig. (4). SDF application in the primary mandibular second molar.

Additionally, the entire dentition may also be treated with 5% sodium fluoride varnish after localized SDF treatment as a preventive measure for the teeth and sites that have not been treated with SDF [7, 8].

SDF Application in Inter-Proximal Areas (Fig. 5)

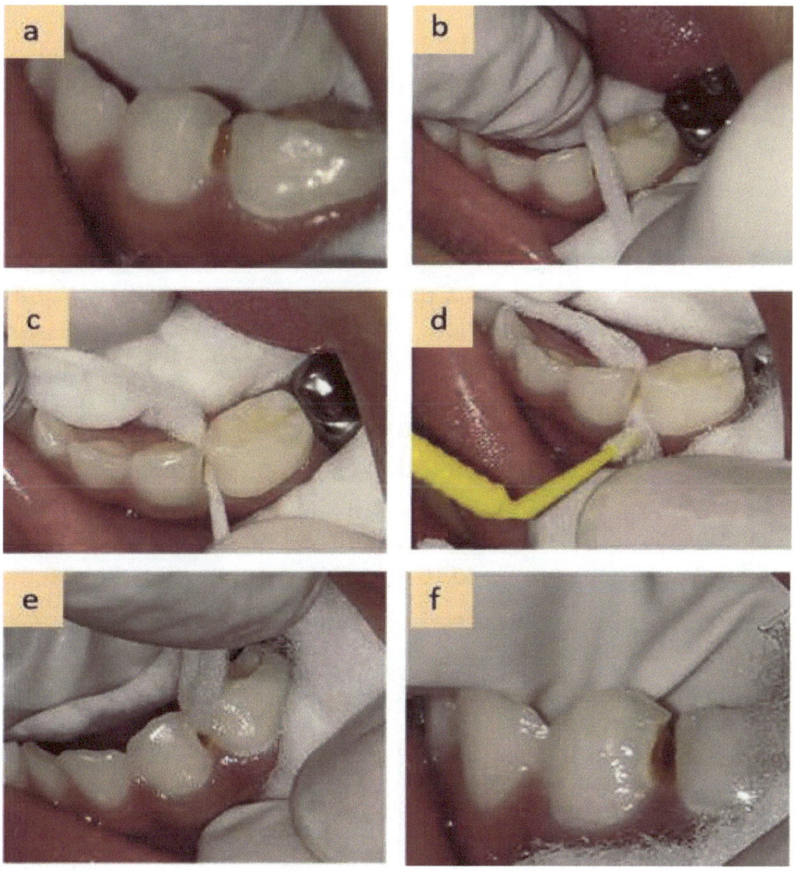

Fig. (5). SDF application on absorbent floss for interproximal areas followed by removal of floss in an occlusal direction.

To apply SDF in proximal lesions, the site is cleaned, isolated and air-dried, and a woven floss may be placed into the contact area. Silver diamine fluoride is applied lingually, buccally, and occlusal to the contact by saturating the floss with the solution using a micro-brush applicator. The floss is left in place for 1-3 minutes. Excess SDF may be dabbed away using a gauze piece. The floss is then removed by holding it by the two ends and pulling it out of the contact area in a gingivo-occlusal direction.

This may also be followed by sodium fluoride varnish application over the tooth.

The floss used for application must be absorbable and non-waxed.

Evidence Supporting the use of SDF as a Non-Restorative Treatment of Caries

The effectiveness of a single application of SDF in arresting carious lesions ranges from 47% to 90%, varying with the cavity size and the tooth location with anterior teeth showing an increased rate of arrest compared to posterior teeth (Fig. **6** and **7**). An umbrella review conducted by Seifo et al. in 2019 comprehensively summarized evidence from 11 systematic reviews on the use of SDF in children and adults [9]. They concluded that SDF effectively arrested coronal caries in the primary teeth and effectively controlled and prevented root caries in adults. However, the usefulness of SDF as a preventive agent in primary and permanent teeth in children was not supported by sufficient evidence. According to a systematic review by Rosenblatt et al., SDF showed a 96.1% caries arresting fraction compared to just 21.3% with fluoride varnishes. Also, the prevention fraction assessed with SDF was seen to be 70.3%. In comparison, it was 55.7% in the case of fluoride varnish, suggesting that SDF was more effective than fluoride varnishes in preventing and arresting carious lesions [10]. A meta-analysis of systematic reviews by Chibinski et al. concluded an overall caries arrestment by 89% at the end of one year compared to other active materials or placebo [11].

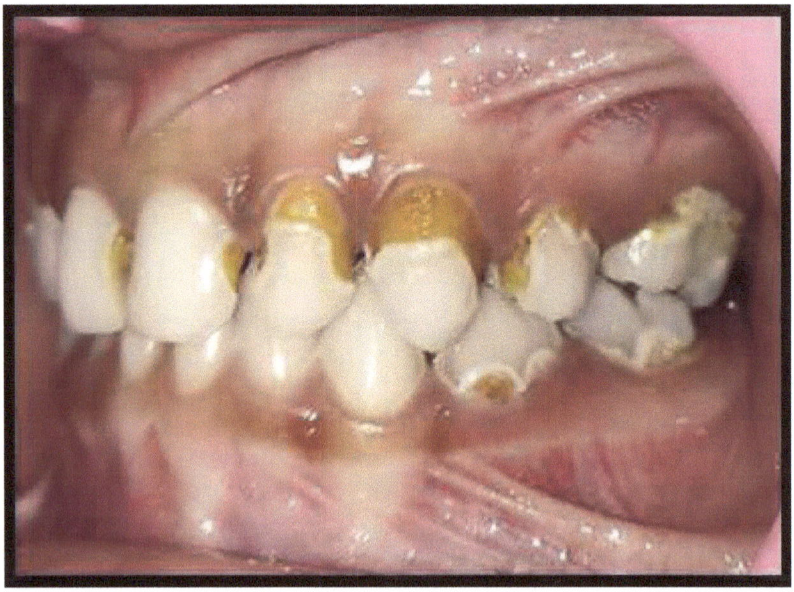

Fig. (6). Preoperative active Carious lesions (Pictures used are original and author's own clinical cases).

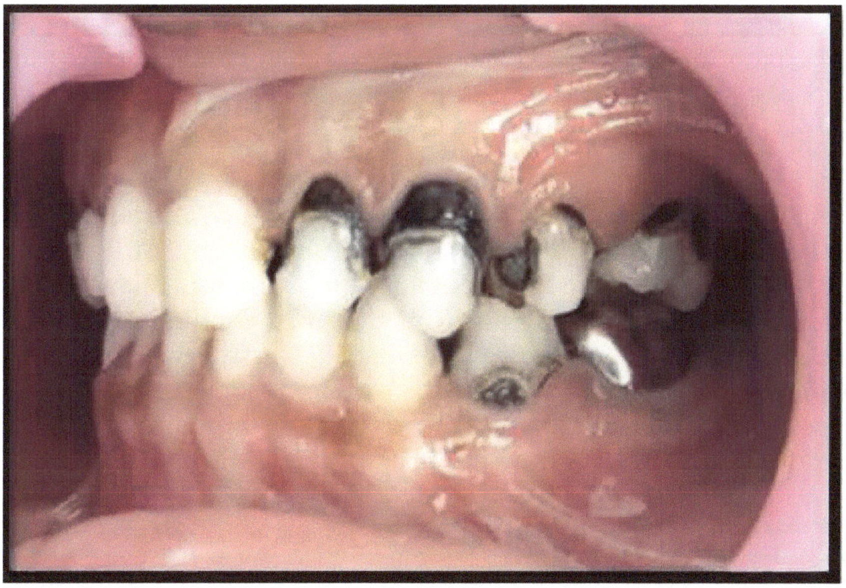

Fig. (7). Postoperative -Arrested carious lesions after SDF application.

The available data on the effectiveness and efficacy of SDF, besides being non-toxic, suggests it to be appropriate as per WHO Millennium Goals and the US Institute of Medicine's key points for 21st-century medical care.

Effectiveness of Silver Diamine Fluoride

The American Dental Association Council on Scientific Affairs and the Centre for Evidence-Based Dentistry also provide a moderate evidence-based strong recommendation for prioritizing bi-annual application of 38% SDF solution for arresting cavitated carious lesions in primary and permanent teeth involving any coronal surface. The 2018 Policy statement by AAPD for the use of SDF in pediatric patients recognizes its use as an optimal caries management strategy focusing on optimized individual patient care as per the aims of a dental home.

Post-Treatment Strategy

The effectiveness of a single application of SDF as an anti-caries agent ranges from 47% to 90%, depending on the cavity size and location. It has been seen that the anterior teeth have a higher rate of caries arrest than posterior teeth. Therefore, regular follow-up and recall of patients for re-evaluation of lesions is advisable.

- A follow-up is advised at 2-4 weeks postoperatively.
- Re-application of SDF may be done when the clinical assessment shows the

absence of caries arrest in lesions that are not visibly dark and hard. Additional SDF application in subsequent follow-up visits can be made as required based on the lesion's colour and hardness or evident sign of caries progression.

SMART Technique

Silver diamine fluoride can also be used as an adjunct to restorative treatment by its application on the carious tooth surface followed by the placement of a restoration. Therefore, it can be used along with atraumatic restorative treatment (also known as **Silver Aided ART or SMART**) or with the Hall technique (Fig. **8**). It can be done immediately after placing SDF or waiting for a few days or weeks post the application of SDF until the carious lesions are arrested. It can also be used for treating dentinal hypersensitivity and symptomatic molar incisor hypo-mineralization (MIH) [12, 13].

Safety Margin and Maximum Dosage

A single drop (25 μl) of SDF solution contains 9.5 mg of silver diamine fluoride and is considered sufficient for treating five teeth. The relative safety margin of using one drop of SDF in an average child weighing 10 kg with early childhood caries is 380 mg/kg LD 50 / 0.95 mg/kg dose = 400-fold safety margin (w) [14, 15].

Adverse Effects

Silver diamine fluoride application may sometimes result in adverse events such as staining adjacent teeth and soft tissues, localized soft tissue irritation, or irritating the pulp. Visible dark staining is a characteristic property of SDF that signifies caries arrest resulting from the formation of metallic silver from silver compounds. There may be no immediate changes in the colour of the lesion; however, it turns dark brown to black over 2-3 weeks. This dark discolouration is permanent unless restored with an aesthetic restorative material (Table **1**). To counteract the staining, the use of potassium iodide (KI) solution over the SDF has been effective. This results in the precipitation of silver iodide components that help remove the ionic silver particles. Despite the stains and discolouration being aesthetically undesirable, many parents prefer this simple option to avoid sedation or general anaesthesia [16].

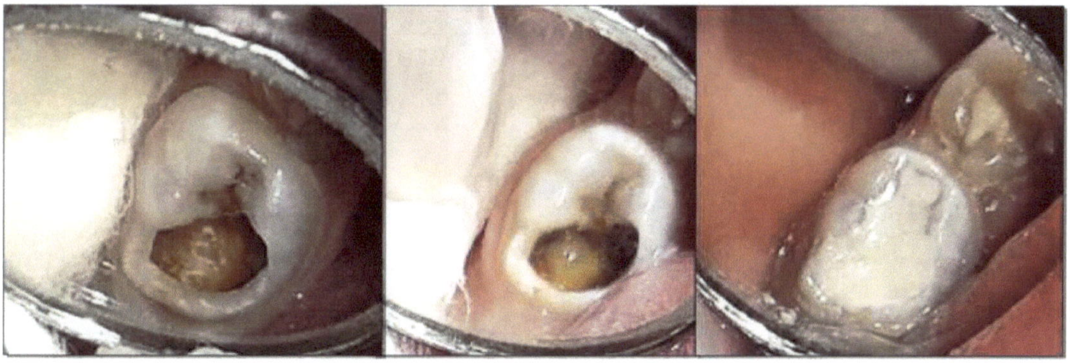

Fig. (8). SMART technique in primary mandibular second molar.

Table 1. Advantages and Disadvantages of SDF.

Advantages	Disadvantages
Disinfects carious lesions.	Permanent black discolouration of carious tooth surface compromising aesthetics.
Atraumatic and minimally invasive.	May inadvertently cause temporary staining of adjacent oral tissues as well as clothes in case of spillage.
Minimal assistance and support are required with no cumbersome armamentarium.	May not always be successful in arresting the lesion as it relies on the compliance with oral hygiene practices by the patient.
Good patient acceptance and cost-effectiveness.	Metallic taste.

CONCLUSION

Silver diamine fluoride is an economical and easy-to-use option for the treatment of dental caries. It is an atraumatic and minimally invasive approach that does not require the aid of additional sophisticated equipment. It also does not require very high precision and is available commercially in ready-to-use containers. The patient acceptance is very high as the patient does not undergo any long and painful procedures. The only drawback of SDF is the blackish staining it produces on the applied tooth surfaces; however, it outweighs its benefits of caries arrest and remineralization. Silver diamine fluoride appears to be an immediate beneficial treatment for children who are unable to receive conventional restorative therapy for the treatment of dental caries and can therefore be widely used for caries control to meet patients' needs.

CONSENT FOR PUBLICATION

Not applicable.

CONFLICT OF INTEREST

The authors declare no conflict of interest, financial or otherwise.

ACKNOWLEDGEMENT

Declared none.

REFERENCES

[1] Clemens J, Gold J, Chaffin J. Effect and acceptance of silver diamine fluoride treatment on dental caries in primary teeth. J Public Health Dent 2018; 78(1): 63-8. [http://dx.doi.org/10.1111/jphd.12241] [PMID: 28749529]

[2] American Dental Association Silver Diamine Fluoride in Caries Management. 2020.https://www.ada.org/resources/research/science-and-research-institute/o-al-health-topics/silver-diamine-fluoride

[3] Nelson T, Scott JM, Crystal YO, Berg JH, Milgrom P. Silver diamine fluoride in pediatric dentistry training programs: survey of graduate program directors. Pediatr Dent 2016; 38(3): 212-7. [PMID: 27306245]

[4] Featherstone JD, Horst JA. Long used in other countries, silver diamine fluoride is now cleared for use in the US While there is an assumption of use for pediatric caries control, here we explore indications for adults 2015; 1-8.

[5] Nuvvula S, Mallineni SK. Silver diamine fluoride in pediatric dentistry. J. South asian Assoc. Pediatr Dent 2019; 2(2): 74.

[6] Wakshlak RBK, Pedahzur R, Avnir D. Antibacterial activity of silver-killed bacteria: the "zombies" effect. Sci Rep 2015; 5(1): 9555. [http://dx.doi.org/10.1038/srep09555] [PMID: 25906433]

[7] Mei ML, Chu CH, Low KH, Che CM, Lo ECM. Caries arresting effect of silver diamine fluoride on dentine carious lesion with S. mutans and L. acidophilus dual-species cariogenic biofilm. Med Oral Patol Oral Cir Bucal 2013; 18(6): e824-31. [http://dx.doi.org/10.4317/medoral.18831] [PMID: 23722131]

[8] Seifo N, Robertson M, MacLean J, *et al.* The use of silver diamine fluoride (SDF) in dental practice. Br Dent J 2020; 228(2): 75-81. [http://dx.doi.org/10.1038/s41415-020-1203-9] [PMID: 31980777]

[9] Seifo N, Cassie H, Radford JR, Innes NPT. Silver diamine fluoride for managing carious lesions: an umbrella review. BMC Oral Health 2019; 19(1): 145. [http://dx.doi.org/10.1186/s12903-019-0830-5] [PMID: 31299955]

[10] Rosenblatt A, Stamford TCM, Niederman R. Silver diamine fluoride: a caries "silver-fluoride bullet". J Dent Res 2009; 88(2): 116-25. [http://dx.doi.org/10.1177/0022034508329406] [PMID: 19278981]

[11] Chibinski AC, Wambier LM, Feltrin J, Loguercio AD, Wambier DS, Reis A. Silver diamine fluoride has efficacy in controlling caries progression in primary teeth: a systematic review and meta-analysis. Caries Res 2017; 51(5): 527-41. [http://dx.doi.org/10.1159/000478668] [PMID: 28972954]

[12] Alvear Fa B, Jew JA, Wong A, Young D. Silver modified atraumatic restorative technique (SMART): an alternative caries prevention tool. Stomatology Edu Journal 2016; 3(2): 243-9. [http://dx.doi.org/10.25241/2016.3(2).15]

[13] Duffin S, Juhl J, Schwab J, Duffin ML. SMART Oral Health: The Medical Management of Caries.

Kindle Direct Publishing, 2019.

[14] Horst JA, Ellenikiotis H, Milgrom PL. UCSF protocol for caries arrest using silver diamine fluoride: rationale, indications and consent. J Calif Dent Assoc 2016; 44(1): 16-28. [PMID: 26897901]

[15] Slayton RL, Urquhart O, Araujo MWB, *et al.* Evidence-based clinical practice guideline on nonrestorative treatments for carious lesions. J Am Dent Assoc 2018; 149(10): 837-849.e19. [http://dx.doi.org/10.1016/j.adaj.2018.07.002] [PMID: 30261951]

[16] Fung MHT, Duangthip D, Wong MCM, Lo ECM, Chu CH. Randomized clinical trial of 12% and 38% silver diamine fluoride treatment. J Dent Res 2018; 97(2): 171-8. [http://dx.doi.org/10.1177/0022034517728496] [PMID: 28846469]

CHAPTER 16

Pit and Fissure Sealants

Vishwas Chaugule[1,*], **Vishwas Patil**[2] and **Shreya Dasgupta**[2]

[1] *Sinhgad Dental College and Hospital, Pune, India*

[2] *D. Y. Patil Dental College and Hospital, Pimpri, Pune, India*

Abstract: Newly erupted posterior teeth in both the primary and permanent dentitions are vulnerable to dental caries attack due to deep, uncoalesced, and not-so-soundly mineralized pits and fissures as compared to their matured counterparts. Therefore, it is more important to "catch them young" before it becomes too late to save them from the deleterious effects of dental caries. Sealing such immature morphological structures with an appropriate sealing material is one of the primary prevention strategies Though this therapy sounds and appears simple, when conducted improperly, it results in the failure of the treatment motto. Hence, there is a need to gain in-depth knowledge of the material, intricacies in the proper selection of the teeth, technique and the behavior of the therapy eventually.

This chapter provides an overview of the historic background and recent evidence-based clinical recommendations for the use of fissure sealants. It describes the different morphological variants of fissures and a wide range of commercially available products with their dispensing means. This writeup also enlightens the conceptual understanding of sealing non-cavitated fissures, therapeutic fissure sealing and smooth surface sealing. Troubleshooting in sealant therapy along with adverse reactions is also described.

Keywords: Dental Sealants, Glass Ionomer Sealants, Occlusal Caries, Pits and Fissures, Preventive Resin Restorations, Primary Prevention.

INTRODUCTION

Oral diseases have a high prevalence in society, the most common being dental caries, which is caused by an ecological imbalance between demineralization and remineralization [1]. The occurrence of dental caries in the oral cavity is more predominant on the occlusal surfaces of posterior teeth, *i.e.,* deciduous molars, premolars and permanent molars. The pits and fissures on these surfaces are inaccessible to conventional oro-physiotherapeutic measures. Hence, there is an

* **Corresponding author Vishwas Chaugule:** D. Y. Patil Dental College and Hospital, Pimpri, Pune, India; E-mail: vbchaugule@gmail.com

Satyawan Damle, Ritesh Kalaskar & Dhanashree Sakhare (Eds.)

accumulation of food remains (debris) and formation of a biofilm. Dental caries is a result of all these events (Fig. **1**) [2]. Even the 21st century statistical data show that 90% of occlusal surfaces of the permanent molars and premolars and 40% of primary molars are affected by caries. Thus, it is a global burden affecting the health and quality of life of children and young adults. Definitive approaches to prevent caries are regular oral hygiene with fluoride-containing toothpaste, a reduction in the intake of cariogenic food, as well as local and systemic fluoridation [3]. Regrettably, fluoride is ineffective in preventing occlusal caries as compared to smooth surfaces as the data from fluoridated communities suggest a low reduction in pit and fissure lesions. Earlier, treatment of caries involved removal of the caries along with healthy tooth structure for the purpose of extension for prevention. Therefore, to prevent and preserve the loss of natural tooth structure, Buonocore in 1955 revolutionized operative dentistry by introducing the concept of "sealing out" caries to prevent the further progress of the carious lesion and thus conserve natural tooth structure [4]. Occlusal sealants are organic polymers which mechanically bind to acid etched enamel. The resin forms an impervious barrier between the occlusal fissures and oral environment, preventing impaction of food debris and ingress of bacteria. If the sealant is present, the occlusal surface is virtually immune to caries attack. The use of sealants focuses on a preventive philosophy, with a desire to preserve tooth structure by preventing or delaying the need for restorative treatment, thus making it a cost-effective treatment. Over the time, various technological advancements led to refinements in the techniques of adhesive dentistry, which enhanced "the power of prevention" [4].

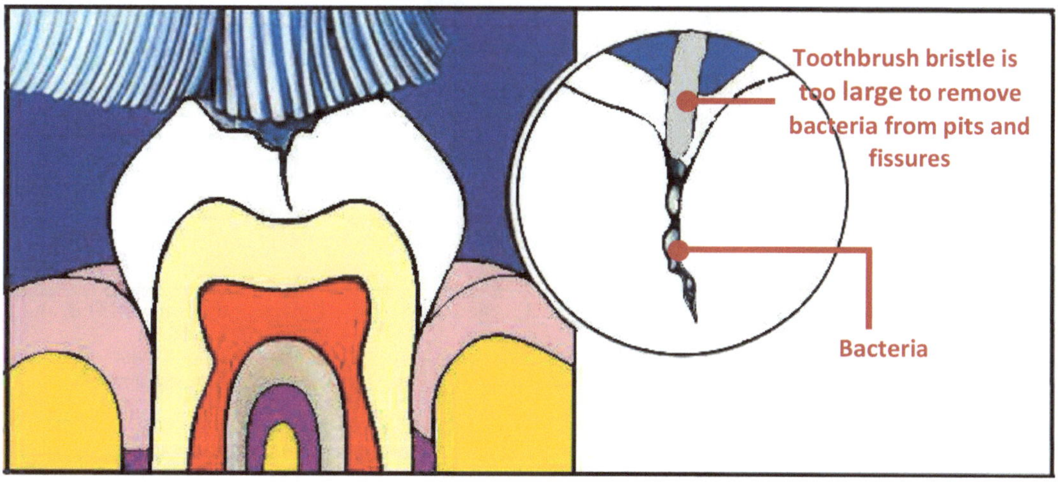

Fig (1). Food and plaque gain access deep into the groove where a toothbrush bristle cannot reach, and a cavity develops easily.

Definition

Pit and Fissure Sealant

According to Simonsen (1978)- the term pit and fissure sealant is used to describe a material that is introduced into the occlusal pits and fissures of caries-susceptible teeth, thus forming a micromechanically bonded, protective layer cutting the access of caries-producing bacteria from their source of nutrients.

Historical Background

Protecting the pits and fissures of newly erupted teeth from caries is not a new concept. Since 1923, when H T Hyatt first suggested prophylactic odontotomy, researchers have put forth different concepts and techniques to decrease caries susceptibility (Table **1**) [5].

Table 1. Landmarks in the history of fissure sealants.

Year	Landmark
1867	Arthur stated that "decay is inevitable, and obliteration of fissures could prevent its occurrence."
1895	Wilson used zinc phosphate cement to seal pits and fissures.
1905	W.D. Miller used silver nitrate for fissure restoration.
1920	Black suggested the conversion of retentive fissures into non-retentive depressions on the occlusal surfaces of teeth to reduce plaque accumulation.
1923	T. P. Hyatt introduced prophylactic odontotomy technique, consisting of restoring the fissures with silver or oxyphosphate cement soon after the eruption of teeth in the oral cavity and later replacing it with amalgam after complete eruption.
1929	Bodecker proposed a technique of converting deep narrow fissures into self-cleansing fissures by performing enameloplasty (fissure eradication).
1939	Gore used polymers (cellulose nitrate in organic solvents) as fissure sealants.
1942	Klein and Knutson used ammoniacal silver nitrate to seal pits and fissures.
1950	Decrease in caries due to fluorides was noticed. But fluorides were found ineffective on occlusal surfaces.
1965	Development of Bis-GMA (Bisphenol A-Glycidyl Methacrylate) by Bowen at the National Bureau of Standards.
1967	First clinical trial by M.G. Buonocore and Cueto using cyanoacrylates as sealants
1968	Rodyhouse used Bis-GMA and MMA (Methyl Methacrylate) with peroxide amines as fissure sealants without etching enamel prior to its application. He reported a 30% decrease in fissure caries using this technique.
1970	Buonocore published his first paper describing the successful use of Bis- GMA resin with ultraviolet light as pit and fissure sealant.
1971	NuvaSeal was the first commercially available pit and fissure sealant.

(Table 1) cont.....

Year	Landmark
1973	Taylor and Gwinnett observed that fissure sites retained debris regardless of the means of prophylaxis.
1974	McLean and Wilson introduced glass ionomer pit and fissure sealants.
1977	Simonsen and Stallard updated the term "Preventive Resin Restoration (PRR)" to "Conservative Adhesive Restoration (CAR)"
1983	The National Institute of Health published a report "Consensus development conference statement on dental sealants in the prevention of tooth decay" which recommended the use of pit and fissure sealants as safe and effective method to prevent decay.
2002	AAPD (American Academy of Paediatric Dentistry) conference paper recommended the use of sealants in permanent molars of children and adolescents.

Trends in Caries Epidemiology in Children

Dental caries and periodontal diseases are pandemics, *i.e.,* affecting all populations irrespective of gender, age or socioeconomic status. There is evidence that the prevalence and severity of cavitated dentine carious lesions among 5- and 12-year-olds have declined over the last decades but the decay component among these age groups is exceedingly high, with a lower prevalence among 12-yea--olds [6]. The pits and fissures of primary molars are also at a risk, since 44% of the surfaces affected by caries in primary teeth are occlusal surfaces despite the occlusal surfaces being flatter and less fissured. Schiffner in 2018 stated that there are strong indications that caries can decline by the placement of fissure sealants [7]. Therefore, pit and fissure sealant therapy form an important part of primary preventive dentistry.

Morphology of Pit & Fissures

Knowledge about the morphology of the pit and fissures is essential to determine the ability of the sealant to effectively seal the occlusal surfaces. It is virtually impossible to determine the anatomical complexity and the depth of a fissure system by direct visual or radiographic examination. Recent studies have revealed that fissure morphology is highly variable, both within the individual tooth and between different teeth [8].

The fissure patterns in the primary teeth were described by Mortimer (1970) as U and V type. Nagano and Gustafson found that in the permanent teeth, the prevalence of 'V,' 'IK,' 'I' and 'U' type was 34%, 26%, 19% and 14%, respectively. Nagano further observed that V and U types were self-cleansing and caries-resistant; however, K-type fissures were very susceptible to caries (Figs **2a** and **b**).

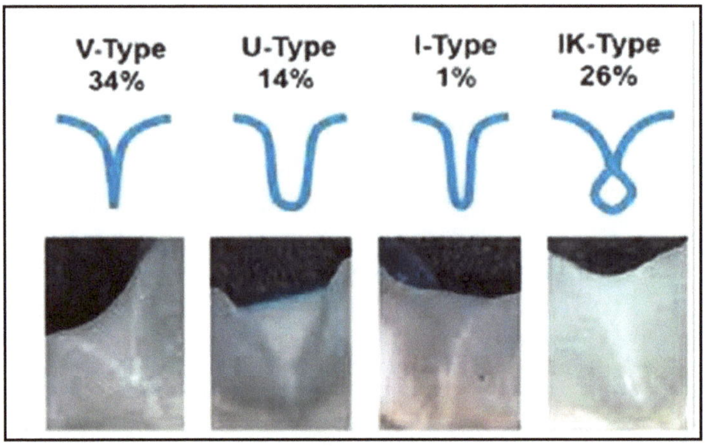

Fig (2a). Types of Fissures - Schematic diagram.

Penetration of the sealant to the base of the fissure occurs more frequently in shallow fissures than in deep fissures. Shallow fissures are more likely to be thoroughly cleaned and etched than deep fissures. Residual material in the depth of the fissure and air entrapment contributes to limiting the sealant penetration into deep constricted fissures resulting in poor retention of the sealant material. An invasive technique for the placement of sealants has been suggested to overcome the problems of deep, constricted fissures. This technique changes the morphology of the fissures from I- and IK-shapes to U- or V-shapes.

It has been observed that the depth of penetration of a sealant material in 'V' and 'U' shaped fissures was comparable to and better than 'I,' 'IK' or 'Y' shaped fissure.

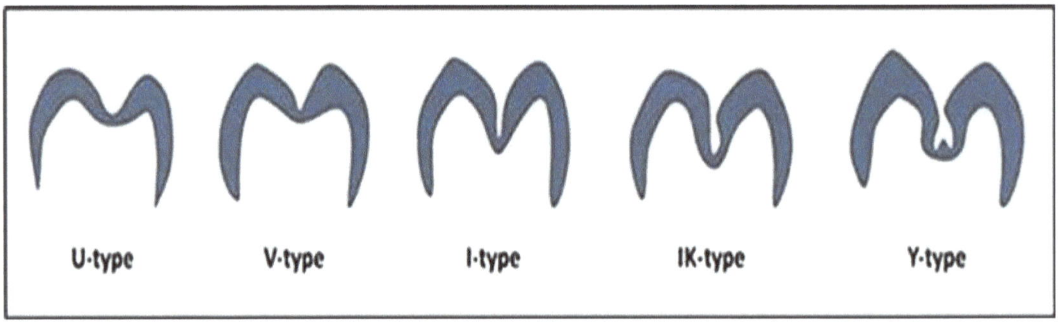

Fig (2b). Types of Fissures - Clinical picture.

Caries Detection Tools

Careful clinical examination happens to be the mainstay in assessing the occlusal surfaces for early caries activity. The visual-tactile technique is the most used and widely accepted method. The use of a sharp probe/explorer has been questioned by many authors, as it can affect the integrity of the thin enamel layer in the fissures. Hence, it is not recommended. Also, the presence of deep fissures which are stained or plugged with organic debris makes it difficult to identify initial caries. This uncertainty leads to disagreement among clinicians about the distinct stages of the caries process. Hence, several clinical visual caries detection systems are suggested [9]. Amongst the several systems, the International Caries Detection and Assessment System and Nyvad systems are the most widely used, in both clinical and epidemiological settings. As per ICDAS, scores 0, 1, 2, 3 are indications for pit and fissure sealant placement while therapeutic fissure sealing can be conducted in teeth with scores 4 and 5. Nyvad classification is another system devised for the detection of activity and severity of carious lesions. According to this classification, scores 0, 1, 2, 4 and 5 should be sealed using fissure sealants.

The diagnosis of pits and fissures indicated for sealant placement is based upon a combination of visual and tactile techniques along with adjunctive advanced caries detecting methods. Of the many new advances in caries diagnosing systems, fluorescence-based systems (Diagnodent and VistaProof) and the use of alternating current impedance spectroscopy (CarieScan system) seem more effective than other systems in diagnosing initial occlusal caries. Diagnodent is a laser fluorescence-based caries detection device. It provides measurement values between 0–99. With values < 20, fissure sealants can be placed, while for lesions scoring 21-30, Preventive Resin Restorations (PRR) may be considered [9, 10]. The final decision is based on the clinician's judgement and experience to select the type and technique of sealant to be applied.

Ideal requisites of pit and fissure sealants [Brauer, 1978; Ngo H, 2012]

- Viscosity allowing penetration into deep and narrow fissures even in the maxillary arch
- Adequate working time
- Rapid cure
- Good and prolonged adhesion to enamel
- Low sorption and solubility
- Resistance to wear
- Minimum irritation to tissues
- Should be able to arrest the carious lesion and stop its progression.

- Easy to manipulate; either the dentist or the auxiliary should be able to apply.
- Should be biocompatible

Classification of Pit and Fissure Sealants (Figs 3a, 3b, 3c)

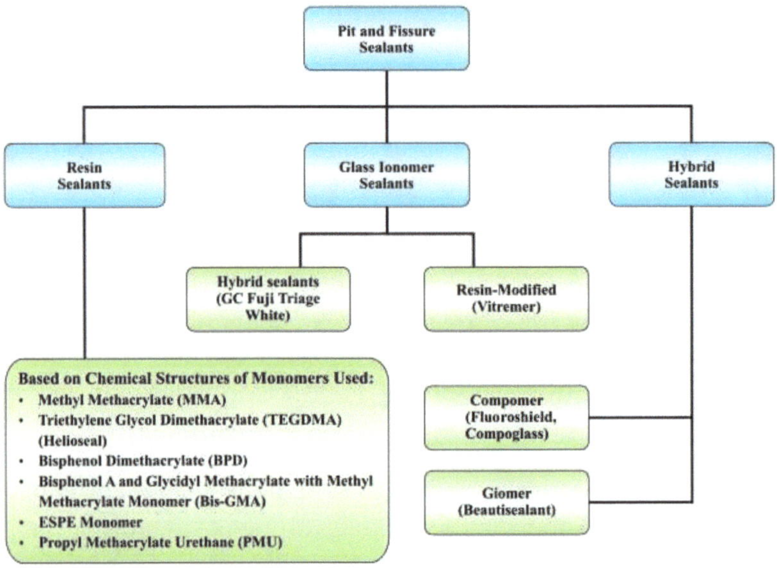

Fig (3a). General classification of sealants.

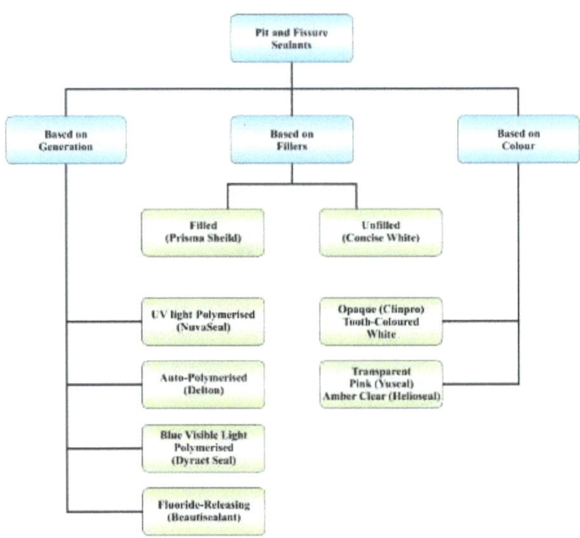

Fig (3b). Classification of pit and fissure sealants based on material.

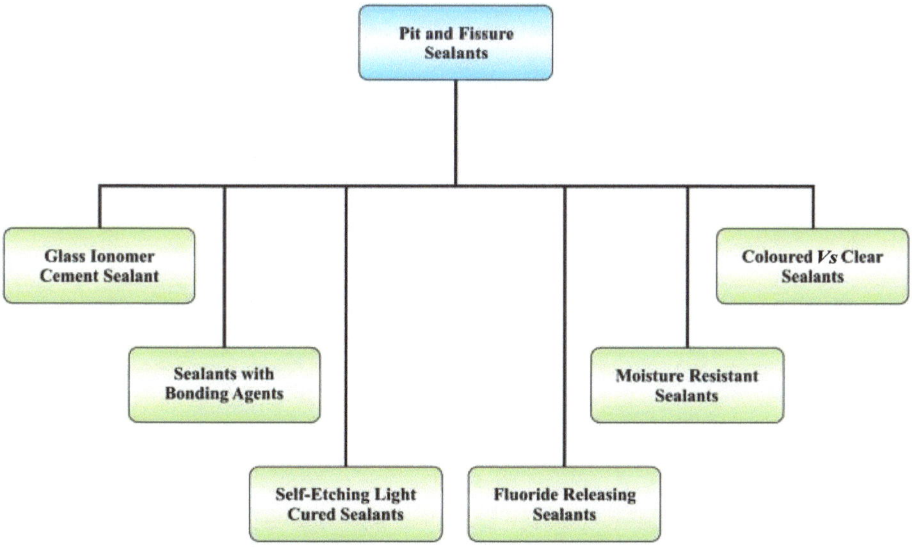

Fig (3c). Classification of pit and fissure sealants according to Norman O. Harris (2014).

Recent Advances

Limitations of Conventional Sealants

- Lack of long-term effectiveness
- Poor retention
- Technique failure attributable to traditional hydrophobic materials
- If sealant fails, sealed in bacteria continue to penetrate deeper into the tooth structures.
- Owing to these difficulties, further search for better material for fissure sealants continued and recently following advances have been introduced in the market.

The conventional materials used as sealants (Fig **4**) had the above limitations. Thus, further research led to the recent advances in sealants as shown in Fig (**5**)

Hydrophilic Sealants

Binds to moist tooth (tooth integrating) and seals against microleakage; works in dry field, *e.g.,* Embrace WetBond Pit & Fissure Sealant Pulpdent.

Self-Etching Sealants

Premier® Enamel Loc™ self-etching pit and fissure sealant eliminates gagging and discomfort from acid- etching and saves time by eliminating a step.

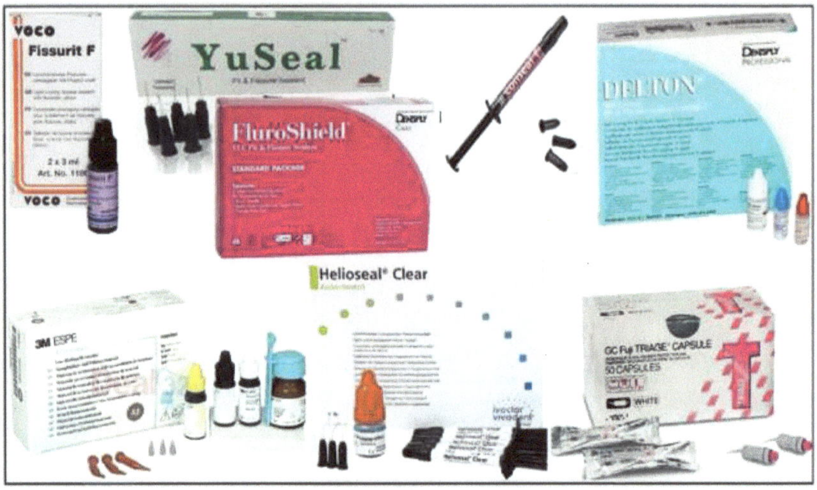

Fig (4). Conventional pit and fissure sealants.

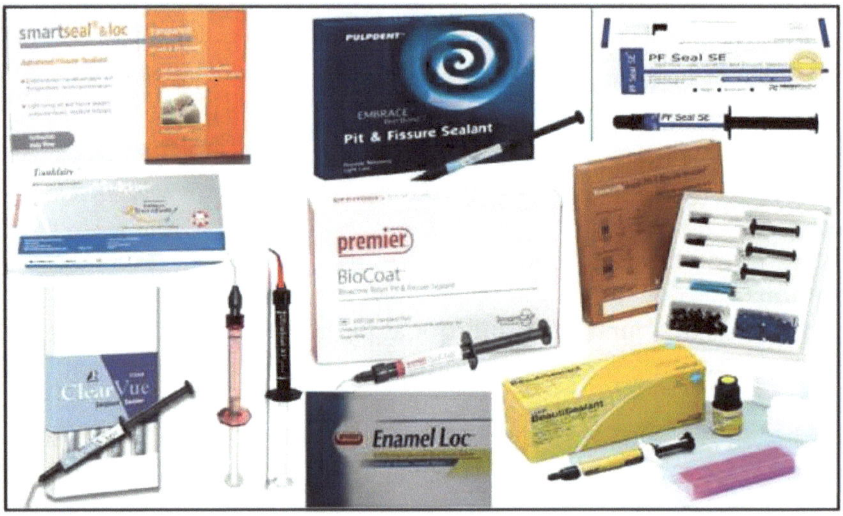

Fig (5). Recent advances in pit and fissure sealants.

Bioactive Resin Pit and Fissure Sealant

These have microcapsules filled with ionic solutions of fluoride, calcium and phosphate. Tooth surfaces, both in contact and adjacent to the sealant, benefit from the extended release of these ions. The demineralization cycle is disrupted, and the remineralization process is continuously supported. The exchange of ions and recharge of microcapsules extends maximum protection without putting the sealant's physical integrity at risk. *e.g.,* BioCoat™, Premier Dental.

Bisphenol-A Free Sealant

Nontoxic, resin-based, light-cured sealant with low viscosity to allow the material to penetrate deep into pits and fissures. *e.g.,* Toothfairy® Pit & Fissure Sealant, Septodont.

Amorphous Calcium Phosphate Releasing Sealant

Self-curing glass ionomer is used as a sealant, liner and surface protector. Features Amorphous Calcium Phosphate nanotechnology to remineralize calcium and phosphate to the tooth structure *e.g.,* Iva Protect SDI.

Indications and Contraindications for Sealant Placement (Table 2)

Table 2. Criteria for identifying teeth to be sealed.

Criteria	Seal	Do not seal
Occlusal morphology	Deep, narrow pits and fissures	Well coalesced pits and fissures Wide easily cleaned groves
Tooth age	Recently erupted teeth	Teeth that have remained caries free for 4 years or longer
General caries activity	Occlusal lesions on other teeth Few or no proximal lesions	Many proximal lesions
Availability of other preventive procedures	Patient receiving appropriate systemic and/or topical fluoride therapy	Patient's water supply is fluoride-deficient, and patient is not cooperating in recommended caries preventive program

Patient Considerations in Sealant Placement

Fig. (**6**) illustrates a decision-making flowchart for selection of patients for applications of dental sealants based on caries risk assessment of the patient, tooth status, patient co-operation and isolation status for the tooth.

In children with bruxism, sealants can be lost by the continuous flexion of the tooth and by occlusal stress [11]. Unfilled resin-based and carbomer-based sealants applied on occlusal surfaces of permanent lower molars were shown to be more effective for preventing caries in child patients with bruxism. Carbomers are a class of glass ionomer-based materials, with the property of gradual mineralization to fluorapatite.

In cases of hypoplastic posterior teeth, sealants have greater retention when applied using fifth-generation adhesive systems prior to the sealant. In case the patient is uncooperative or has extreme sensitivity, glass ionomer fissure sealants can be considered [12].

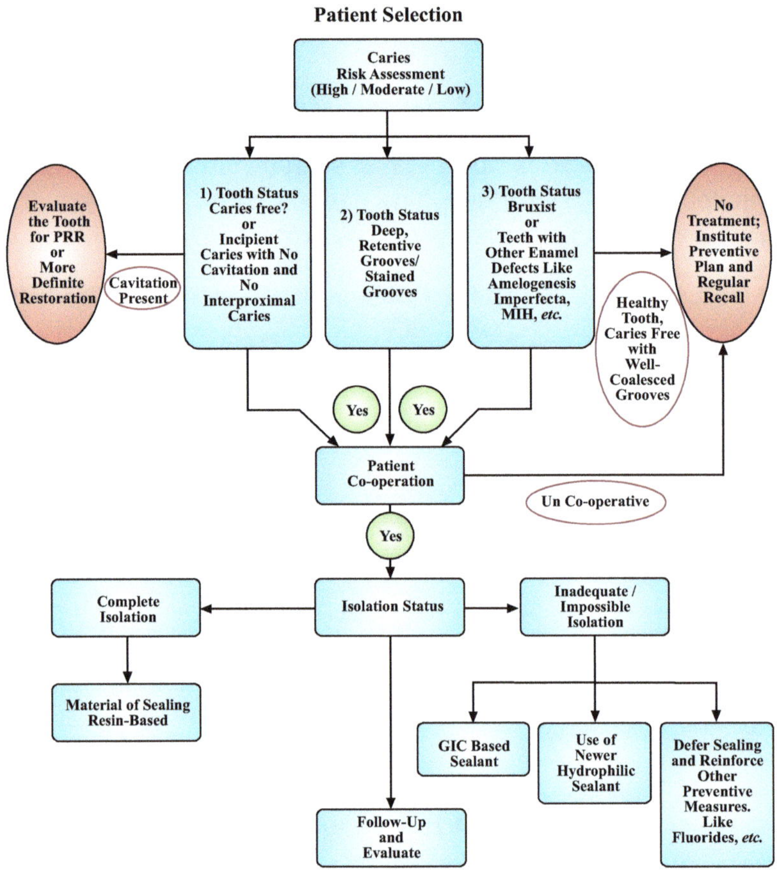

Fig (6). Decision making flowchart for patient selection.

Dispensing and Delivery Systems of Sealants

Sealants have proven to be an important adjunct in patient care. However, many clinicians avoid the use of sealants due to products that fail to produce predictable, consistent results. One of the reasons for the failure of sealants is the delivery systems of sealants to the tooth.

Requisites of Ideal Delivery Systems

- Provide a delivery system for a flowable/ liquid material.
- It should be particularly adaptable for the delivery of the materials.
- It should be simple to operate and inexpensive.

- After the application of the sealant, the tip should instantaneously get ejected upon the mere application of slight excessive pressure to a plunger member; such a system is safe, aseptic and convenient.
- The system should not be such that the tip requires manual removal, subjecting the operator to encounter the sealant, necessitating time consuming and annoying removals thereof.

Currently Available Dispensing and Delivery Systems for Sealants

Dental sealants may be applied by any one of the several types of applicators such as brushes, sponges, cotton pledges held with tweezers, or dispensers with disposable tips made of plastic tubing. Each one offers certain advantages depending upon the nature of the sealant being applied and the dexterity of the operator.

Brushes

- Only a small amount of sealant is carried and hence it is time consuming.
- Resultant concomitant fatigue to the operator
- Uniform application on the posterior teeth is difficult
- Accidental misapplication on the soft tissues can cause irritation

Plastic sponges and cotton pledgets

- Both are picked from small boxes with a tweezer.
- Very frequently sponges cling together due to static electric charges thereon.
- With cotton pledges, the intermingled fibrils cause undesirable clinging.
- Both soak large quantities of sealant
- It may leave lint embedded in the sealant on the tooth surface leading to clinical failure.

Dispenser

- A small tube/tip of plastic is inserted into the dispenser head.
- Heads are many times bulky.
- Obstructs unobstructed vision of the dentition, especially in children.
- Often pose difficulties in avoiding the flow of the sealant during application to the maxillary dentition
- After sealant application, the tip must be removed manually
- Contents tend to continue to flow after the action of the dispensing plunger on the delivery piston has ceased. This continued flow is due to the reservoir cylinder of the cartridge, which "breathes" when dispensing dental materials like fissure sealants require specialised practices and equipment, as the materials get affected by light, temperature, etc. Hence, they are stored in small bottles made

of dark glass. The delivery tip with a spiral passageway around the bristles helps in sheer thinning of a thixotropic sealant and provides a high degree of precision.

Armamentarium and Technique

The application of pit and fissure sealants, while inherently simple, is very technique sensitive, requiring attention to detail at all stages. Before commencing the procedure, all the necessary instruments and equipment should be arranged. The armamentarium included is determined based on the operator's preference and delivery system of the sealant material to be used. Fig. (**7**) displays the armamentarium and Figs. (**8a** and **8b**) show the steps in sealant placement and PRR, respectively.

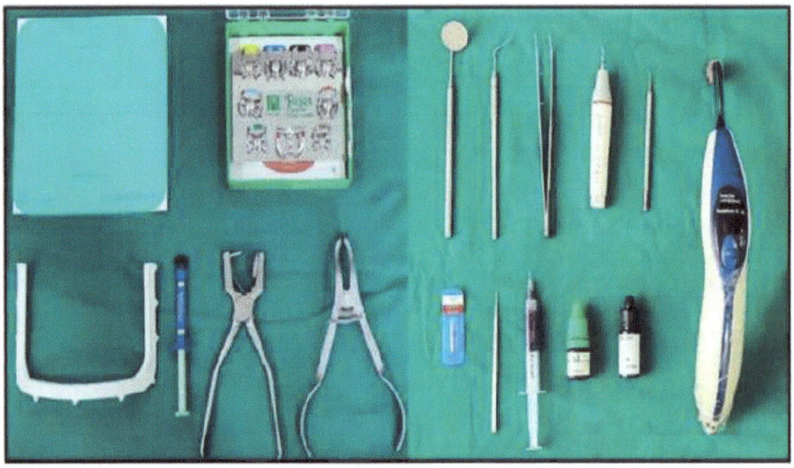

Fig (7). Armamentarium required for pit and fissure sealants.

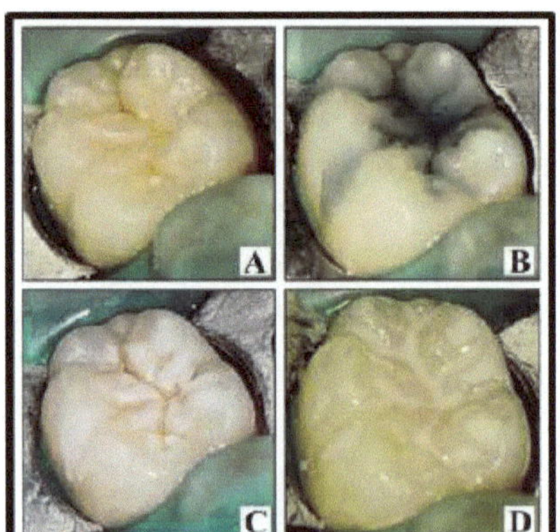

Fig (8a). Pit and fissure sealant placement; **A**- pre-operative, **B**-etching, **C**- post etching, **D**-post sealant application.

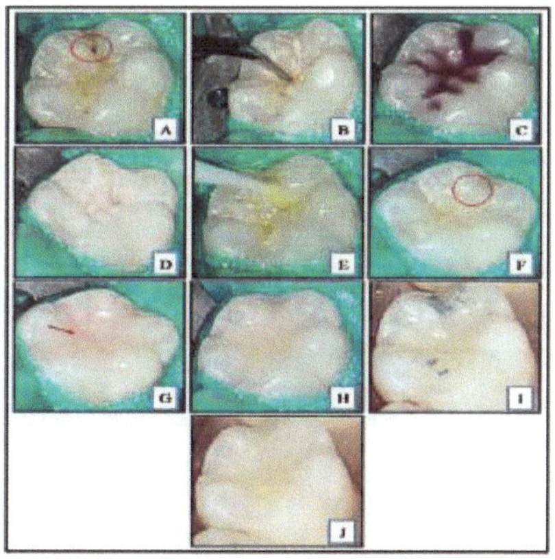

Fig (8b). Steps in preventive resin restoration (A-J); **A-** pre-operative, **B-** cleaning, **C-** etching, **D-** post etching, E- bond application, **F**-cured resin restoration, **G-** sealant application, H-post curing, **I-** evaluation of high points, **J-** post operative.

Four Handed Versus two Handed Application Techniques

When possible, a four handed technique should be used for the placement of pit and fissure sealants (Fig. **8a**, **b**).

Cleaning

Cleaning the tooth facilitates the removal of debris and deposits prior to sealant application. It can be done by using a rubber cup and prophy paste or a bristle brush and dentifrices. The tooth can also be cleaned with a dry bristle brush in a slow-speed handpiece. While using prophy paste or dentifrices, it is advisable to use non-fluoridated paste, since fluoride might interfere with acid etching. Another available cleaning method is an air polisher with sodium bicarbonate in a water slurry. However, this raises the pH of the tooth, making it imperative to etch and rinse twice to neutralize the higher pH and effectively etch the tooth.

Centric Stop Registration

This step is done with the help of articulating paper. The excess flow of sealant in these areas can cause occlusal interference, eventually leading to sealant failure. This step can be done prior to the isolation of the tooth.

Isolation

Isolation of the tooth is mandatory prior to sealant application. It can be achieved using either rubber dam or cotton rolls with an effective saliva ejector.

Mechanical Preparation

Enameloplasty can be performed using fissurotomy shallow taper fissure and narrow taper fissure or a small one-quarter round bur. It is considered a simple, cost-effective and easily accessible method with acceptable sealant retention. The air abrasion system uses a stream of aluminium oxide particles which abrade the tooth surface resulting in roughening of the enamel, removal of suspected caries, and cleaning pits and fissures. The use of lasers to roughen enamel is also suggested as a pre-treatment method. The main advantage of laser etched surface is the resistance of enamel to caries. A systematic review in 2016 stated that tooth preparation prior to sealant application increases sealant retention; however, these methods cannot be used as an alternative for conventional acid etching [13].

Self-etch Versus Acid Etch

The use of no rinse, self-etching bonding agents instead of acid etching prior to sealant application is not recommended. These agents may provide lesser retention than that obtained by acid etching.

Enamel Preparation

Acid etching with 35–37% phosphoric acid followed by rinsing and drying of the tooth is the accepted method of preparing enamel prior to sealant application. The most critical step in sealant application is acid conditioning or acid etching (Table 3).

Table 3. Acid etching, washing and drying times for primary and permanent teeth. (IADR sealant symposium recommendations, 1991).

Step	Primary tooth (seconds)	Permanent tooth (seconds)
Acid etching	30	20
Wash	30	30
Dry	15	15

Increased Etching Time for Deciduous Teeth is Attributed to Several Reasons

- Deciduous teeth have less mineral and more organic material in the enamel
- Deciduous teeth have a larger internal pore volume and thus more exogenous organic material.
- Deciduous teeth have more prismless enamel on their surface than permanent teeth.
- The prism rods in deciduous teeth approach the surface at a greater angle and thus are more difficult to etch.

Washing and Drying

- The tooth must be washed and cleaned with water for 30 seconds after etching, to remove all the acid etchant residues.
- Following this, the tooth must be dried for 15 seconds.
- Optimally etched enamel has a chalky white frosty appearance.
- If salivary contamination occurs, re-etch for 10 seconds and repeat the procedure.

Bonding Agent Application

Feigal et al. in 1993 suggested using a bonding agent under the sealant. They used hydrophilic bonding materials to aid the bond strength when the sealant is applied in a moist environment. A recent systematic review evaluated sealant retention with or without adhesive systems. Adhesive systems had a positive effect on retention of sealants. It also stated that 4th and 5th generation adhesives (etch and rinse type) had better sealant retention than self-etch adhesives, *i.e.,* 6th and 7th generations [14].

Sealant Application

Apply the minimum amount sealant required to cover the pit and fissure network. Remove any air bubbles or voids before curing. During sealant application, all the susceptible pits and fissures should be sealed for maximum caries protection. In the mandibular teeth, apply the sealant distally and allow it to flow mesially, while in the maxillary teeth it should be allowed to flow distally.

Polymerization

Position the light curing tip as close to the surface being sealed as possible and cure for at least the recommended curing time. If more than one surface of the same tooth is being sealed, *e.g.,* occlusal and buccal/palatal, cure each surface separately. Protocols for evaluating the light output and curing performance of the unit should be implemented in accordance with the manufacturer's instructions.

Testing Retention

Sealant retention should be checked with a probe after application and if necessary, the sealant should be re-applied, repeating each step of the procedure.

Inadequate Moisture Control

In a cooperative patient, if a resin-based sealant is indicated, but moisture control is difficult to achieve, resin-based sealants should be attempted and reviewed within 6 months. Where adequate moisture control cannot be achieved, newer hydrophilic sealants can be applied. Glass ionomer sealants may be considered on a case-to-case basis, as an interim preventive measure when there are indications for placement of a resin-based sealant but concerns that moisture control may compromise such placement.

Follow Up and Recall

Sealants should be checked when the patient is recalled and if necessary, repaired or replaced. The recall interval for high-caries-risk children should not exceed twelve months. If there is a particular concern about sealant retention, recall within 6 months is appropriate. The CCC Sealant Evaluation System is a simple, legitimate and reproducible method to detect sealant integrity since it determines all the three factors responsible for sealant retention like- Colour, Coverage and Caries.

Effectiveness and Retention of Sealants

Pit-and-fissure sealants are one of the most effective, yet underutilized interventions for preventing caries, especially in children. The effectiveness over time depends on the correct execution of the clinical protocol [1].

Upon comparing various fissure sealant materials with respect to adherence to the enamel surface, penetration, and risk of retention loss, minimal difference has been observed between the sealant materials. However, resin-based sealants have been found to be more effective than Glass ionomer sealants. In addition, unfilled sealants had better penetration into fissures than filled sealants, due to their lower viscosity [15].

Assessment of the Marginal Seal Integrity for Retentiveness [16]

It is performed by a tactile-visual method by using a mirror and #5 explorer

Objective is to clinically evaluate the retentive areas by probing the marginal surface of the applied sealing material in different directions, suggestive of areas of plaque accumulation.

Evaluation is Performed in Four Directions

1. Mesial to distal

2. Distal to mesial

3. Buccal to lingual / palatal

4. Lingual /Palatal to buccal

Scores are as follows

- non retentive
- retention in one direction
- retention in two directions
- 3 - retention in three directions
- 4 - retention in four directions

It has also been classified as “intact sealant,” “partial loss,” and “complete loss.”

Sealant longevity

Another predictor of success for fissure sealants is their longevity. Although sealants do wear naturally and get damaged over time, they usually last between 5 to 10 years. Longevity is dependent upon the sealing material used. Resin sealants have been shown to have superior retention than Glass ionomer sealants [16].

Sealing Non-Cavitated Carious Lesions

Sealants are viable treatment options for controlling non-cavitated lesions on the occlusal and proximal surfaces when there is no significant breach in the surface integrity of the tooth. These are initial caries lesions without any cavitation. They are characterized by a change in colour, surface structure and glossiness due to the demineralization before macroscopic breakdown occurs. It is difficult to diagnose such lesions. So, these lesions may get sealed inadvertently [16]. AAPD guidelines support sealing of occlusal non-cavitated early carious lesions under regular observation and repair. Resin infiltration is suitable for preventing caries progression when applied to occlusal non cavitated pits and fissures.

Therapeutic Pit and Fissure Sealing (TFS)

Whereas the classic preventive pit and fissure sealing is defined as microinvasive sealing of caries-free or stained fissures, therapeutic pit and fissure sealants always involve some minimal cutting action to exclude dentin caries. The access must be just as wide as a dental probe needs to explore the dentin beneath. It is therefore the primary solution for small, minimally carious lesions and represents the first step of a minimally invasive restorative concept, *i.e.,* preventive resin restoration. Teeth having ICDAS scores of 2–5 are indicated for this treatment.

Materials for Therapeutic Fissure Sealing: Adhesive Sealing, flowable composites, sculptable composites.

Therapeutic Fissure Sealing involves opening of dentin; therefore, etching with phosphoric acid alone is not enough for overall pre-treatment. Since occlusal load also comes into play, classical low filled sealing materials fall short from a material science view. The restorations are conducted with totally bonded low viscosity resin-based composites (Smart and Bioactive materials) [3].

Troubleshooting in Sealant Therapy [4]

Dental sealants are one of the most universally used safeguarding materials, as well as the most inadvertently misused products today. Too often when a sealant fails "the virgin tooth goes into a diseased one." Improper application is the leading cause of sealant failure.

Sealant failures

- The success of a sealant does not always go unhitched. Hence sealants are underused.
- The resin cannot flow into the fissure to form tags if remnants of debris are present. Therefore, it is necessary to clean the fissures before sealant placement.
- Saliva contamination- remains a problem, with a resultant decrease in retention and thus, reduced effectiveness.
- If isolation is inadequate, viscous saliva gets into the porosities and if the sealant is flown after drying the surface, it floats as saliva from porosities does not get eliminated. So, one must re-etch the surface and repeat the process in a completely isolated environment.
- The penetration of the sealant is, on average, 17% of the depth of the groove. Therefore, additional placement steps such as priming and drying may be necessary to place a hydrophobic sealant.
- The use of a proper dispensing /delivery system for a selected resin sealant is also essential.
- High viscosity sealants may not be able to fully penetrate even in enamel that has been properly etched. For this reason, some of the researchers recommend using 4th and 5th generation dental adhesives to improve the adhesion and adaption of sealants to the morphology of molars.
- Failure of the marginal integrity of pit and fissure sealants would result in demineralisation and finally decay under the leaking sealant. This can be damaging to the sealed tooth. Therefore, it would be helpful to have the ability to diagnose sealant leakage before extensive demineralisation. A diagnostic tool like Diagnodent would be useful. It will exhibit fluorescence proportionate to the degree of caries, resulting in elevated scale readings on its display.
- Allergic reactions to sealants - though rare the patient may develop signs and symptoms like asthmatic reactions and urticaria. So, unlike the routine line of

treatment for such allergic reactions, removal of the sealants from the affected patient's teeth have shown to be effective in controlling these reactions.

Safety of Sealants

Dental Sealants: Are they Safe?

Dental sealants are completely safe for children. However, rumours, fears, and doubts still pop up. Hence, many parents are naturally concerned. This is largely since they are not aware of the studies and findings concerning dental sealants.

A Controversial Concern: Bisphenol A (BPA)

Some researchers have condemned dental sealants for increasing exposure to BPA. According to the National Institute of Environmental Health Sciences, it is a chemical produced in enormous quantities for use primarily in the production of polycarbonate plastics and epoxy resins. Many dental sealants do contain a miniscule amount of BPA, which happens as a by-product of their manufacturing process. Pure BPA is rarely present in a sealant. A transient presence of BPA in saliva has been reported immediately following placement of some resin-based sealants. The longest duration of salivary BPA was 3 hours after the placement. Thus, there is negligible risk of chronic low dose of BPA exposure. Currently available evidence suggests that there are no oestrogen-like side effects with resin-based sealants.

Probable Causes of Degradation

a. Excessive placement of a sealant without checking the premature contacts.
b. Excessive bruxism.
c. Rough, sticky candy.
d. Inadequate curing

Care to be Taken

a. Use of a proper delivery and dispensing system for the specific sealant used.
b. Proper curing light
c. Adequate curing of the placed sealant.
d. Check for the premature contacts upon occlusion.
e. Immediate cleaning of the sealed surface or removal of the oxygen inhibition layer of the unreacted monomer, which is present on the outer layer of the sealant surface to reduce the amount of unreacted monomer using pumice or rotary rubber cup is recommended.

The potential exposure to BPA after using dental sealants in a child of average weight is 0.037 mg/kg body weight. This exposure level is more than 50,000 times lower than the LD50 values that have been reported for BPA. Thus, the actual exposure to BPA is less than the maximum acceptable dose of 0.05 mg/kg body weight/day [17]. To date, there is no evidence that sealants lead to patient harm, while there is considerable evidence of benefits.

Role of Parental Education and Socio-Economic Status

Parental Attitude [18]

- India, a land of diversity, has many religions, communities, cultures and socio-economic strata.
- Parental education and family income have a direct impact on children's teeth.
- Parental attitude towards the importance of oral hygiene plays a key role in the preservation of healthy teeth in children.
- Low-income families do not pay enough attention to the preventive dental health of children.
- Many surveys have shown that parents do not have sufficient knowledge about the benefits of sealants in keeping their child's molars healthy.
- Countries that successfully implemented preventive programs up to the age of 18 years, achieved satisfactory results in the field of dental caries.
- Parental decisions are influenced by their attitudes which reflect on children's oral health practice.
- Many parents feel that sealant therapy is expensive in India. Moreover, insurance companies do not offer compensation for sealants.
- Attitude towards fissure sealants is related to the parent's gender and to the mother's level of education.
- Mothers were found to be more positive about fissure sealant application for their children than fathers.
- Most of the parents have a low level of knowledge about fissure sealants.
- The relationship between the mother's knowledge and the number of children exhibits a weak positive correlation.

Reasons Cited by the Dentist

- Despite supportive investigations and encouragement for the use of sealants from the scientific community adoption of this preventive agent by dentists has progressed slowly.
- Patients have difficulty in understanding the value of sealants.
- Patients are unwilling to pay.
- Uncertainty due to the absence of surveys about this preventive agent.
- Paucity of information for the public.

- One of the Indian studies revealed that 62.8% of dentists working at private clinics apply fissure sealants infrequently, because they believe it wears easily.

Possible Solutions

- Dental clinics are the primary source of information about sealants. Increasing the acceptability of sealant therapy would be more if it gets reimbursed.
- Media should play a vital role in conveying the importance of sealant therapy to the public at large.
- Paediatric dental health care attitude and practice among parents in relation to sealant therapy needs to be revisited by accelerating the efforts of paediatricians, paediatric dentists and allied healthcare professionals.
- Conducting programs in schools, publishing articles in the media in regional languages, distributing handout bulletins and pamphlets, and establishing kiosks in Primary Health Care Centres may be considered for promoting effective sealant therapy.
- Therefore, to enhance the utilisation of dental sealants, strategies to encourage dentists to promote them with the patient and the public should be included.
- Educating potential consumers about the benefits of dental sealants and to promote greater insurance coverage for oral health care including sealants.

Sealants in Primary Molars

There is no concrete evidence to support sealing fissures in primary molars. Further investigations are required to assess the role of sealants in preventing/arresting non-cavitated carious lesions in primary molars.

Why is there Poor Emphasis in Children?

1. Less prominent occlusal fissure morphology of primary molars.

2. Uncooperative behaviour displayed by young paediatric patients.

3. Moisture control.

4. Inconsistent and low-quality results.

5. Dental patient reported outcomes of paediatric patients including pain, anxiety and diminished oral health related quality of life may have a prolonged negative impact leading to dental anxiety and treatment avoidance.

6. Long term retention rate of glass ionomer cement is poor.

Hence, high quality clinical trials are required in future to generate reliable evidence in primary molars.

Primary and permanent teeth differ in pit and fissure anatomy, enamel demineralization susceptibility and dentin microstructures. Sealing primary molars is more costly initially but reduces subsequent dental treatment. Sealing of fissures in primary molars is an effective method for preventing and arresting caries. However, regular check-ups must be conducted to avoid advanced tooth decay attributable to leakages in the sealing [15].

Patient Centred Benefits of Sealing Primary Molars

1. Healthier population
2. Long term cost savings
3. Does not require local anaesthesia
4. Lesser period of patient co-operation required
5. No anxiety, phobia and dentist avoidance behaviours.

Alternative Techniques

Preventive resin restoration (Fig. 9)

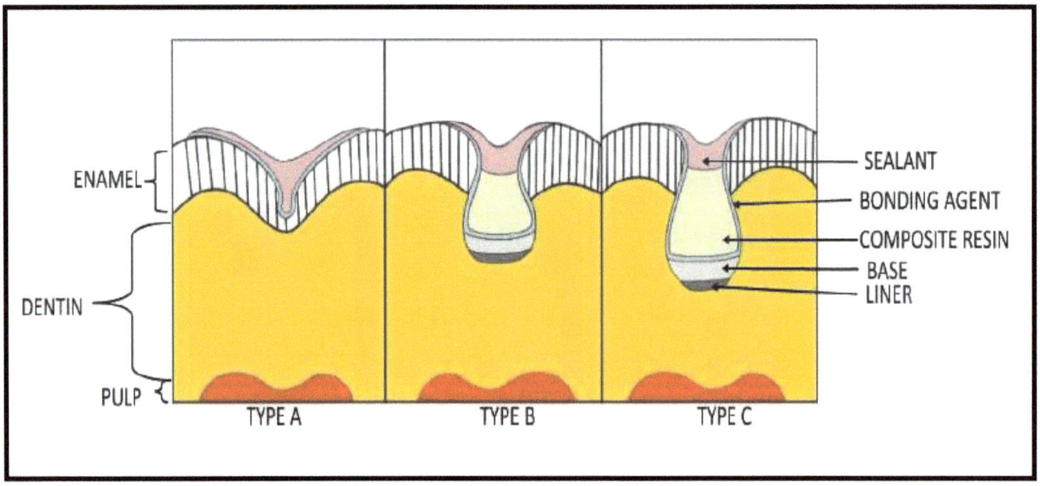

Fig (9). Preventive resin restoration.

They are the natural extension of the use of sealants. It is an integration of the preventive approach of sealants for caries susceptible pits and fissures and the therapeutic restoration of incipient caries. It is a conservative answer to the conventional ‘extension for prevention’ philosophy of G.V. Black.

Based on the extent and depth of the caries as determined by exploratory preparation, PRR is classified into three types:

- **Type A:** Suspicious pit and fissures where caries removal is limited to the enamel. A slow speed ½ or ¼ carbide round bur is used to remove decalcified enamel. Sealant is placed.
- **Type B:** Incipient lesion in dentin that is small and confined. An appropriate base is placed in the areas of dentin exposure, the composite resin is placed, and the remaining pit and fissure are covered with a sealant.
- **Type C:** Lesions are larger and deeper than in type B. It includes extensive dentinal involvement and requires restorations with posterior composite material. An appropriate base is placed over the dentin. Pits and fissures are covered with sealant; local anaesthesia is required only in these cases.

Pre-Fissure Sealant Application

For overall caries prevention, it is now accepted that a preventive regimen should commence as soon as the tooth starts erupting. In molars, the eruption process is lengthy, and the enamel surface is immature and susceptible to acid attack. The operculum covering the erupting tooth is an anatomical barrier that prevents cleaning of the enamel surface due to lack of access. This is an important risk factor to be considered.

Obtaining a dry field on such partially erupted is not possible and hence conventional glass ionomer cement is the only material that can be used for this purpose. Its properties like fast-setting, high fluoride release and less moisture sensitivity make it appropriate for use in these teeth.

Application of glass ionomer cement under the operculum is known as the "pre-fissure sealant" technique. It was designed by Hein Ngo in 2012 to provide protection to molars during the period of eruption. It can be later replaced with a long-term sealant after the complete eruption of the tooth [19].

Smooth Surface Sealant

This concept utilizes low viscosity resins to seal initial proximal lesions. It is an alternative therapeutic approach to prevent further progression of enamel lesions. Achieving access to these lesions is quite difficult.

Hein Ngo in 2012 suggested an alternative procedure that provides easy access to the proximal surface before the contact with adjacent tooth develops [19].

Technique

a. Isolate tooth using a rubber dam
b. Clean exposed surfaces using an abrasive strip
c. Apply 37% phosphoric acid on all proximal surfaces for 20 seconds
d. Rinse and dry the surfaces
e. Apply hard-wearing nano filled resin and light cure
f. Evaluate the surfaces for any material overhangs

Resin Infiltration

A recent micro-invasive technique called as 'Resin Infiltration' has been introduced, which uses a special low viscosity resin (Icon), that penetrates the porous body of an initial carious lesion in the enamel, blocking the diffusion of acids into the lesion, thereby slowing or arresting the lesion progression. In contrast to conventional sealants, which adhere to the enamel surface, resin infiltration penetrates inside the initial carious lesion. It uses 15% HCl for etching the surface, which aids in better penetration of the resin.

Advantages of the Resin Infiltration Technique

a. Mechanical stabilization of demineralized enamel.
b. Permanent obturation of superficial porous and demineralized areas.
c. Preservation of sound, hard substance.
d. Arrest of lesion progress by increasing resistance to demineralization.
e. Minimized risk of secondary caries development
f. High patient acceptance.

SUMMARY

Dental sealants are an evidence based clinical practice and are recommended by federal agencies as well as professional organisations like ADA and AAPD as an effective preventive method to avoid decay in primary and permanent molars in children.

It is advisable to use modern caries detection tools as an adjunct to clinical decisions made in the conventional manner for early caries detection.

- Sealants are effective in minimising the progression of non-cavitated occlusal carious lesions.
- In comparison to two-handed dentistry, four-handed delivery is associated with an increase in the retention rate of sealants.
- Preventive sealants should be placed with low viscosity resin composites.

- For erupting teeth and in case of problems with moisture control, glass ionomer sealants may be preferred.
- The ability of a sealant to prevent dental caries is highly dependent on its ability to be retained on the tooth surface.
- Recently it has been demonstrated that the use of an adhesive system before applying a sealant improves its retention.

CONCLUSION

The main principle underlying the use of sealants is "Prevention is better than cure." Non-diseased teeth, even though sealed with pit and fissure sealants, are more valuable than meticulously restored teeth. Hence, adults as well as children should receive sealants when a tooth or the patient is at risk of experiencing caries. In case of a clinical condition wherein a restoration is not yet warranted, the practitioner should err on the side of placing a sealant rather than monitoring the lesion. Sealants are cost-effective, as they directly save the cost of materials, administrative time, and procedure time. In return, this gives benefits such as a reduction in caries, number of dental visits and procedures. Research studies conducted by the Centre of Disease Control conclude that sealants are safe and effective and reduce tooth decay and help to shield fissures of teeth, where fluoride toothpaste is not protective. Maximizing the cost effectiveness of this preventive approach is the key to the success of pit and fissure sealants.

CONSENT FOR PUBLICATION

Not applicable.

CONFLICT OF INTEREST

The authors declare no conflict of interest, financial or otherwise.

ACKNOWLEDGEMENT

Declared none.

REFERENCES

[1] Evidence-based clinical practice guideline for the use of pit-and-fissure sealants. Pediatr Dent 2016; 38(6): 263-79.
[PMID: 27931466]

[2] Elmarakby AM. Why Pits and Fissures Remain a Challenge in Prevention of Caries Lesion? J Oral Med 2017; 1: 1-2.

[3] Cvikl B, Moritz A, Bekes K. Pit and Fissure Sealants—A Comprehensive Review. Dent J 2018; 6(2): 18.
[http://dx.doi.org/10.3390/dj6020018] [PMID: 29895726]

[4] Wells MH. Pit and fissure sealants: scientific and clinical rationale. Pediatr Dent 2019; 1: 461-481.e2. [http://dx.doi.org/10.1016/B978-0-323-60826-8.00033-X]

[5] Khetani P, *et al.* History and Selection of Pit and Fissure Sealants – A Review. Quest Journals. Journal of Medical and Dental Science Research 2017; 4: 5-12.

[6] Frencken JE, Sharma P, Stenhouse L, Green D, Laverty D, Dietrich T. Global epidemiology of dental caries and severe periodontitis – a comprehensive review. J Clin Periodontol 2017; 44 (Suppl. 18): S94– S105.

[7] Schiffner U. Trends in Caries Epidemiology in Children. Pit and Fissure Sealants 2018; 1-10. [http://dx.doi.org/10.1007/978-3-319-71979-5_1]

[8] Hirsch C. Pit and fissure sealants. Bekes K, editor. Springer International Publishing; 2018 Feb 27.

[9] Melo M, Pascual A, Camps I, Del Campo Á. *In vivo* study of different methods for diagnosing pit and fissure caries. J Clin Exp Dent 2015; 7(3): e387-91. [http://dx.doi.org/10.4317/jced.52347] [PMID: 26330935]

[10] Tassoker M, Ozcan S, Karabekiroglu S. Occlusal Caries Detection and Diagnosis Using Visual ICDAS Criteria, Laser Fluorescence Measurements, and Near-Infrared Light Transillumination Images. Med Princ Pract 2020; 29: 25-31. [http://dx.doi.org/10.1159/000501257] [PMID: 31158839]

[11] Bechir ES, Suciu M, Bechir F, Berneanu FD, Bechir A, Tohati A. Clinical Trial Concerning the Effectiveness of Two Types Dental Sealants in Children with Bruxism. Mater Plast 2020; 57(1): 191-6. [http://dx.doi.org/10.37358/MP.20.1.5326]

[12] Patel A, Aghababaie S, Parekh S. Hypomineralisation or hypoplasia? Br Dent J 2019; 227(8): 683-6. [http://dx.doi.org/10.1038/s41415-019-0782-9] [PMID: 31654000]

[13] Bagherian A, Sarraf Shirazi A. Preparation before acid etching in fissure sealant therapy: yes or no? J Am Dent Assoc 2016; 147(12): 943-51. [http://dx.doi.org/10.1016/j.adaj.2016.08.003] [PMID: 27666005]

[14] Bagherian A, Sarraf Shirazi A, Sadeghi R. Adhesive systems under fissure sealants: yes or no? J Am Dent Assoc 2016; 147(6): 446-56. [http://dx.doi.org/10.1016/j.adaj.2016.01.014] [PMID: 26993212]

[15] Naaman R, El-Housseiny A, Alamoudi N. The use of pit and fissure sealants— A literature review. Dent J 2017; 5(4): 34. [http://dx.doi.org/10.3390/dj5040034] [PMID: 29563440]

[16] Anauate-Netto C, Borelli Neto L, Amore R, Di Hipólito V, D'Alpino PHP. Caries progression in non-cavitated fissures after infiltrant application: a 3-year follow-up of a randomized controlled clinical trial. J Appl Oral Sci 2017; 25(4): 442-54. [http://dx.doi.org/10.1590/1678-7757-2016-0633] [PMID: 28877284]

[17] Rathee M, Malik P, Singh J. Bisphenol A in dental sealants and its estrogen like effect. Indian J Endocrinol Metab 2012; 16(3): 339-42. [http://dx.doi.org/10.4103/2230-8210.95660] [PMID: 22629496]

[18] Tahani B, Yadegarfar G, Ahmadi A. Knowledge, attitude, and practice of parents of 7–12-year-old children regarding fissure sealant therapy and professional fluoride therapy. J Educ Health Promot 2017; 6(1): 106. [http://dx.doi.org/10.4103/jehp.jehp_17_17] [PMID: 29296607]

[19] Ngo H, Seow K. Two compliance-free and site-specific caries control techniques: pre-fissure and proximal sealants. International Dentistry South Africa 2012; 2(1): 38-42.

CHAPTER 17

Vaccination in Children/Caries Vaccine

Nilima Thosar[1,*], **Shailja Chatterjee**[2] and **Priyanka Bhaje**[3]

[1] *Department of Pediatric and Preventive Dentistry, Sharad Pawar Dental College, and Hospital, Wardha-442107, Maharashtra, India*

[2] *Yamuna Institute of Dental Sciences and Research, Yamuna Nagar, India*

[3] *Rungata College of Dental Sciences and Research, Bhilai, Chhattisgarh 490024, India*

Abstract: Vaccination is an important measure that is undertaken to provide an individual with acquired immunity against a variety of diseases which may result in significant morbidity and sometimes, may even result in mortality. The vaccination program undertaken by Government has helped in containing many diseases which were responsible for many fatalities in the past. Like any other branch of science, vaccines are also evolving with continuous advancements in their mode of synthesis as well as the method of delivery.

Even though various approaches to caries prevention are available, dental caries is still considered to be an irreversible, and a prevalent disease among humans mankind. *Mutans streptococci* are responsible for such activity. Biofilm is formed on the tooth surface due to everyday diet consumption followed by the role of mutans streptococci through the entry into biofilm on the tooth surface. Most treatment options or medications work for the disposal or destruction of this microorganism. The concept of immunization can be the alternative that works on either inactive or passive grounds. Certain molecular determinants of *mutans streptococci* are studied and considered for caries formation. Therefore, their use in the preparation of the caries vaccine is widely researched.

Keywords: Advancements, Caries Vaccine, Immunization, Mutans Streptococci, Vaccine.

INTRODUCTION

The term "vaccine" originated from the Latin words 'Variolae vaccines or cowpox. Edward Jenner was the first person to demonstrate the concept of vaccination in 1795 by injecting sera from cowpox to prevent chickenpox. A "Vaccine" may be defined as 'A biologically derived product that can provide

* **Corresponding author Nilima thosar:** Department of Pediatric and Preventive Dentistry, Sharad Pawar Dental College, and Hospital, Wardha-442107, Maharashtra, India; E-mail: drnthosar@rediffmail.com

adaptive immunization against a specific organism or disease'. Various routes of its administration are oral, intranasal, or injectable routes [1].

Vaccines are of two types:

- Prophylactic vaccines- to prevent disease
- Therapeutic vaccines -used for treating disease

The etiologic agent for dental caries is *mutans streptococci*. There are various approaches for the prevention of dental caries such as fluorides, pit and fissure sealants, and synthetic and mechanical plaque removal agents.

Dental caries like other diseases occurs on tooth surfaces that are covered by saliva in which antibody immunoglobulin secretory IgA (SIgA) is present. Therefore, immunization procedures using salivary SIgA antibodies help to induce caries immunity. Salivary IgA antibodies have the potential to inhibit the accumulation of *mutans streptococci* on the teeth.

VACCINES FOR CHILDREN

Classification of Vaccines

a. Live-attenuated vaccines: Mumps, measles, rubella, and Varicella zoster.
b. Inactivated vaccine: Influenza, Hepatitis A, Pneumococcal polysaccharide.
c. Recombinant sub-unit: Hepatitis B.
d. Toxoids: Diphtheria; Tetanus.
e. Conjugated polysaccharides with protein: Hemophilus influenza, Meningococcus, Pneumococcus.

Constituents of a Vaccine

Vaccines contain therapeutic agents or drugs and are generally derived from either killed or attenuated forms of micro-organisms, toxins, or surface proteins. A vaccine is constituted of- an antigen, solvent (water or saline), additives, preservatives, and at times, adjuvants. All of these ingredients of a vaccine are collectively termed as 'excipients [2].

Preservatives: Preservatives ensure vaccine sterilization due to their shelf-life. These prevent container contamination and also aid in protecting from microbiological contamination. These are non-toxic in quantities used and do not diminish their potency. The most commonly used preservatives in various kinds of vaccines are as follows:

- Phenol: It is used in vaccines against typhoid and pneumococcus.
- Benzalkonium chloride: It is used in the Anthrax vaccine.
- 2-phenoxyethanol: It is a preservative used in inactivated polio vaccines.
- Thimerosal: It is effective against the influenza virus.

Adjuvants: These agents act by enhancing the immunological effects of the antigenic component in a vaccine. However, these do not act as antigens. The most commonly used adjuvants in vaccines are Aluminium salts. Vaccines that contain adjuvants show slightly higher adverse reactions such as pain at the site of injection, fever, and malaise. Examples of adjuvant containing vaccines are- Hepatitis A and B, DPT (Diphtheria, Pertussis, and Tetanus), HPV vaccine, Japanese encephalitis (all of these contain Aluminium salts as adjuvants) whereas for the H1N1 vaccine, an adjuvant used is MF59 which is an emulsion of oil in water.

Antigens: Antigens are those components of a microorganism or any vaccine that triggers the host's immunological response. These cause the production of antibodies. Sometimes, these vaccines can produce serious side effects or clinical outcomes.

VARIOUS VACCINES FOR CHILDREN

There are various vaccines used for various systemic diseases [3]. Vaccines for various medical conditions have been summarized along with their type and year and depicted in Table **1**.

Table 1. Summary of various vaccines used in routine immunization.

Name of the disease	Vaccine type	Year in which developed
	Viral	
Smallpox	Live attenuated	1798
Rabies	a) Inactivated vaccine b) Inactivated form derived from cell culture	1885 1976
Yellow fever	Live attenuated	1932
Influenza	a) Inactivated vaccine b) Live attenuated	1936 2003
Polio	a) Inactivated vaccine b) Live attenuated	1955 1062
Mumps	a) Inactivated vaccine b) Live attenuated	1948 1967
Rubella	Live attenuated	1969
Varicella	Live attenuated	1974

(Table 1) cont.....

Name of the disease	Vaccine type	Year in which developed
Herpes zoster	Live attenuated	2005
Rotavirus	Live attenuated	2006
Japanese encephalitis	a) Inactivated vaccine b) Live attenuated	1935 1988
Tick-origin encephalitis	Inactivated vaccine	1937
Hepatitis A	Inactivated vaccine	1995
Hepatitis B	a) Plasma-derived b) Recombinant protein	1981 1986
Human Papilloma Virus	Recombinant protein	2006
Bacterial		
Cholera	a) Inactivated (injectable) b) Inactivated/recombinant protein c) Inactivated (oral dose)	1896 1991 1997
Typhoid	a) Inactivated form b) Live-attenuated c) Polysaccharide d) Conjugated protein	1886 1983 1994 2008
Plague	Inactivated vaccine	1897
Diphtheria	Toxoid	1923
Tetanus	Toxoid	1926
Pertussis	a) Inactivated vaccine b) Purified protein form	1914 1981
Tuberculosis	Live attenuated	1921
Pneumococcal	a) 23 valency polysaccharides b) Conjugated protein	1983 2000
Meningitis	a) Protein polysaccharide b) Conjugated protein	1971 1994
Anthrax	Protein	1954

TYPES OF VACCINES AND THEIR MECHANISM OF ACTION

Live-attenuated vaccines [2, 4, 5]: These vaccines act by simulating infectious processes within the body, thereby, boosting the host's immune status. Their effect lasts life-long. Examples include- mumps, measles, rubella, varicella, herpes zoster, typhoid, etc. The first attenuated vaccine was developed for rabies.

Inactivated vaccines [6]: These vaccines are made up of inactivated or whole-killed micro-organism. These act by promoting the synthesis of antibodies, but no cell-mediated immunity is produced. These vaccines require booster dosages to sustain the immunological response; for example, hepatitis A, rabies, polio, and influenza.

Sub-unit or conjugated vaccines [4]: These vaccines are produced in case there is a known antigen. These vaccines are of three types-

- Those derived from capsules (capsular vaccines) - Haemophilus, typhoid, pneumococcus, typhoid.
- Those derived from toxins (toxin-derived or toxoids): diphtheria, tetanus, pertussis.
- Those comprising neutralizing antigens (mainly, cell surface components) - hepatitis B, human papillomavirus, and pertussis.
- Protein-based subunit vaccines: These are a variety of subunit vaccines wherein the disease-causing protein portion is used.

Polysaccharide-Based Vaccines [7, 8]: In these vaccines, a portion of pathogenicity-inducing polysaccharides contains a capsule or the sugar coat of a cell membrane. However, this vaccine induces a very minimal inflammatory response.

Modes of Vaccine Delivery

The various modes of vaccine delivery include- oral route, injectable or nasal/mucosal sprays [9]. Targeting of mucosal tissues whether nasal or oral can act as an easy target for inducing body defense by promoting mucosal IgA antibodies production and maybe the production of secretory IgG antibodies. However, there are certain challenges in delivering vaccines via the oral route such as- there are various physiological restrictions that can hamper the therapeutic effects via this route. For instance, the low pH conditions existing in the stomach, intestinal conditions, different proteolytic enzymes such as chymotrypsin and trypsin apart from mucinous barrier; retention period in intestines and adsorption rates. This impacts the half-lives of the vaccines, thus decreasing their efficaciousness.

Immunization Schedule: The immunization schedule which is followed in India [10] is depicted in Table **2** which shows the name of the vaccine, its time of administration along with the dose, route, and site.

Table 2. Immunization schedule as per the National Immunization Schedule in India.

Name of vaccine	Time of administration	Dose	Route of administration	Site of administering the vaccine
For Infants				
BCG	At birth or as till one year	0.1ml (0.05 ml till 1 month)	Intra-dermal	Left Upper Arm
Hepatitis B	At birth or within 24 hours	0.5 ml	Intramuscular	Antero-lateral mid-thigh
Oral Polio Vaccine -0	At birth or within 15 days	Two drops	Oral	Oral
Oral Polio Vaccine: 1, 2 and 3	At 6, 1, and 14 weeks (can be administered till 5 years)	Two drops	Oral	Oral
Pentavalent 1, 2 and 3	At 6, 10, and 14 weeks (can be given till one year of age)	0.5 ml	Intramuscular	Antero-lateral mid-thigh
Rotavirus	At 6, 10, and 14 weeks (can be given till one year)	5 drops	Oral	Oral
IPV	Two fractional doses were administered at 6 and 14 weeks	0.1 ml	Intra-dermal administration in two fractional doses	Right upper arm
Measles or Measles/Rubella (MR) (First Dose)	On completion of 09 to 12 months (can be administered till 5 years)	0.5 ml	Subcutaneous	Right upper arm
Japanese Encephalitis - 1	On completion of 09 to 12 months.	0.5 ml	Subcutaneous	Left upper Arm
Vitamin A (Primary dose)	After 9 months along with measles-Rubella	1 ml (1 lakh I.U.)	Oral	Oral
For Children				
DPT (First booster dose)	16 to 24 months	0.5 ml	Intramuscular	Antero-lateral mid-thigh
Measles/ MR (Second dose)	16 to 24 months	0.5 ml	Subcutaneous	Right upper arm
Oral Polio Vaccine (booster dose)	16 to24 months	2 drops	Oral	Oral
Japanese Encephalitis-2 (Selected endemic districts)	16 to 24 months	0.5 ml	Subcutaneous	Left Upper Arm

(Table 2) cont.....

Name of vaccine	Time of administration	Dose	Route of administration	Site of administering the vaccine
DPT Booster-2	5 to 6 years	0.5 ml	Intramuscular	Upper Arm
TT (Tetanus toxoid)	10 and 16 years	0.5 ml	Intramuscular	Upper Arm

CARIES VACCINE? PRESENT AND FUTURE

Dental Caries Vaccine

Etiology

Mutans streptococci have been introduced by Clarke and are considered as one of the causative agents for smooth surface caries. In 2002, the genomic arrangement of this microorganism was studied [11].

Mutans Streptococci Action

There are 2 important properties of mutans streptococci

- Acid-producing capacity - Acidogenic
- Tolerating acidic environment – Aciduric [12]

Chart 1: Mechanism of action of mutans streptococci

- Dietary carbohydrates are utilized by oral microorganisms for their metabolic activities. After consumption of dietary carbohydrates such as sucrose, due to the microbial action of mutans streptococci, it is split into either glucose/ fructose or extracellular polysaccharides due to enzymatic action which is responsible for adherence to tooth structure through plaque which is tenaciously adherent on the tooth. Once deposited on the tooth surface, due to metabolic activities of bacteria, glucan/ fructan is rapidly absorbed using "phosphor pyruvate-mediated phosphotransferase sugar uptake system (PEP-PTS)" and lactic acid is formed which can cause tooth dissolution (Chart **1**, Figs. **1** & **2**).
- Lactose is directly converted into lactic acid. In case of depletion of extracellular polysaccharides, intracellular polysaccharides or intracellular storage compounds act as energy sources for microbial activities.

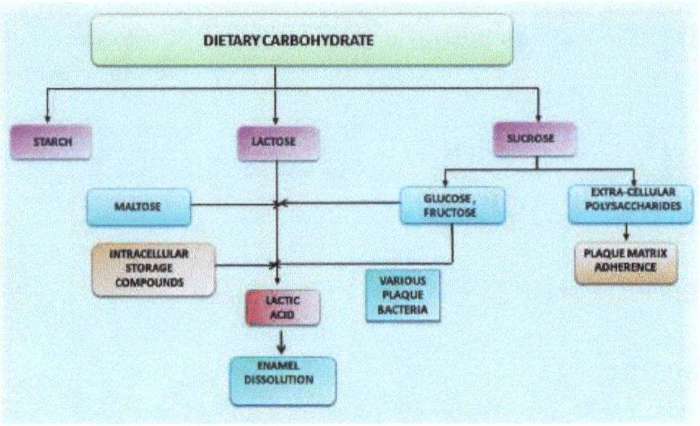

Fig. (1). *Mutans streptococci* action for the acid formation and tooth demineralization.

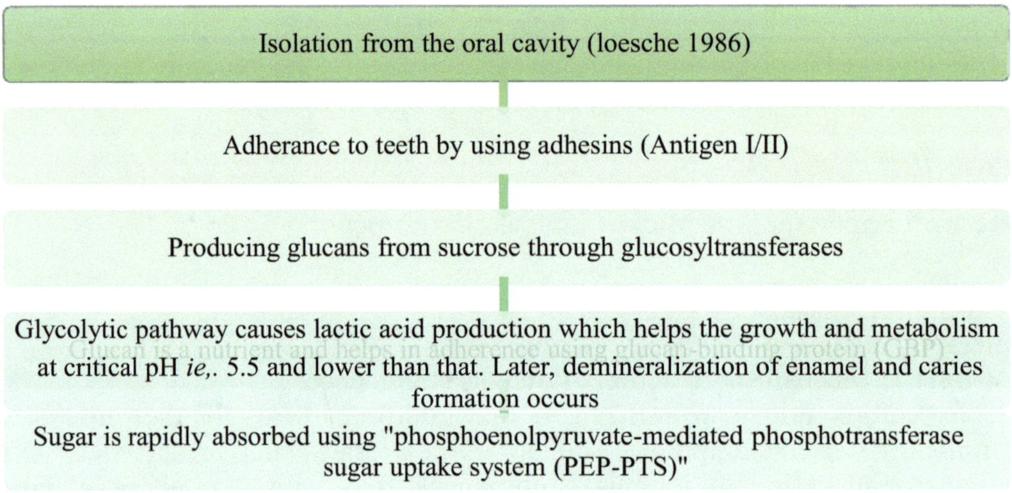

Fig. (2). Utilization of dietary carbohydrates for microbial activities.

Immune Response of Caries Vaccine

It is an immune and biological formulation that helps to protect against the disease and acts by giving an immune response (Chart 2,3) [11, 12].

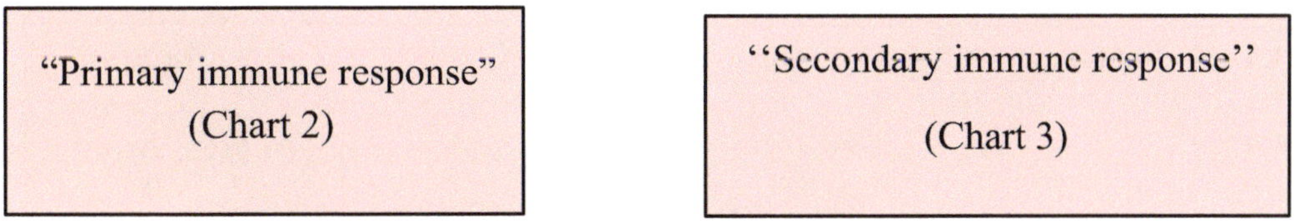

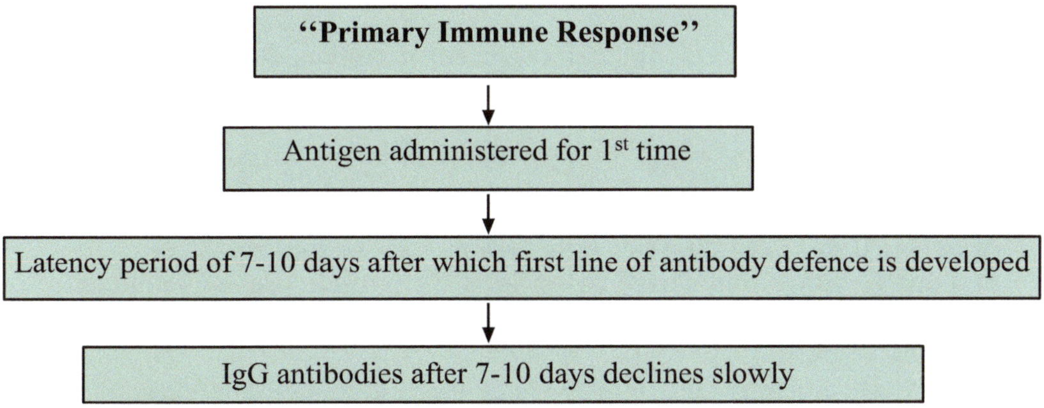

Chart. (2). Primary immune response.

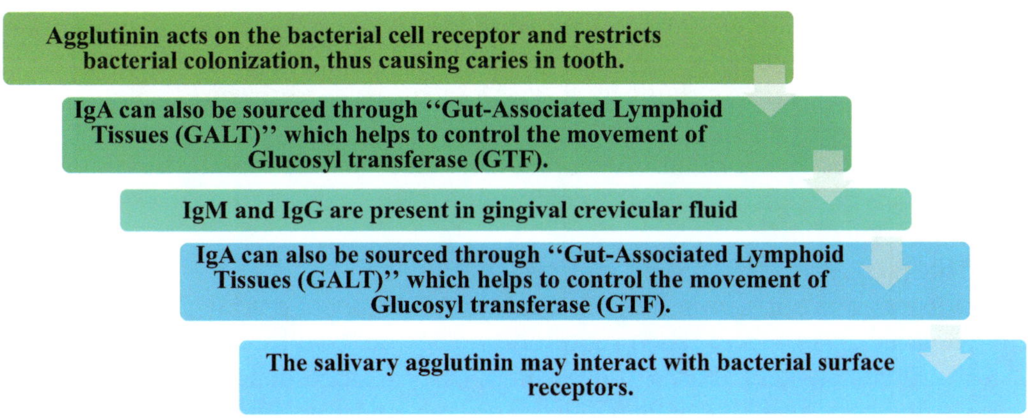

Chart. (3). Secondary immune response.

The Secondary Response (Booster)

- Secondary response is in the form of a booster (Chart 3)
- There is a surge in both IgM and IgG antibodies.
- Collaboration is necessary between the B and T lymphocytes to have immunological memory.
- This collaboration of primary and secondary responses is referred to as immunological memory.

- Salivary S-IgA is an essential immunoglobulin available in saliva.
- Other important immunoglobulins include IgG and IgM, the source of which is from the gingival fluid.
- Other cellular structures of gingival fluid include Lymphocytes, Macrophages, and Neutrophils

Molecular Targets

Following molecular targets are responsible for the mechanism of bacterial adherence (Chart **4**, Fig. **3**).

1. Adhesins: [12-14]
   - It contains a polypeptide chain having 1600 molecules
   - Antigen I/II discovered on the surface of *mutans streptococci*
   - Immune response transferred to Antigen I/II particle prevents adherence of *mutans streptococci*
2. Glucosyltransferases (GTFS): [12-14]
   - *Mutans streptococci* and *S. Sobrinus* have glucosyltransferases in their structure.
3. Glucan-binding proteins: [12-14]
   - *Mutans Streptococci* have "glucan-binding proteins" on their surface and pass to receptor cells.
   - *Mutans streptococci* cannot bind with glucans due to the presence of "cell-divider related glucan-restricting proteins (Gbps)".
   - *Mutans streptococci* and *Streptococcus sobrinus* as well have various proteins with "glucan binding" potentialities.
4. Dextranases: [12-14]
   a. This protein is prepared by *mutans streptococci.*
   b. If used as an antigen, it helps in *mutans streptococci* colonization in plaque.
   c. *Mutans streptococci* when required crushes dextran by providing chemical dextranase to keep stores of dextran in early formed dental plaque.
      - Adhesion Ag I/II, GBPs, GTFs, Enolase, and Phosphate-binding protein are used for the preparation of the dental vaccine.
      - Dental vaccine initiates the formation of specific antibodies which helps to hamper the function of these virulence factors. Therefore, it helps to reduce counts of *mutans streptococci* of plaque and prevent the development of dental caries.

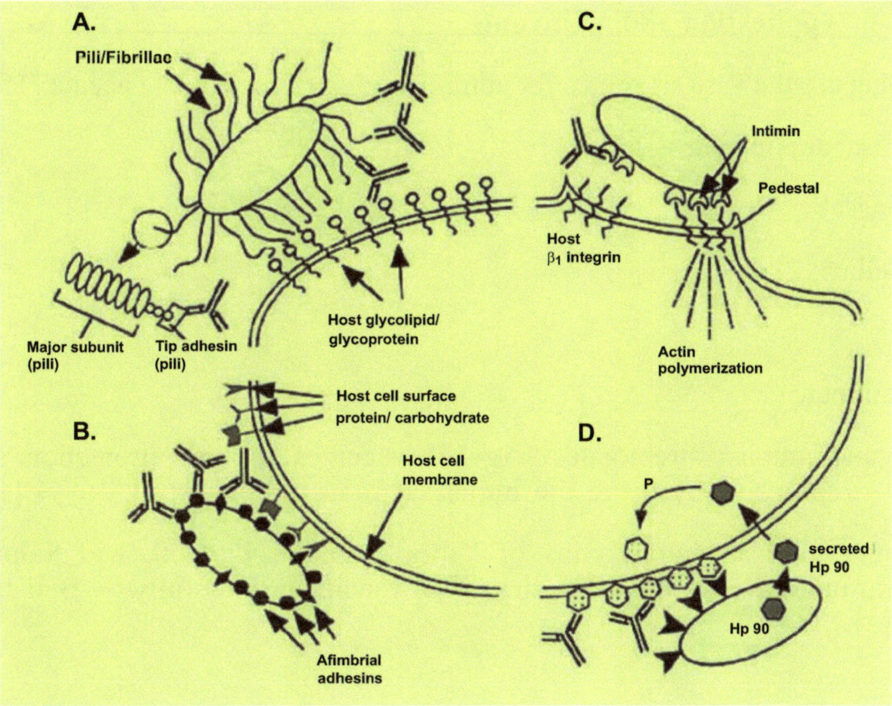

Chart. (4). Mechanism of bacterial adherence.

- •Fimbrillae or pilli present on bacterial surface act as proteinaceous appendage. They bind to host cell such as carbohydrates by adhesins which are present on distal side of pilus or fibrilla. Antibodies which are targeted towards adhesins protein interfere and block the interaction between bacteria and host.
- •Similar action as mediated by afibrial adhesion proteins. Here, antibodies not only block the bacterial attachment but also impedes the bactrial colonization by iinterfering its ability to associate with mucosal tissues.
- •There is ability of some bacteria to have association with eukaryotic cells by using intimin proteins. It results in host cell signaling, cytoskeletal rearrangements, internalization of bacteria, and in certain situations, systemic disease.Therfore strategy is to block block initmate association and adherance and orevent infections.
- •Receptor protein is secreted by bacteria themselves. It gets internalized by targeted host cell, phosphorylated, and embedded in eukaryotic cell as a new receptor for its binding firmly by the bacterium.

Fig. (3). Mechanism of bacterial adherence.

Routes of Application and Adjuvants

Following are the various routes for administration of the caries vaccine [15]:

1. Mucosal application

2. Intranasal

3. Tonsillar

4. Oral

5. Rectal route

GBPB and mutans streptococci Ag I/II vaccines showed protection against *mutans streptococci* by using the intranasal route. (Smith et al. 1997) [15].

Adjuvants such as enterotoxins of Vibrio cholera, E. Coli, and Salmonella Typhimurium have been used in the caries vaccine successfully by Batista et al. 2017 [15].

Routes of Administration – Caries Vaccine (Fig. 4)

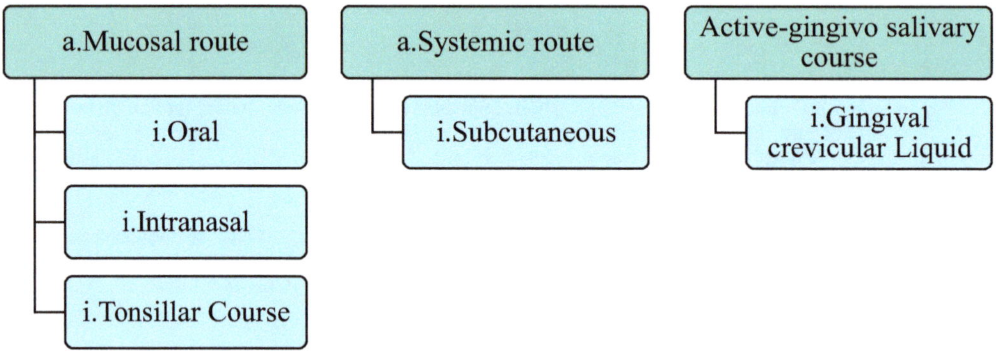

Fig. (4). Different routes of administration.

1. Active vaccination:
2. Passive Immunization: Supplementation provided from outside sources can help to acquire immunity (Fig **5**).

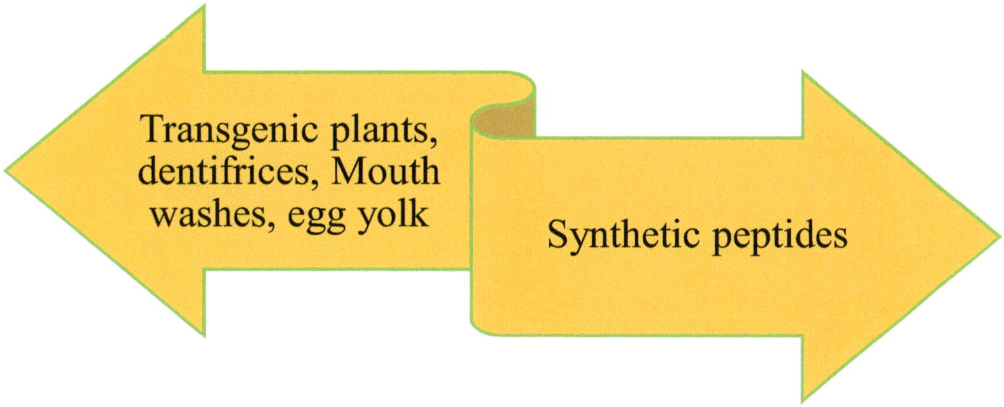

Fig. (5). Supplementation from outside sources to provide passive immunization.

Appropriate Time for Caries Vaccine Administration in Children

- Period of **the** window of infectivity ranges from between 19-33 months during which chances of teeth getting infected with mutans streptococci are more (Fig **6**).
- Appropriate and beneficial time for vaccination against dental caries is infancy before teeth eruption.
- During this time, colonization of mutans streptococci is delayed on tooth surface due to inhibition of their adherence by the action of S-IgA antibodies.
- During the window of infectivity, early tooth colonizers are responsible for creating a synergistic effect toward the suppression of mutans streptococci.
- A booster dose of caries vaccine will be required at the time of the first permanent molar eruption.

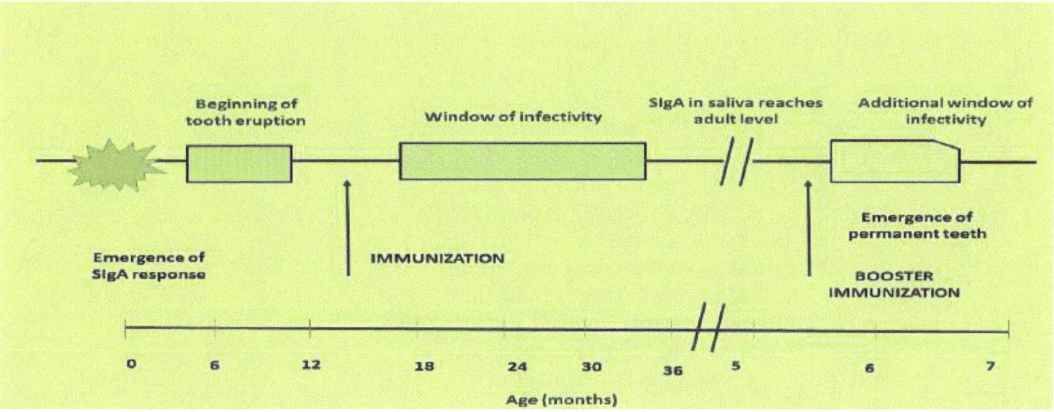

Fig. (6). Window of infectivity.

Advantages of Caries Vaccine (Fig. 7)

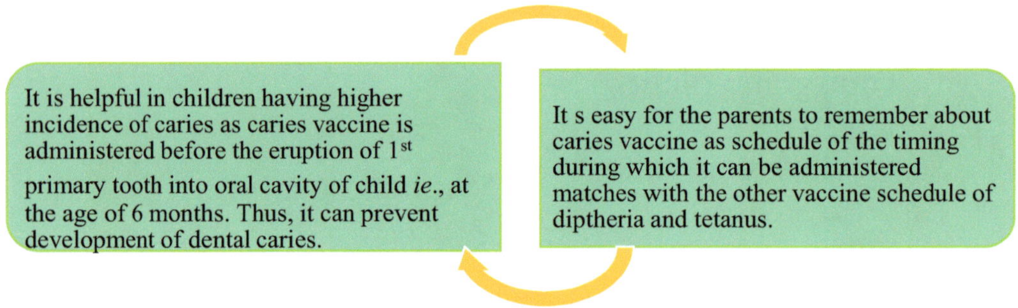

Fig. (7). Advantages of caries vaccine.

Following are the advantages of the caries vaccine [1].

Limitations of caries vaccine (Fig. 8)

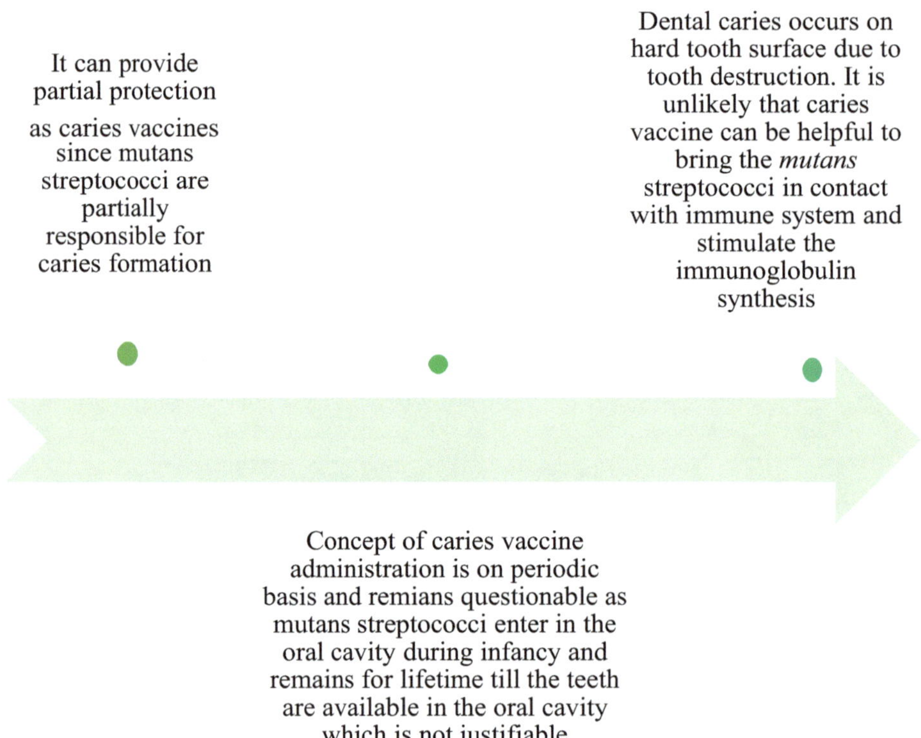

Fig. (8). Limitations of caries vaccine.

Future Trends of Vaccines

DNA vaccines [2, 3]: Gene derived from bacteria or viruses are used for the preparation of DNA vaccines (Chart **5**).

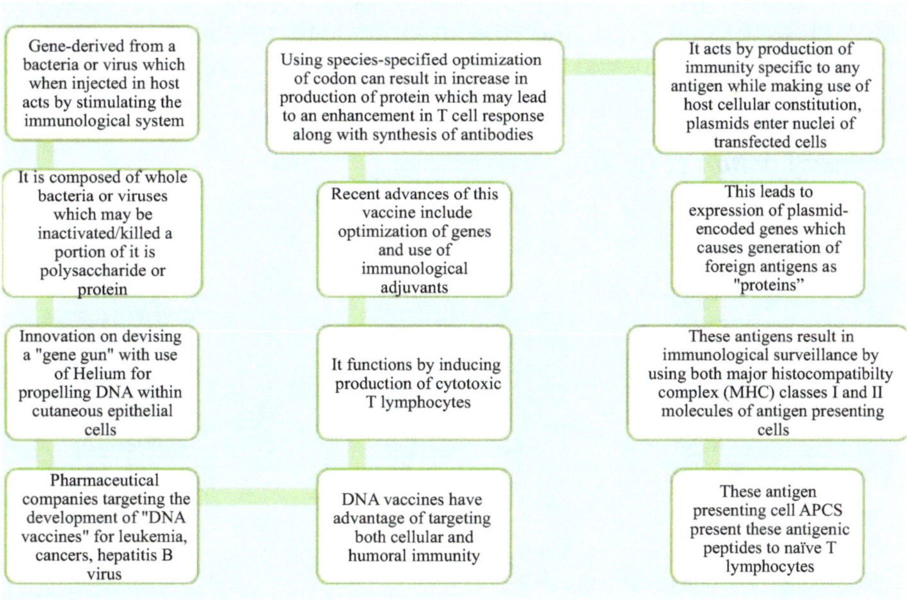

Chart. (5). Mechanism of DNA vaccine.

Anti-HIV DNA Vaccine

It utilizes the concept of a combination of HIV and DNA vaccines together (Fig 9) [2, 3].

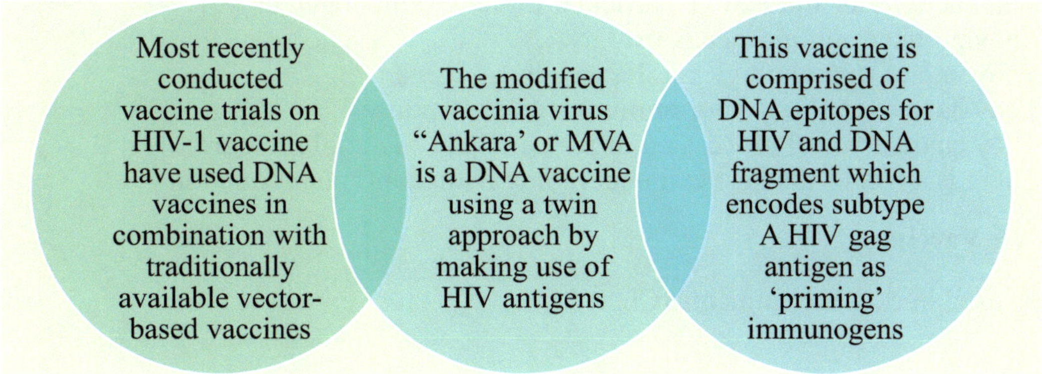

Fig. (9). Anti-HIV DNA vaccine.

DNA vaccines in Cancer Immunotherapy

Newer approaches for promoting DNA vaccines in cancer therapy have been proposed which include- electroporation which is used for the delivery of antigens or cytokines within tumors. Advantages of DNA vaccines include- their relative safety, easy storage conditions, and ease in large-scale production. These vaccines are used for encoding bacterial or viral antigenic immunogenic mechanisms by involving different immunological mechanisms [2, 3].

Mechanisms of action (Fig. 10)

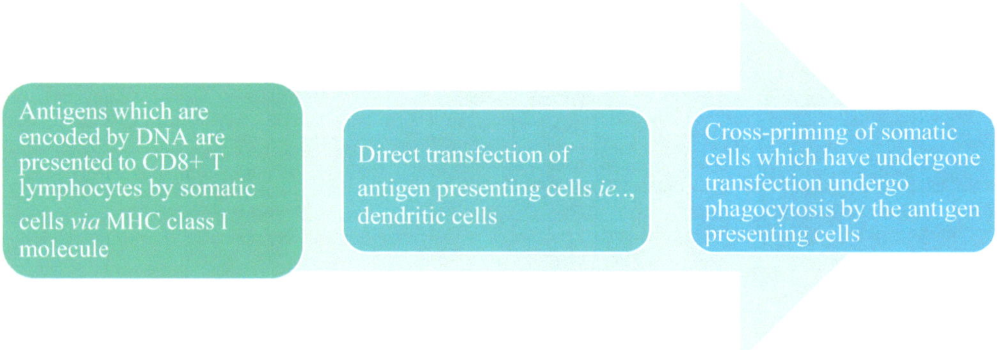

Fig. (10). Mechanism of action of DNB vaccine.

There are three mechanisms.

Disadvantages of DNA Vaccines

- Their activity is limited to a particular protein immunogen only.
- They produce antibodies against DNA.
- They induce immunological tolerance by antigens.
- They have a relatively poor immunological response
- They cause atypical processing of parasitic and bacterial proteins
- There is a risk of the host cell undergoing malignant transformation

RNA Vaccines

It is used in cancer treatments (Chart **5**).

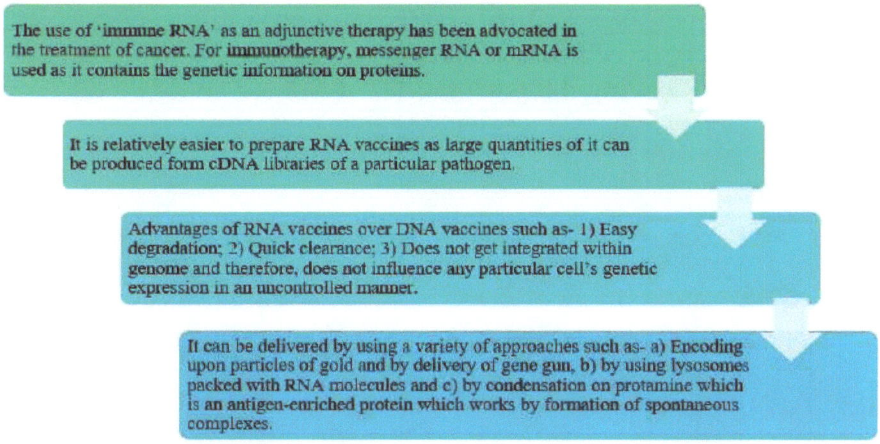

Chart. (6). RNA vaccine.

Recent Advances in Caries Vaccine Production (Fig. 11)

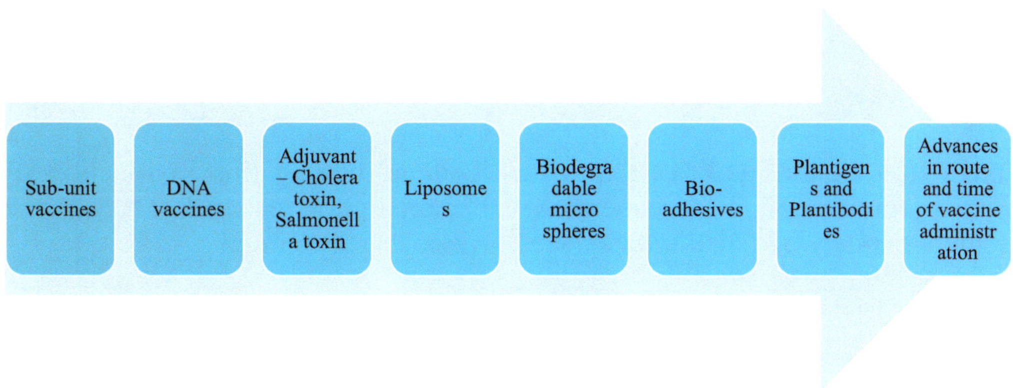

Fig. (11). Advances in caries vaccine.

1. Subunit Vaccine [13, 14]

The whole vaccine when introduced into the host produces an antibody response. But it can cause cross-reaction with heart muscles. So, a specific protein unit of an organism acts as an antigen. Sub-unit vaccines consisting of synthetic peptides based on putative functional domains of glucosyltransferase are developed. They attack directly on the antigen surface.

- It contains structural elements of the Ag I/II adhesins family, Gifs or gbps
- It contains single/ multiple copies of epitopes of domains associated with salivary binding, catalytic processes/ glucan binding activities.

- Homologous sequences induce cross-reactive response influencing colonization, attachment/ accumulation of microbiota.
- It excludes sequences having the potential for unwanted antibody responses.

Types: Synthetic peptide vaccines (Fig. **12**), Recombinant vaccines/ attenuated expression vectors

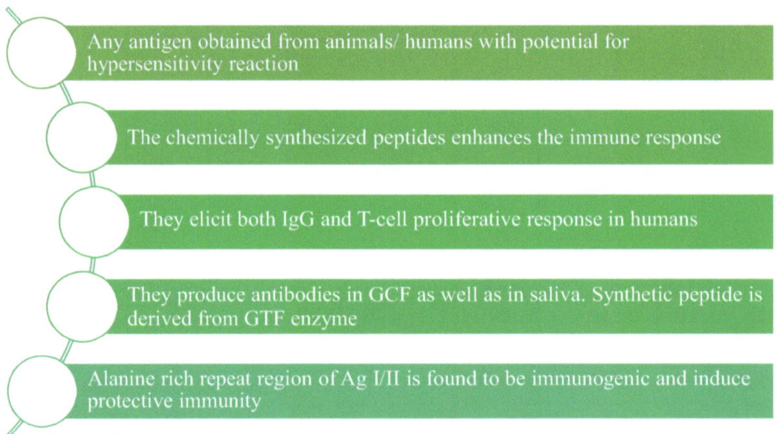

Fig. (12). Synthetic peptides.

2. Conjugate Vaccine [13, 14]: It is the chemical conjugation of functionally associated protein/peptide components with bacterial polysaccharides. It enhances the immunogenicity of T-cell independent polysaccharide entities.

Recombinant bacterial vector (Fig. **13**).

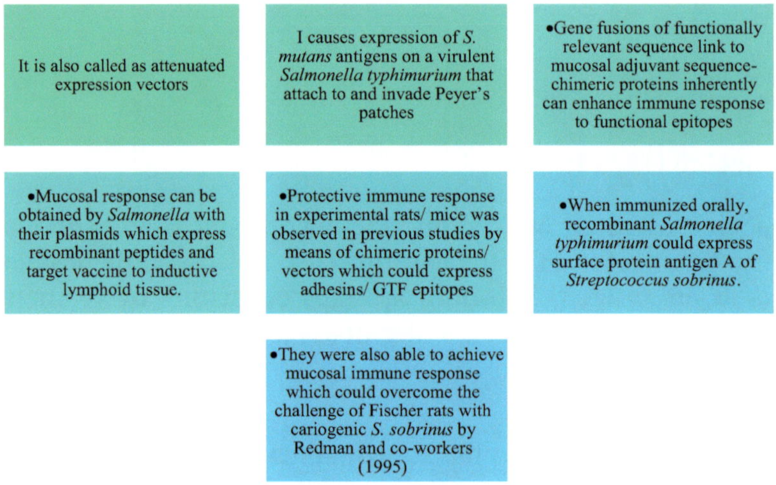

Fig. (13). Recombinant bacterial vectors.

DNA Vaccine [13 - 15]

- It makes antigenicity long-lasting. It is the bacterial plasmid that expresses genes for the antigen of interest in the cells of the host.
- Anti-caries DNA vaccine, pCIA-P, encodes 2 highly conservative regions of PAc, could induce protective anti-caries immune responses.
- When specific DNA is administered, the host starts synthesizing protein components coded by DNA.
- Cell wall protein antigen of mutans streptococci is considered a virulence factor as it favors its initial attachment to the tooth. Anti-caries DNA vaccine acts on such cell wall protein.
- Its long-term effect is like that of natural protein.
- It induces both cellular and humoral immunity.

Adjuvants [13 - 15]

- These are the molecules to which antigenic peptides are attached to produce a potent immune response.
- They act as a reservoir where the antigen is released progressively.
- They present the antigen directly to immune-competent cells.
- Certain adjuvants act as chemical immune stimulators of lymphoid cells.
- Some adjuvants which are tried for long are Freund's incomplete adjuvant-aluminum hydroxide or phosphate, Freund's complete adjuvant-Freund's incomplete adjuvant with a suspension of killed tubercle bacilli, Silica particles, Beryllium sulfate, Endotoxins.
- Adjuvants used with caries vaccine antigens recently are: Mucosal adjuvant e.g., cholera toxin- A1 subunit of cholera toxin, coupling with carrier microparticles, Live bacterial vectors are, Attenuated Salmonella, BCG, normal oral flora, etc., Live viral vectors e.g., Vaccina, adenovirus, and polio replicons.

Liposomes [15]

- Jackson *et al.,* 1990 had conducted a study using Liposomes Containing Anti-Idiotypic Antibodies: An Oral Vaccine which could induce protective immunity to dental caries via the mucosal introduction of the vaccine.
- These are lipid vesicles lined by external liposomal membranes and are composed of similar lipids of the cell membrane.
- Any liposoluble antigen can be incorporated into the lipid membrane and any hydro soluble antigen in the internal cavity of the liposome.
- Change in lipid composition can alter the particle size of liposomes. Initially, a small liposome delivers the antigen rapidly, while the larger liposome releases

the antigen slowly. Thus, sustained release of antigen can be shown.

ISCOM

- ISCOM vaccine can elicit a mucosal and systemic immune response by either mucosal or parenteral route as suggested by Childers NK et al, 2002
- These are solid particles produced by attaching antigen with a biocompatible detergent and adjuvant which gives rise to minute structures of 35 nm.
- Protein antigens of caries vaccine can be included.

Bio gradable Micro-sphere

- It is used by Eldridge JH et al, 1989 after its use by oral route
- Its composition is similar to that of surgical sutures.
- Antigens are incorporated in microspheres which are released by non-enzymatic rapid hydrolysis.
- Microspheres can be kept in host tissue which causes the sustained and long-term release of antigen.

Bio-adhesive

- Smith DJ *et al.,* 2001 had successfully used bio-adhesive: GTF peptide constructs to induce levels of salivary IgA antibody by an intranasal route which was selected, as this route has nasal-associated lymphoid tissue (NALT)
- Various bio-adhesives which can be used for caries vaccine include bio-adhesive poly D, L-lactide-coglycolide (PLGA) microparticles and Liposomes, biospheres, and bioadhesives which have shown efficacy in delivering antigen

Plantigens and plantibodies [15]

- This is the newer technology used for producing antigen and antibody action against cariogenic pathogens sourced from plants. These have been shown to give better results against dental caries without showing side effects.
- Plants cells have protein synthesis machinery similar to humans and are useful to synthesize plantings which are antigens and plantibodies which act as antibodies.
- Research was conducted on transgenic plants in 1983 by using tobacco plants. Later such research works extended to plants producing fruits and vegetables.
- CARO Rx is the first clinically tested plantibody. After professional cleaning of teeth, it was applied over two weeks. Antibody produced prevents the attachment of S. mutans to the tooth. It was observed that subjects treated with this, remained caries-free for 6 months in phase I clinical trials.

CONCLUSION

A vaccination program for children in India for various medical conditions is already in existence. Animal and various in vitro experimental studies concerning the *mutans streptococci* and its molecular determinants responsible for dental caries formation are available in the literature. Its recent advances also have been explored. Human trials concerning the dental caries vaccine are lacking. Despite the vast discussion on the dental caries vaccine, its use is still questionable. Therefore, the dental caries vaccine should be given due importance like other vaccines to prevent the incidence of dental caries in children. Its usage and feasibility in Indian children should also be explored.

CONSENT FOR PUBLICATION

Not applicable.

CONFLICT OF INTEREST

The authors declare no conflict of interest, financial or otherwise.

ACKNOWLEDGEMENT

Declared none.

REFERENCES

[1] Ozawa S, Clark S, Portnoy A, *et al.* Estimated economic impact of vaccinations in 73 low- and middle-income countries, 2001–2020. Bull World Health Organ 2017; 95(9): 629-38. [http://dx.doi.org/10.2471/BLT.16.178475] [PMID: 28867843]

[2] Minor PD. Live attenuated vaccines: Historical success and current challenges. Virol 2015; 497-486: 379-92.

[3] World Health Organization. Global Health sector strategy on viral hepatitis 2016-2021. Towards ending viral hepatitis. WHO/HIV/2016.06

[4] https://www.historyofvaccines.org/content/articles/different-types-vaccines (Last updated 17 January 2018) (Last accessed on 18/04/21)2018.

[5] Hasan MN, Shahriar SMS. Oral vaccines- Types, delivery strategies, current, and future perspectives. Biomed J Sci Tech Res 2018; 11(2): e8398-405. [http://dx.doi.org/10.26717/BJSTR.2018.11.002075]

[6] Rydig S, Coveney S. What is an Inactivated Vaccine? (news-medical.net) https://www.news-medical.net/health/What-is-an-Inactivated-Vaccine.aspx (Last accessed on 18/04/21)

[7] Sun B, Yu S, Zhao D, Guo S, Wang X, Zhao K. Polysaccharides as vaccine adjuvants. Vaccine 2018; 36(35): 5226-34. [http://dx.doi.org/10.1016/j.vaccine.2018.07.040] [PMID: 30057282]

[8] Cordeiro AS, Alonso MJ, de la Fuente M. Nanoengineering of vaccines using natural polysaccharides. Biotechnol Adv 2015; 33(6): 1279-93. [http://dx.doi.org/10.1016/j.biotechadv.2015.05.010] [PMID: 26049133]

[9] Garg N, Aggarwal A. Advances Towards Painless Vaccination and Newer Modes of Vaccine Delivery. Indian J Pediatr 2018; 85(2): 132-8.
[http://dx.doi.org/10.1007/s12098-017-2377-2] [PMID: 28620730]

[10] https://drtrinadh.wordpress.com/2020/06/07/2420/

[11] Gupta DC, Mankel DH. Caries Vaccine: An Overview. Saudi Journal of Oral and Dental Research 2020; 5(5): 250-3.
[http://dx.doi.org/10.36348/sjodr.2020.v05i05.003]

[12] Shah V, Chovateeya S, Patel DK, Suthar N, Shah A, Patel J. Vaccination against Dental Caries – Possibilities, Prospects & Dangers. J Adv Med Dent Scie Res 2018; 6(5): 9-11.

[13] Sharma Y, Chaudhary D, Nagpal R, Bishnoi A, Trinath T, Rapsang E. Dental Caries vaccine – a Change. Acta Scientific Dental Sciences 2.10, 2018: 41-44.

[14] Patel M. Dental caries vaccine: are we there yet? Lett Appl Microbiol 2020; 70(1): 2-12.
[http://dx.doi.org/10.1111/lam.13218] [PMID: 31518435]

[15] Chatterjee K. Caries Vaccine: The Journey So Far. Acta Scientific Dental Sciences 3.1 (2019): 111-115.

CHAPTER 18

Post COVID-19: Changing Perspective of Pediatric Dentistry

Ritesh Kalaskar[1,*], **Shailja Chatterjee**[2] and **Priyanka Bhaje**[2]

[1] *Sinhgad Dental College and Hospital, Pune, India*

[2] *Dr. D. Y. Patil Dental College and Hospital, Pimpri, Pune, India*

Abstract: Novel coronavirus disease (COVID-19) is one of the worst pandemics known to mankind. It affects people of all age groups. The children may present with milder symptoms and may also be asymptomatic. In the current scenario, pediatric dentists pose a high risk of the disease due to close contact with not just children but also with their parents. Additionally, the majority of pediatric dental procedures advocate the use of an air rotor that generates massive aerosol increasing the transmission risk by a manifold. This, necessitates a change in dental practice protocol to adapt to the new routine. It requires modification in behaviour management techniques, tele-triaging of patients, stringent infection control, minimization and replacement with minimally invasive techniques along with the use of adequate isolation.

Keywords: Coronavirus Disease, Children, Pandemic, Pediatric Dental Clinic, Tele Dentistry.

INTRODUCTION

The current pandemic of COVID 19 is a serious problem to mankind in terms of health and economy. The world is facing an unprecedented threat from the coronavirus (COVID-19). The World Health Organization (WHO) has characterized COVID-19 as a pandemic and the virus has now spread to several countries and territories [1]. The disease can get transmitted through direct contact with persons, touching surfaces contaminated with the virus or through respiratory droplets of an infected person. This virus can survive on surfaces for several hours, but simple disinfectants can kill it. Although cases of COVID-19 appear to be fewer among children, national responses to the pandemic had kept the children away from school and health services to prevent transmission and to reduce the impact of this epidemic.

* **Corresponding author Ritesh Kalaskar:** Sinhgad Dental College and Hospital, Pune, India; E-mail: riteshpedo@gmail.com

Satyawan Damle, Ritesh Kalaskar & Dhanashree Sakhare (Eds.)

The disruption and closure of schools and health services around the world compromise the children's right to education and health facilities. Learning about COVID-19 is the only way to diminish fears and anxieties related to the disease.

What is COVID-19?

COVID-19 is a disease caused by a new coronavirus called SARC –CoV-2. On 31st December 2019, a cluster of pneumonia cases, caused by a newly identified β-coronavirus, was observed in Wuhan, China. This coronavirus was initially named the 2019-novel corona-virus (2019-nCoV) on 11 February 2020 by WHO. The World Health Organization officially named the disease corona-virus disease 2019 (COVID-19). The Chinese scientists rapidly isolated a SARS-CoV-2 from a patient within a short time and came up with genome sequencing of the SARS-CoV-2 [2, 3].

Virology (Table 1)

Table 1. Classification of Corona-viruses.

Name	Found in
Alpha coronaviruses	Bats, rodents, civets, and humans
Beta coronaviruses	Bats, rodents, civets, and humans
Gamma coronaviruses	Birds
Delta coronaviruses	Birds
Omicron	White-tailed deer

Coronaviruses (CoVs) comprise a large family of enveloped, single-stranded, zoonotic RNA viruses belonging to the family Coronaviridae, order Nidovirales. They can infect a variety of animals (including livestock, companion animals and birds), which can cause serious respiratory, enteric, cardiovascular, and neurologic diseases. In humans, CoVs mostly cause respiratory and gastrointestinal symptoms ranging from the common cold to more severe diseases such as bronchitis, pneumonia, severe acute respiratory distress syndrome (ARDS), coagulopathy, multi-organ failure and death [3].

It was found that the genome sequence of SARS-CoV-2 is 96.2% identical to a bat CoV RaTG13, whereas it shares 79.5% identity with ARS-CoV. Based on the virus genome (Fig. **1**) sequencing results and evolutionary analysis, the bat has been suspected as the natural host of virus origin, and SARS-CoV-2 might be transmitted from bats *via* unknown intermediate hosts to infect humans. It is clear now that SARS-CoV-2 could use angiotensin-converting enzyme2 (ACE2), the same receptor as SARS-CoV, to infect humans [3, 4].

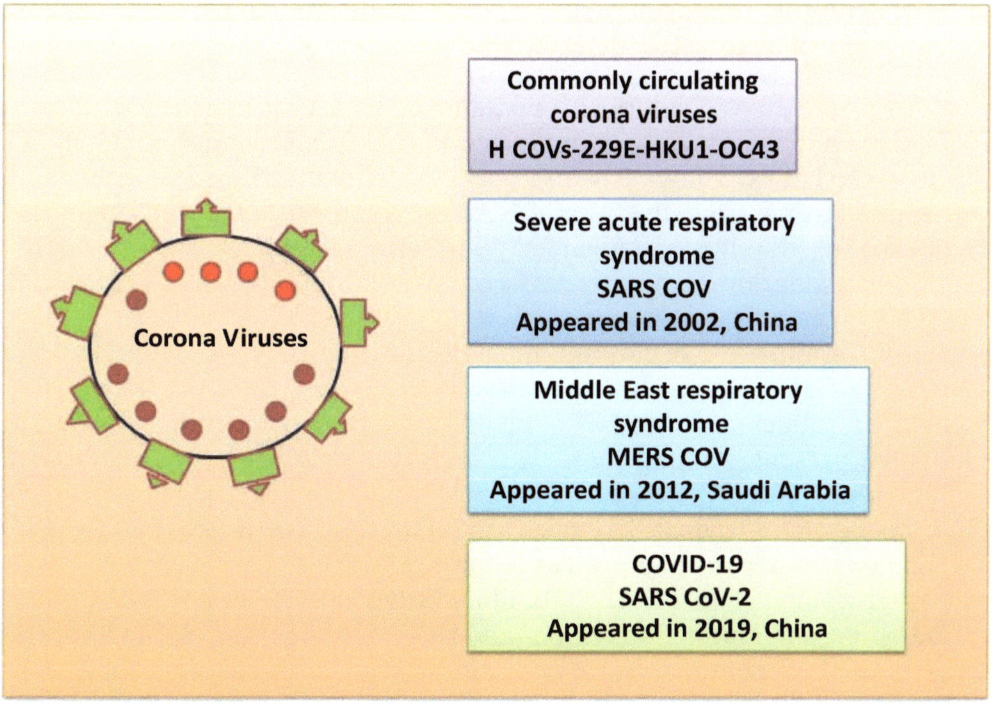

Fig (1). Summary of Corona-viruses disease.

Pathogenesis & Pathophysiology

COVID-19 infection is transmitted through:

- Large droplets generated during coughing and sneezing by symptomatic or asymptomatic patients
- Touching surfaces contaminated by the virus and then touching the nose, mouth, and eyes.
- Use of contaminated water *via* aerosolization
- Fecal-oral route is also postulated.
- As per current information, transplacental transmission from pregnant women to their fetuses has not been described. However, neonatal disease due to postnatal transmission is also a possible mode of transmission.
- Patients can be infectious for as long as the symptoms last and even during clinical recovery [5].

The virus can remain viable on surfaces for days in favourable atmospheric conditions but is destroyed in less than a minute by common disinfectants like sodium hypochlorite, hydrogen peroxide, etc. The incubation period varies from 2 to 14 days (median 5 days) [6, 7].

Coronaviruses are enveloped, positive-stranded RNA viruses with nucleocapsid. In CoVs, the genomic structure is organized in a +ssRNA of approximately 30 kb in length — the largest known RNA viruses — and with a 5′-cap structure and 3′-poly-A tail. Starting from the viral RNA, the synthesis of polyprotein 1a/1ab (pp1a/pp1ab) in the host is realized. The transcription works through the replication-transcription complex (RCT) organized in double-membrane vesicles and *via* the synthesis of subgenomic RNAs (sgRNAs) sequences. Of note, transcription termination occurs at transcription regulatory sequences, located between the so-called open reading frames (ORFs) that work as templates for the production of subgenomic mRNAs. In the atypical CoV genome, at least six ORFs can be present. Among these, a frame shift between ORF1a and ORF1b guides the production of both pp1a and pp1ab polypeptides that are processed by virally encoded chymotrypsin-like protease (3CLpro) or main protease (Mpro), as well as one or two papain-like proteases for producing 16 non-structural proteins (nsps). Apart from ORF1a and ORF1b, other ORFs encode for structural proteins, including spike, membrane, envelope, and nucleocapsid proteins and accessory proteic chains. Different CoVs present special structural and accessory proteins translated by dedicated sgRNAs [2, 4, 8].

Pathophysiology and virulence mechanisms of CoVs and SARS-CoV-2 have links to the function of the non-structural and structural proteins. For instance, research underlined that nsp is able to block the host's innate immune response. Among functions of structural proteins, the envelope has a crucial role in virus pathogenicity as it promotes viral assembly and release. Among the structural elements of CoVs, there are spike glycoproteins composed of two subunits (S1 and S2). Homotrimers of S proteins compose the spikes on the viral surface, guiding the link to host receptors. Scientific evidence suggests that SARS-CoV-2 spike proteins interact with the human angiotensin-converting enzyme 2 (ACE2) to bind to the host cell. The interaction between the viral protein and its cell membrane receptor is a critical step in the replication cycle. SARS-CoV-2 has two loops around the receptor-binding domain which might be promoting the interaction with the human ACE2 receptor thus improving the binding to this receptor by increasing the number of atoms involved. Neonates, infants, and children are less likely to be affected by SARS-CoV-2. The possible reasons could be the SARS-CoV-2 receptor and angiotensin-converting enzyme 2 (ACE2) is reduced in the respiratory tract of children; coronaviruses associated with common colds may offer some protection; T helper 2 immune responses are protective in children; eosinophilia, which is associated with T helper 2 may be protective; and children reduce the levels of inflammatory cytokines [2 - 4, 7, 8].

General Clinical Features of COVID-19

The clinical features of COVID-19 are varied, ranging from an asymptomatic state to acute respiratory distress syndrome and multi-organ dysfunction including the heart and kidney in particular.

The most common symptoms are

- Dry Cough
- Fever
- Fatigue

Other symptoms that are less common but may affect some patients are: loss of taste or smell, sore throat, headache, fatigue, myalgia, nasal congestion, conjunctivitis, skin rashes muscle or joint pain and diarrhoea. Thus, they are indistinguishable from other respiratory infections. In a subset of patients, by the end of the first week, the disease can progress to pneumonia, respiratory failure, and death. This progression is associated with an extreme rise in inflammatory cytokines including IL2, IL7, IL10, GCSF, IP10, MCP1, MIP1A, and TNFα. The median time from the onset of symptoms to dyspnea is 5 days, hospitalization: 7 days and acute respiratory distress syndrome (ARDS): 8 days. The median duration of hospital stays in those who recovered was 10 days. Adverse outcomes and death are more common in the elderly and those with underlying co-morbidities such as diabetes, hypertension, and asthma. The reported data rates due to coronavirus disease vary from country to country, in India it is less (1.5%) as compared to other countries [7, 8].

Symptoms in Children

Children are less commonly affected by SARS-CoV-2. The most common symptoms are fever (50%) and cough (38%) in a mild form of COVID-19. In low to moderate form fever, rhinitis, cough, fatigue, headache, and diarrhoea are present and in more severe cases dyspnea and cyanosis might be present. Recently WHO reported multisystem inflammatory syndrome (MIC-C) in children affected with SARS-CoV-2. In this, different body parts can become inflamed, including the heart, lungs, kidneys, brain, skin, eyes, or gastrointestinal organs. Children with MIS-C may have a fever and various symptoms, including abdominal (gut) pain, vomiting, diarrhoea, neck pain, rash, bloodshot eyes, or feeling extra tired. Additional symptomatic children may develop radiologic ground-glass lung opacities which can be observed on chest Computed Tomography Scans. Most infected children recover 1–2 weeks after the onset of symptoms [4, 7 - 9].

According to the latest report of the National Institute of Health, published in the scientific journal, Nature Medicine, nearly half of the coronavirus patients suffer from oral symptoms during the infection. Since these infections may not be very visible and can go unnoticed by people. The report suggests that these symptoms are even present in most of the asymptomatic cases of coronavirus. While the study to determine the oral symptoms are still underway, here are some of the symptoms that the scientists believe can be an indicator of COVID-19 infection in your body.

Dry mouth: Dry mouth is very common in most viral infections and recent studies have pointed out that the COVID-19 virus can also cause this. In a dry mouth, the body fails to produce saliva which protects the mouth from bad bacteria and other pathogens and helps in the process of digestion. Patients feel dryness or stickiness in their mouth and the saliva becomes thicker. They may feel difficulty in chewing food and speaking and experience a harsh burning sensation. Bad breath may also be a sign of dry mouth.

Lesions: Most viral infections including COVID-19 can cause a sensation of widespread inflammation in patients' mouths. This happens when the virus attacks muscle fibers and oral linings. The inflammation may result in a lesion and painful bump in the mouth which can put an individual off on some foods. For some people, it can also cause mouth ulcers.

COVID Tongue: This is a very common talked symptom of COVID-19. According to studies, COVID-19 causes a burning sensation on the surface of the tongue. Many experts also link it to the skin rashes that COVID-19 patients get.

Changes in the colour of the tongue: COVID-19 can cause effects in the mouth that results in a change in the colour and texture of the tongue. mouth irritation, swelling and multiplication of the pathogen near oral cavities can make the tongue feel weird. It can also cause mouth irritation, make lips and tongue tingle, or cause a lot more irritation than it usually should be. It can also cause a colour change or would be used to seeing.

One of the most useful ways to beat the coronavirus is the early detection of the virus in the body. If a patient feels any of the common or oral symptoms of the coronavirus, getting it checked can help him in the fight against the virus.

Differential Diagnosis of COVID-19 (Table 2, Fig 2)

The symptoms of the early stages of the disease are nonspecific. Differential diagnosis should include the possibility of a wide range of infectious and non-infectious (*e.g.,* vasculitis, dermatomyositis) common respiratory disorders.

- Adenovirus
- Influenza
- Human metapneumovirus (HmPV)
- Parainfluenza
- Respiratory syncytial virus (RSV)
- Rhinovirus (common cold)

Table 2. Diagnosis of COVID-19.

Clinical features	• Mild case-fever, cough • Mild to moderate case- fever cough, rhinitis, fatigue, headache, and diarrhoea • Severe case- fever cough, rhinitis, fatigue, headache, diarrhea, breathlessness and cyanosis
Laboratory findings	• White blood cell count- normal or reduced • Neutrophil and/or lymphocyte counts- decreased • C-reactive protein and procalcitonin levels- normal • D-dimer- elevated • Abnormal coagulation and thrombocytopenia may occur
Radiographical observation	• Bilateral multiplepatchy, nodular pulmonary ground-glass opacities • Speckled ground-glass opacities • Infiltrating shadows in the middle and outer zone of the lung or under the pleura. (*These findings are unspecific and milder compared with those in adults.*)
Molecular test	• Real-time polymerase chain reaction (RT-PCR) on upper or lower respiratory secretions. • Rapid antigen detection

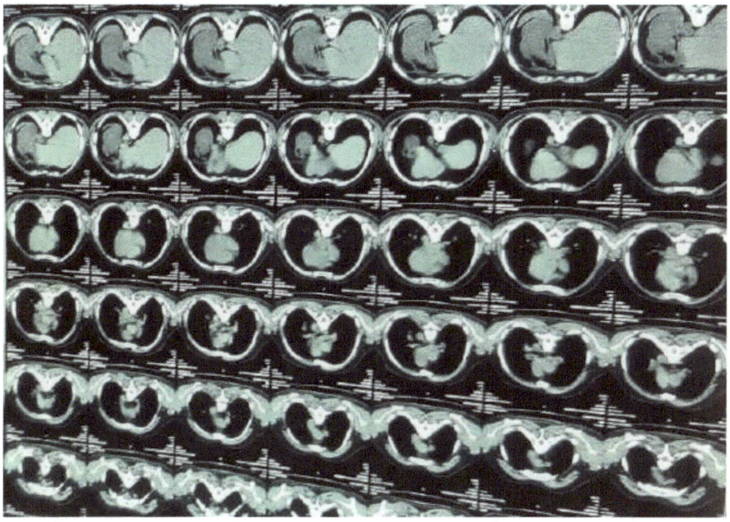

Fig (2). CT Chest showing radio opacities in COVID-19 patients.

For suspected cases, rapid antigen detection, and other investigations have to be adopted for evaluating common respiratory pathogens and non-infectious conditions.

COVID Tongue – Similar to coetaneous infection, patients with COVID-19 also showed raised bumps on the tongue, followed by inflammation and redness of the tongue and canker sores. It was common for those patients who felt a burning sensation in their mouth and loss of taste. There are lots of ACE receptors in the tongue so the virus heavily concentrates in this region giving rise to bumps and swelling (Fig. **3**).

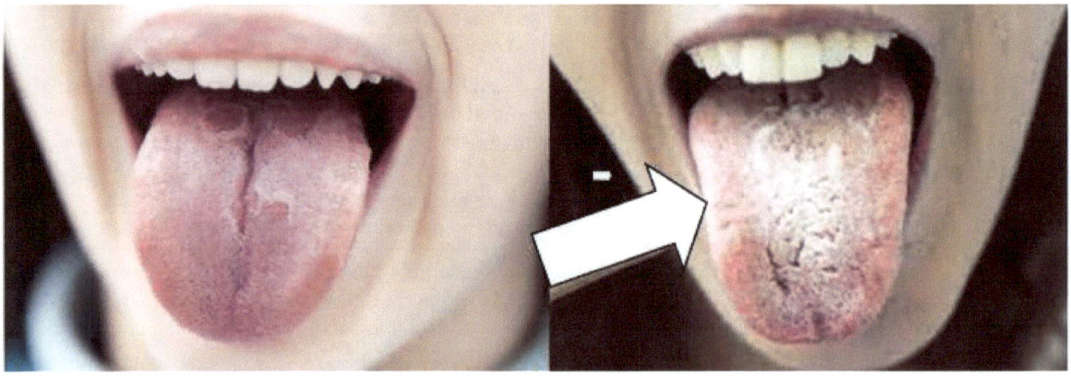

Fig (3). COVID tongue.

Management of COVID-19

There is no treatment for COVID-19; Prevention is the best method to eradicate the disease from this planet. **HUM** principles are followed to curb the disease

- Hand sanitizing or washing at regular interval
- Use Mask regularly

Maintain distance with others (6 feet)

Management of COVID-19 in Pediatric Dental Setting

A pediatric dentist takes care of the dental health of the vulnerable population in society i.e children. Children are mostly accompanied by parents so there is an increase of cross-transmission of infection either from dentist/oral health care worker to children/parents or vice versa. Therefore, a precisely planned protocol has to be drawn for the dental management of pediatric patients in this pandemic and there off.

Dental management in COVID-19 pandemic can be classified as follows:

1. Preventive measures to be followed by patients and their family.

2. Measures to be taken by oral health care providers.

3. Preventive measures were undertaken by the Government.

Preventive Measures to be followed for Patients and their Family

As the saying goes "charity starts at home" preventive measures should start at the patient's home by following all the general guidelines given by the state or central government.

- Avoid/restrict unnecessary travel.
- Avoid crowded places and organize events.
- Maintain at least 4-6 feet distance from anyone who is coughing or sneezing.
- Avoid handshaking
- Avoid touching eyes, mouth, or nose
- Following good respiratory hygiene. This means covering one's mouth and nose with bent elbow or tissue when one cough/sneezes. Then disposing of the used tissue immediately preferably in a closed container.
- Regularly and thoroughly cleaning hands with an alcohol-based hand rub containing 70% alcohol, when the hand is visibly clean or wash them with soap and water for at least 20 seconds especially after coming from outside, after going to the toilet, before preparing food and before eating.
- Suspected infected surface should be clean with a simple disinfectant to kill the virus.
- A regular diet which includes fruits, vegetables, etc. to stay healthy.
- Consult your family doctor and self-isolate by avoiding human contact for clinical symptoms of respiratory infection if there is a travel history to a Coronavirus-affected area and close contact with an infected person.
- Updates on the latest information from trusted sources, such as WHO or respective local and national health authorities [10, 11].

Preventive Measures to be Undertaken by the Oral Health Care Provider

During this pandemic, only emergency dental treatment is allowed because the majority of the dental procedures are aerosol-generating which endanger oral health care provider, parents, and children due to risk for COVID-19 infection.

General Guidelines to be Followed by Pediatric Dental Clinic

- Appointment schedule should be followed to avoid the rush in the dental clinic.
- Patients should wait in their car if they arrive early or undergoing treatment is delayed.
- Signboard ought to be placed at the clinic entrance instructing parents to reschedule dental visits telephonically if they had any symptoms of COVID-19 or if they had travelled to the cOVID affected area or had come in contact with COVID-19 positive people.
- Schedule minimum appointments during the day.
- Telephonically appoint patients and triage (to decide the order of treatment) them according to their level of dental care, i.e., emergency, urgent and elective care.
- In case any patient needs aerosol-based treatment, then need to take a detailed medical history and contact history. We need to follow guidelines for throat swab sample collection as per local government standard guidelines.
- Avoid non-emergency or cosmetic treatment to the patients and defer the same.
- Take temperature readings as part of the routine assessment of patients before initiating any interactions prior to registration for dental procedures. Record the temperature at every visit.
- Take the contact and address details of treated patients.
- Install physical barriers (*e.g.,* glass or plastic windows) at reception areas to limit close contact with any potentially infectious patients.
- Ask patients to wear surgical or similar masks at all times, wash hands prior to entry and remove footwear.
- Ask patients to tie their hair and avoid wearing earrings, finger rings and carrying bags.
- Make sure the personal protective equipment being used is appropriate for the procedures being performed.
- Physical/Social distancing should be maintained in clinical areas and patient appointments should be strictly followed.
- Pre-procedure rinses with 1% hydrogen peroxide (15mL of the solution for 30 seconds). Do not use a spittoon. Use the same sink that had been used for washing the hands and face.
- Clean and disinfect waiting and operating areas frequently, including door handles, chairs, and washrooms.
- All payments should be done preferably through online mode or while making cash transactions, take the appropriate care in handling the cash, as it may be contaminated too [11, 12].

Preventive Measures Undertaken by the Government

Since there is no specific treatment available at the moment, governments all over the world have taken stringent measures to prevent the spread of this highly infectious disease by locking down the city/country. The lockdown restricts people from stepping out of their homes. All transport services–roads, air and rail are suspended, with exceptions for transportation of essential goods, fire, police, and emergency services (Table **3**). Educational institutions, industrial establishments and hospitality services are also suspended. Services such as food shops, banks and ATMs, petrol pumps, other essentials, and their manufacturing are exempted [12].

Table 3. Emergency and Urgent Care for Pediatric Patients during Pandemic.

Emergency Dental Care	Urgent Dental Care for Children and Adolescent
• Fast spreading infections of facial spaces such as Ludwig's angina, acute cellulitis of dental origin and acute trismus • Uncontrolled bleeding of dental origin • Severe uncontrolled dental pain, not responding to routine measures • Trauma involving the face or facial bones • Radiographs like PNS, OPG, CBCT in facial trauma and medico-legal situations	• Acute pulpitis • Dental abscess • Dento-alveolar trauma • Pain of cavitation needing temporization • Unavoidable Dental Extractions • Orthodontic procedures – Orthodontic appliances impinging oral mucosa, orthodontic treatment causing iatrogenic effects, delivery of clear aligners and patients on skeletal anchorage • Management of infants with cleft lip and palate

Management of children in pediatric dental practice can also be classified as:

- Children who have not been exposed to COVID-19: this will include management based on unconfirmed COVID-19 cases as presented in the above flowchart (Fig. **4**).
- Children who are presently COVID-19 positive: Similar to the above flowchart.
- Children who have recovered from COVID-19: Includes psychological changes in children and behaviour management approach following prolonged isolation or hospital stay due to COVID-19. Also, children's reactions to oral health care workers wearing PPE based on past experiences may have a profound effect on children's behaviour in the dental office [13].

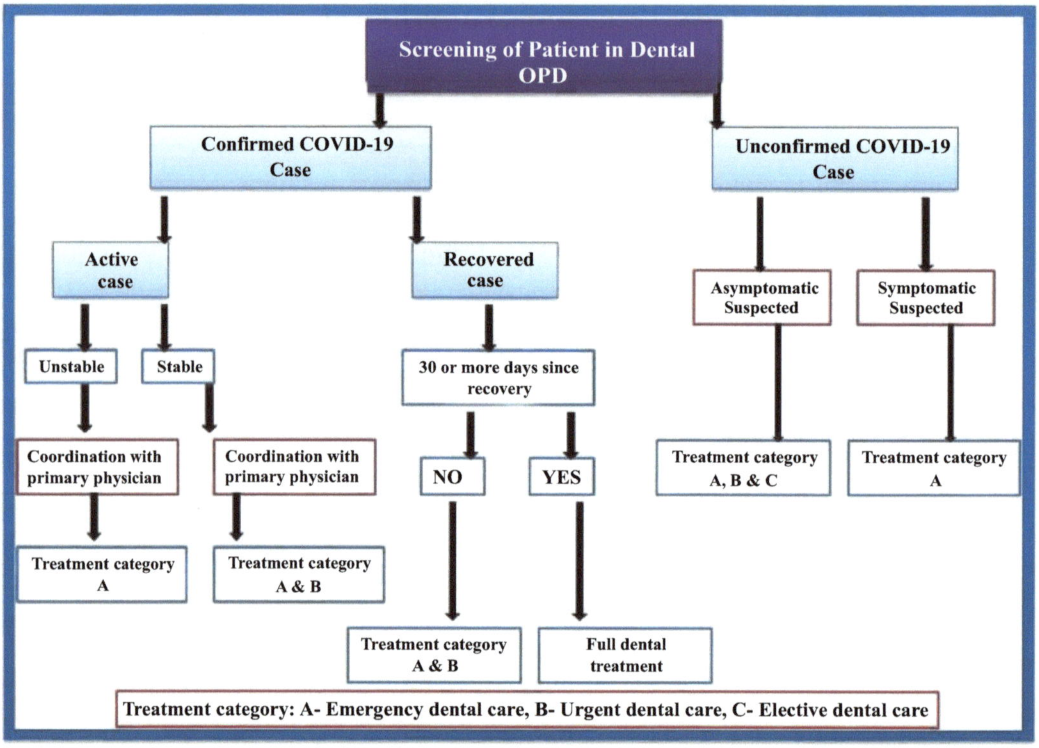

Fig (4). Screening of COVID-19 patients at the dental clinic.

Changing Perspective of Pediatric Dental Practice Due To COVID-19 Pandemic

Dentistry is considered the number one profession for transmitting infections. This explains the gravity of the situation and how essential it is for us as healthcare professionals to protect ourselves, our families, and our patients. Recently, WHO feared about this virus becoming just another endemic virus in our community and may never go away. Therefore, if these speculations are to be believed, the dental practice will have to reorganize itself using innovative solutions to continue the provision of dental care with minimal risk of cross-infection. This requires us to amend our practice based on the guidelines issued by various authorities keeping in mind the best of our patient's interests and also how far it is practical to implement them.

Tele-dentistry

Considering the ongoing circumstances of COVID-19, the main aim of pediatric dentistry is to avoid contact between persons as far as possible and Tele-dentistry can cater to the current need of social distancing. Tele-dentistry offers a wide range of applications such as

- Teleconsultation
- Telediagnosis
- Teletriage
- Telemonitoring
- Telecommunication

Teleconsultation allows the parents to take advice from oral health care providers *via* telecommunication. The majority of dental conditions can be diagnosed directly; therefore, dental photography can reduce the need for close communication. Online telediagnosis can be used not only to diagnose the lesion but also to differentiate it from other lesions. Tele triaging allows timely and appropriate disposition of patient symptoms *via* smartphone. Telemonitoring allows the regular follow-up of patients thus avoiding physical visits to hospitals and allowing virtual visits for evaluating and monitoring patients' disease. Telecommunication allows enquiring patients regarding any history of travel or symptoms indicative of COVID-19 and also allows scheduling of appointments to permit fewer crowds in the waiting area [13, 14].

Use of Personal Protective Equipment (PPE)

These protective gears are designed to safeguard healthcare workers by minimizing exposure to a biological agent. These protective gears are donned based on the risk of the procedure performed mainly for aerosol-generating procedures (AGPs). It comprises a head cover, face shield, goggles, masks, gloves, coverall/gowns, and shoe cover.

Based on the possibility of the spread of COVID-19 infection, three-level protective measures for dental professionals are recommended for specific situations.

- Primary protection (standard protection for staff in clinical settings). Wearing a disposable working cap, disposable surgical mask, and working clothes (white coat), using protective goggles or face shield, and disposable latex gloves or nitrile gloves if necessary.
- Secondary protection (advanced protection for dental professionals). Wearing a disposable head cap, disposable surgical mask, protective goggles, face shield, and working clothes (white coat) with disposable isolation clothing or surgical clothes outside, and disposable latex gloves.
- Tertiary protection is strengthened protection when contact patient is suspected

or confirmed COVID-19 infection. Although a patient with COVID-19 infection is not expected to be treated in the dental clinic, in the unlikely event where it occurs, and the dental professional cannot avoid close contact, special protective outwear is needed. If protective outwear is not available, working clothes (white coat)with extra disposable protective clothing outside should be worn. In addition, disposable head caps, protective goggles, face shields, disposable surgical masks, disposable latex gloves, and impermeable shoe covers should be worn [15].

Component of PPE Kit

Face Shield and Goggles

- To prevent contamination of eyes, nose and mouth by droplets generated during coughing or sneezing of an infected person or during aerosol-generating procedures carried out in a clinical setting.
- To prevent contamination of eyes/nose/mouth inadvertently touching with a contaminated hand.

Masks

- It prevents the contamination of nasal or oral airways from the particulate matter generated by droplets or aerosols. Two types of masks are recommended for various categories of personnel working in hospital or community settings.
- Triple-layer surgical mask- A triple-layer surgical mask is a disposable mask; fluid resistance protects the wearer from droplets of infectious material emitted during coughing or sneezing.
- N-95 Respirator mask- An N-95 respirator mask is a respiratory protective device with high filtration efficiency to airborne particles. To provide the requisite air seal to the wearer, such masks are designed to achieve a very close facial fit. Such mask should have high fluid resistance, good breathability (preferably with an expiratory valve), clearly identifiable internal and external faces, duckbill/cup-shaped structured design that does not collapse against the mouth. If correctly worn, the filtration capacity of these masks exceeds those of triple-layer medical masks. Since these provide a much tighter air seal than triple-layer medical masks, they are designed to protect the wearer from inhaling airborne particles.

Gloves

- To prevent contamination of nose, mouth, and eyes through hands which can inadvertently come in contact with contaminated surfaces. Nitrile gloves are preferred over latex gloves because they resist chemicals, including certain disinfectants such as chlorine. There is a high rate of allergies to latex and contact allergic dermatitis among health workers. However, if nitrile gloves are not available, latex gloves can be used. Non-powdered gloves are preferred to powdered gloves.

Coverall/Gowns

- Coverall/gowns are designed to protect the torso of healthcare providers from exposure to viruses. Coveralls typically provide 360-degree protection because they are designed to cover the whole body, including the back and lower legs and sometimes head and feet as well.
- Coveralls and gowns are deemed equally acceptable as there is a lack of comparative evidence to show whether one is more effective than the other in reducing transmission to health workers. Gowns are considerably easier to put on and remove . An apron can also be worn over the gown for the entire time the health worker is in the treatment area. Coveralls/gowns have stringent standards that extend from preventing exposure to biologically contaminated solid particles to protecting from chemical hazards.

Shoe covers

- Shoe covers should be made up of impermeable fabric to be used on overshoes to facilitate personal protection and decontamination.

Headcovers

- Coveralls usually cover the head. Those using gowns should use a headcover that covers the head and neck while providing clinical care for patients. Hair and hair extensions should fit inside the headcover.

Steps of Donning and Doffing of PPE

Donning of PPE

- Before donning PPE all jewellery should be removed and head hairs should be tied properly.
- Ensure appropriate size PPE is selected based on the care of the patient.
- Wash the hand for 40-60 seconds or sanitize the hands with alcohol-based scrub before donning.
- Check for tear or damage to PPE and ensure all the straps are tied properly.
- Place N95 mask over nose and mouth and ensure it is proper fit so that no air escapes from the nose of the mask. Do not touch the mask after securing it in place, if at all it is needed, then wash the hands before touching the mask.
- Face shields or goggles are placed in a position to protect the eyes.

- Thereafter wear the gloves and make sure that they are over the PPE cuff so that no part of the skin is exposed.
- Always take the help of your colleague for the proper and correct wearing of PPE.

Doffing of PPE (Fig 5)

- Removal of PPE poses the highest risk of transmission of infection to healthcare workers, therefore it is done with utmost care. Avoid any contact with the contaminated PPE with clothes, skin and especially face.
- First remove the gloves and discard them safely, thereafter, remove the PPE slowly by pulling it out of the body and ensuring there is no contact with the clothes and surrounding environment. Turn the PPE inside out and dispose it of safely in the garbage.
- Wash the hand before removing the face shield, head cap, shoe cover or eye protector and mask should be removed last. Remove them carefully and discard them [15, 16].

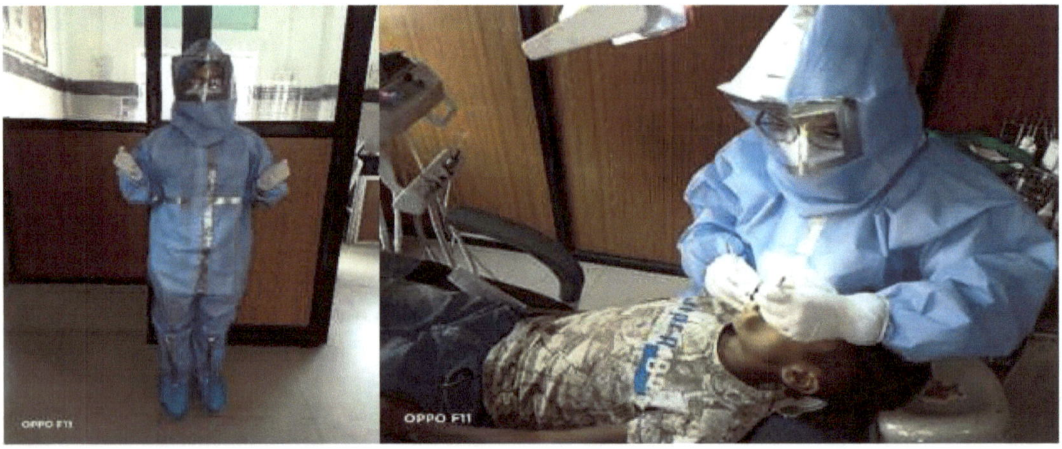

Fig (5). PPE Kit: A- Oral health care worker in PPE kit, B- Oral health care worker in PPE kit while working on patient.

Behaviour Management

Behaviour management is the cornerstone of pediatric dentistry. Apart from the above-stated challenges, other obstacles can encounter while managing children in the current situation.

- Firstly, parental presence in the operatory is not advised to prevent crowding in compact places. Hence, children need to be adequately trained to cooperate in the absence of parents.

- It is advocated to perform maximum treatments in single appointments based on the child's cooperation to minimize their visits.
- Children who are extremely uncooperative or require protective stabilization should be postponed from treatment as far as practically viable.

Patient Entry and Discharge Protocol

- On entry to the dental clinic patients and their parents should sanitize their hands and are not allowed to touch any surfaces as far as possible.
- There temperature should be monitored at the entry of the clinic using an infrared thermal scanner or any suitable device.
- Apart from obtaining dental history, parents should be enquired regarding symptoms of COVID-19 or Severe Acute Respiratory illness.
- After the first visits, patients are encouraged to visit the dental clinic on the scheduled date and time.
- In case of emergency before visiting the dental clinic, the parent is encouraged about enquiring about the availability of appointment and after reaching the dental clinic they should preferably wait in their cars till their turn comes.
- Clinical examination including oral examination should be done preferably on a dental chair taking all the standardized safety precautions as mentioned by local/state or central government.
- Patients are advised to perform pre-procedural rinse with 10 ml of 0.5% povidone-iodine solution.
- As far as possible, non-aerosol generating, and emergency treatment should be performed.
- Cash handling should be avoided as it can be contaminated, therefore digital transactions are preferred [17].

Modification in a Pediatric Dental Clinic Setup

Actually, no modifications are required in the dental clinic/dental hospital in view of COVID-19 because these requisites are supposed to be present in the dental clinic/dental hospital. Although some aspects of this protocol have been neglected in practice but now, considering the current situation, it has become mandatory.

- The operatory room should be well ventilated and regular servicing of the air conditioner ought to be done.
- Dental clinic should be equipped with an HEPA filter and a UV light system.
- Playroom should have limited toys which can be sanitised and should be placed at a distance.
- Dental chairs should be placed at a distance of 6 feet apart if more than one chair is present.

- Suction machine or saliva ejectors should be installed with each dental chair.
- Changing areas should be available in dental setups for proper donning and doffing.
- Washrooms should be installed with either sensor taps or taps with elbow handle.
- Automatic sanitiser dispenser should be installed in the dental clinic at entry and in the working area.
- If possible, use directional airflow, such as from fans to ensure ventilation.
- There should be sufficient space available for storage in the dental clinic/dental hospital.
- Dental clinics should have a separate area for sterilization purposes.
- Whenever possible only child patients should be allowed in the operatory. Mask and face shield should be supplied if the accompanying person enters the operatory room.
- Limit paperwork in the operatory clinic
- Training of auxiliary staff on how to follow established protocols.
- Signage boards indicating symptoms of infectious disease and its preventive strategies can be placed in the waiting area [17].

Disinfection of Pediatric Dental Clinics

Stringent infection control practices are the need of the hour.

- Patient waiting room and operatory room should be fumigated daily
- After completion of treatment, the areas/parts of the dental chair which are most likely to get contaminated should be disinfected.
- Regularly wipe all the touchable areas such as tables, chair arms, doorknobs, light switches hangers, TV remote, etc with disinfectants.
- After completion of treatment, the instruments should be cleared away immediately for rinsing followed by sterilization or disinfection.
- If the floor is dirty, it should be cleaned using a detergent or soap and water prior to disinfection.
- Four-handed or six-handed dentistry should be practiced avoiding cross-transmission of infection.
- Cover the keyboard of a computer with a disposable, flexible, clear barrier (*e.g.*, plastic wrap) and change between patients.
- All dentists and support staff should wash their hands thoroughly with soap and water and follow up with alcohol-based hand sanitizers before and after screening or interaction with each and every patient.
- Oral health care providers and support staff should wear at least 3 ply masks, face shields, suitable head cap and shoe cover all the time.

- Three in one syringe, water lines, suction pipes should be flushed with disinfectant after every patient.
- Before the start of treatment, patient is recommended to rinse with 1% hydrogen peroxide to reduce the number of microbes in the oral cavity.
- Rubber dams and high-volume saliva ejectors should be preferably used to help minimize aerosol or spatter in dental procedures [15, 16].

Negative Pressure Isolation for Dental Clinic

Dental professionals are at high risk of getting infected through saliva and blood-contaminated aerosol. Centre for diseases control, United States recommended negative pressure dental clinics to prevent infection in the dental clinic. For negative pressure rooms, the sum of the mechanically exhausted air must exceed the sum of the mechanically supplied air. In a negative pressure room, air should flow from hallways and corridors into the isolation rooms. This prevents cross-contamination and the spread of viruses, bacteria, and fungi. The exhausted air must be directly funneled to the outside of the building. If this is not possible then air should be passed through the high-efficiency particulate air filter (HEPA) before recirculation. If the air gets recirculated, then high-density HEPA filters with a minimum efficiency reporting value of 8 or higher should be available which capture almost 97.77 per cent of particles whose diameter is greater than 0.3μm. Entry and exit to the room should be minimized.

Protocol for Health Workers on Reaching Home

- Oral health care providers and other staff of the hospital/clinic are advised to wear the PPE in the operatory and change just prior to leaving the clinic.
- Hand washing should be done thoroughly before leaving the clinic/hospital.
- On reaching home, all personal belongings should be kept in a box outside which should be sanitized.
- Shoes should be removed outside and hands to be sanitized before entering the house.
- It is highly recommended to not touch anything or come in contact with family members before taking a shower which should be done immediately after entering the house [15].

New Normal in the Therapeutic Approaches

It is a well-established fact that prevention is better than cure and is much cheaper and more stable. In this pandemic, the use of such preventive strategies had gained momentum and is directed towards a more patient-centered approach. Worldwide research on the management of early carious lesions concluded that non-cavitated lesions can be managed non-invasively by incorporating a low cariogenic diet, appropriate management of the biofilm, home as well as dental office application of fluorides and sealing techniques.

- The main aim of the management of carious lesions is to minimize aerosol-generating procedures (AGPs) as far as possible. Biological treatment alternatives for asymptomatic teeth and teeth showing signs of reversible pulpitis range from atraumatic restorative technique (ART), interim therapeutic restorations (ITR), indirect pulp therapy (IPT), hall technique (HT) to the use of silver diamine fluoride (SDF). Research has shown that both biological methods of caries management comprising HT and IPT and conventional methods of complete caries removal or pulpotomies are equally successful in managing carious lesions in primary teeth.
- SDF has become a significant change in the current pandemic. Numerous systematic reviews substantiate the efficacy of SDF in managing carious lesions in young children and those with special health care needs. It arrests caries by hampering bacterial metabolism due to the presence of Ag and by enhancing remineralization. American Dental Association recommends using SDF to arrest advanced cavitated carious lesions on any coronal surface of primary and permanent teeth. They suggest clinicians prioritize the use of 38% SDF solution (biannual application) over 5% NaF varnish. However, its biggest drawback is the blackish discoloration resulting in an unaesthetic appearance and metallic taste which makes it unacceptable. But it has been observed that restoration with glass ionomer cement (GIC) and composites completely masks the black discoloration.
- Pit and fissure sealant is recommended to arrest or reverse the non-cavitated carious lesions on the occlusal surfaces of both primary and permanent teeth.
- Atraumatic restorative technique (ART) can be an invaluable, effective evidence-based alternative to conventional methods in the post-COVID-19 era for treating and preventing carious lesions in both primary and permanent teeth.
- The interim therapeutic restoration can also be an alternative in this pandemic to restore and prevent further decalcification and caries in young patients, uncooperative patients, or patients with special health care needs. It can also be used when conventional cavity preparation or placement of conventional dental restorations is not feasible and dental care needs to be postponed.
- In a few cases, the use of handpieces is inevitable; hence the use of micromotor or anti-retraction handpieces is advocated in such scenarios.
- Additionally, the use of rubber dam isolation and suction is mandatory for any type of procedure.
- Certain practitioners have also explored the use of extraoral suction device since it aids in removing toxic products and preventing cross-contamination among

the patient and dentist and also works as an air sterilizer in the operatory. (Fig. **6**, Table **4**).

- Extraoral dental radiographies, such as panoramic radiography and cone-beam computed tomography (CBCT), are appropriate alternatives during the outbreak of COVID-19 as intraoral dental imaging stimulates saliva secretion and coughing [15, 16].

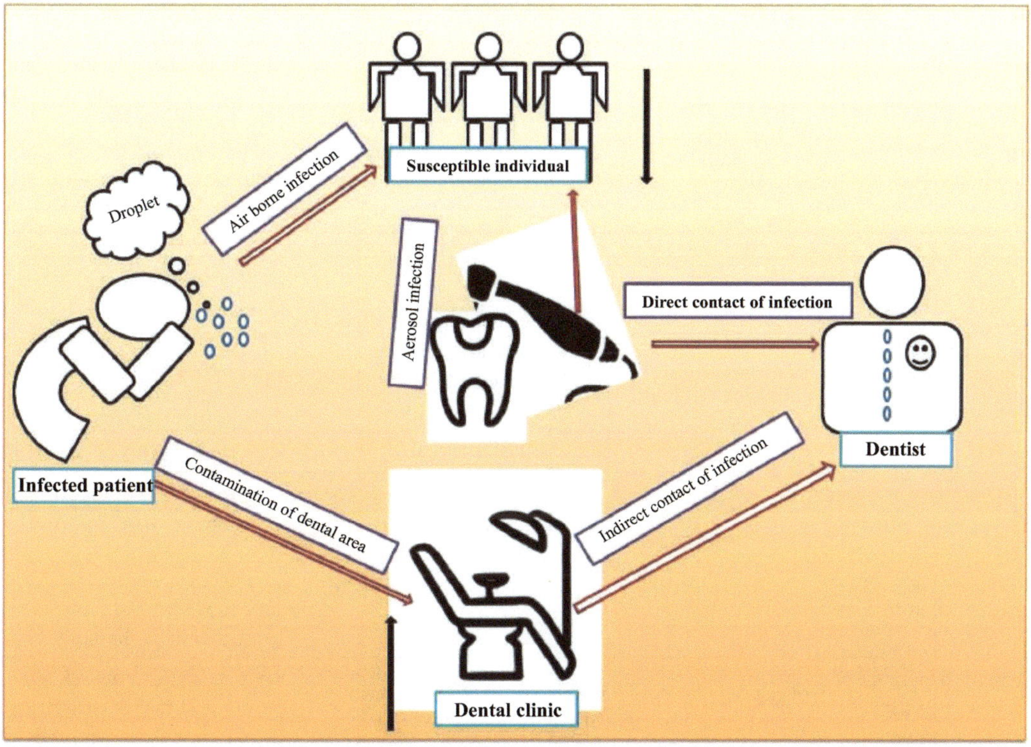

Fig (6). COVID-19 infection transfer process in dental clinic.

Table 4. Myths and facts related to COVID-19 disease.

Myths	Facts	Myths	Facts
Only older adults and young people are at risk of COVID-19.	COVID-19 can affect people of any age. However, older adults and adults with pre-existing health conditions are more likely to become severely ill.	Spraying chlorine or alcohol on the skin kills coronavirus in the body.	Applying alcohol or chlorine to the body can cause harm, especially if it enters the eyes or mouth. Although people can use these chemicals to disinfect surfaces, they should not use them on the skin. These products cannot kill viruses within the body.

(Table 4) cont.....

Myths	Facts	Myths	Facts
Antibiotics are effective in preventing and treating the new coronavirus.	No, antibiotics do not work against viruses, only bacteria. The new coronavirus (2019-nCoV) is a virus and therefore antibiotics should not be used as a means of prevention or treatment.	Coronavirus cannot be transmitted in areas with hot and humid climates.	Coronavirus can be transmitted in all areas including areas with hot and humid weather.
Hand dryers are effective in killing coronavirus.	No Hand dryers are not effective in killing coronavirus.	Eating garlic helps prevent infection with the new coronavirus.	Garlic is a healthy food that may have some antimicrobial properties. However, no evidence from the current outbreak that eating garlic has protected people from the new coronavirus.
Regularly gargling with salt water or saline can prevent corona-19 infection	No evidence that regularly gargling has protected people from coronavirus infection. While this may help soothe a sore throat.	Non-vegetarian food (meat) consumption can lead to coronavirus infection.	It has been established that the novel coronavirus has jumped from an animal to a man and is originally a zoonotic disease. However, no known animal species have been known to carry this virus as of yet.
Once you get COVID-19, you cannot recover from the disease	The majority of people do recover from coronavirus infection within 10-15 days	Drinking alcohol reduces the risk of infection	Not drinking alcohol doesn't reduce the risk of COVID-19 infection. Alcohol can disinfect the skin; it does not work in the same way inside the body.
Adding pepper to meals helps in preventing Coronavirus disease	Hot peppers in food can be tasty but do not protect against coronavirus disease.	COVID-19 infection is transmitted through house flies.	To date, there is no evidence to suggest that coronavirus infection is transmitted through house flies.
Vitamin C supplements will stop you from catching the COVID-19 infection	Researchers are yet to find any evidence that vitamin C supplements can render people immune to COVID-19 infection	The novel coronavirus can be transmitted through mosquito bites	To date, no evidence suggests that coronavirus can be transmitted through mosquito bites.
Small children can't get infected with COVID-19	Children can get infected with coronavirus	You are free from coronavirus if you can hold your breath for 10 seconds or more?	No this is not true The best way to confirm COVID-19 is a laboratory test.

(Table 4) cont.....

Myths	Facts	Myths	Facts
Ultraviolet disinfection lamp kills the coronavirus	Yes, UV light kills the coronavirus on surfaces and not from the skin. UV lights should not be used to sterilize hands or other areas of skin as they may damage the skin.	You should not breastfeed your baby if you had a coronavirus infection.	As per WHO women with COVID-19 should be supported to breastfeed safely. Because mother milk provides all the necessary nutrition and strengthens a baby's immune mechanism.
Face masks always protect against coronavirus	Disposable and cloth masks can protect against droplets, but not against aerosolized particles. The CDC recommends that all people should wear a cloth face mask in public places where it is difficult to maintain a 6 feet distance	Drinking silver kills the coronavirus	No evidence drinking silver in the prevention of coronavirus disease but rather can lead to kidney damage.

Challenges for Dental Education

The current scenario has taken a major toll on both undergraduate and postgraduate teaching curricula. During this pandemic, it is highly encouraged to continue the online lectures and seminars with the use of existing smart devices and applications which have made it possible for students to review lectures whenever and wherever possible. Additionally, patient-based learning and practical procedures have taken a huge setback for students. Case studies and problem-based learning on online platforms need to be encouraged. With the advent of 3D printing technology, it is possible to print 3D faces, teeth, dental arch etc. to provide practical learning to the student with the sense of performing it on real patients. These changes could be adapted to continue the curriculum for students and prevent the impact of the current situation on their future [17].

COVID-19 VACCINES

There are four categories of vaccines in clinical trials: Some of them try to smuggle the antigen into the body, and others use the body's cells to make the viral antigen

- Whole virus
- Protein subunit
- Viral vector
- Nucleic acid (RNA AND DNA) [4, 9, 10].

COVAXIN® is India's first Indigenous COVID-19 vaccine developed by Bharat Biotech in collaboration with the Indian council of medical research and the National Institute of virology. It has been developed using Whole-Virion Inactivated Vero Cell-derived platform technology. Inactivated vaccines do not replicate and are therefore unlikely to revert and cause pathological effects. They contain dead viruses, incapable of infecting people but still able to instruct the immune system to mount a defensive reaction against an infection.

COVISHIELD

The Oxford-AstraZeneca vaccine is being manufactured locally by the Serum Institute of India, the world's largest vaccine manufacturer. The vaccine is made from a weakened version of a common cold virus (known as an adenovirus) from chimpanzees. Vaccine after injecting inpatient stimulates the immune system to start antibodies production and aims to fight against corona-19 infection. The vaccine is given in two doses between 8-12 weeks apart.

SPUTNIK V is a Russian-made vaccine developed by Russia's Gamaleya National Research Center of Epidemiology and Microbiology and the Russian Direct Investment Fund. It is based on two adenovirus vectors; Recipients generated robust antibody responses to the spike protein, which included neutralizing antibodies, the proportion of the total immunoglobulin that inhibits the virus binding to its receptor. They also showed evidence of T-cell responses, consistent with an immune response that should not quickly wane. The interim report of the phase 3 data is now presented. The efficacy trial on Sputnik V showed 92% efficacy.

The Caravan is an MRA- based vaccine. CVnCoV and CV07050101 are the other names for this vaccine. It is manufactured by a German biopharmaceutical company known as CureVac N.V. The country of origin of this vaccine is Europe, being the Netherland as its headquarters. The route of administration of this vaccine is Intra-muscular (IM). Two doses of this vaccine are administered. The duration between 2 doses is 28 days. This vaccine is having an efficacy of 95%.

The Pfizer Vaccine was developed by Pfizer, Inc., and BioNTech, Germany. It was developed under the name BNT162b2. The vaccine works by introducing a molecule to cells, known as messenger RNA (mRNA). This molecule teaches cells to make a protein from the virus that causes COVID-19, which is SARS-CoV-2. The body detects this protein and triggers an immune response. This creates antibodies, as well as longer-lasting immunity that can fight off future SARS-CoV-2 infections. It is advocated to take 2 shots of this vaccine intramuscularly at an interval of 21 days. Based on this, the vaccine was 95% effective at preventing laboratory-confirmed COVID-19 illness in people without evidence of a previous infection. The local side effects reported with this vaccine are pain, redness, swelling and general side effects are tiredness, headache, muscle pain, chills, fever, and nausea.

The CoronaVac Vaccine is manufactured by Sinovac Biotech Ltd. China. It is a two-dose vaccine, after the first dose, the second dose is taken after half a year or 6 months. It is an inactivated virus COVID-19 vaccine (Ad5-nCoV vaccine). It has an 80-90% efficacy rate within 2 months after 2 shots.

Janssen COVID-19 vaccine is manufactured by Janssen Pharmaceuticals Companies of Johnson & Johnson, Netherland. It is the only single-dose vaccine. It is an inactivated virus COVID-19 vaccine (Ad5-nCoV vaccine). The J&J/Janssen vaccine was 66.3% effective in clinical trials (efficacy) and is given to people who had no evidence of prior infection 2 weeks after receiving the vaccine. People had the most protection 2 weeks after getting vaccinated.

COVID 19 Vaccine by Moderna codenamed as mRNA -1273, developed by National Institute of Allergy and Infectious Diseases, Biomedical Advanced Research and Developed Authority and Moderna. It developed in the USA. It is an RNA vaccine composed of nucleoside-modified RNA encoding a spike protein of SARS-CoV-2 which is encapsulated in lipid nanoparticles. It is given in 2 doses with an interval of 4 weeks in between. The route of administration of 0.5 ml vaccine is intramuscular having an efficacy of approximately 94%.

CONCLUSION

Keeping in mind the unique environment of the dental clinic, the risk of COVID-19 transmission is very high. With the continuing increase in COVID-19 cases, it is viable for pediatric dentists to be well informed regarding its signs and symptoms and follow stringent infection control protocol considering every patient as potentially infected with the virus. Guidelines issued by authorities cannot cover all the possible clinical situations, hence exercising professional judgment becomes crucial on whether to provide treatment or not based on the circumstances. It is viable for pediatric dentists to adapt to the new normal and utilize opportunities to encourage preventive approaches for dental diseases. It is highly recommended to minimize or attempt to eliminate aerosol-generating procedures during this pandemic and even after easing restrictions in the future. Attempts should be made to replace them with more biological and minimally invasive options.

CONSENT FOR PUBLICATION

Not applicable.

CONFLICT OF INTEREST

The authors declare no conflict of interest, financial or otherwise.

ACKNOWLEDGEMENT

Declared none.

REFERENCES

[1] Chilamakuri R, Agarwal S. COVID-19: Characteristics and Therapeutics. Cells 2021; 10(2): 206. [http://dx.doi.org/10.3390/cells10020206] [PMID: 33494237]

[2] Chen Y, Guo Y, Pan Y, Zhao ZJ. Structure analysis of the receptor binding of 2019-nCoV. Biochem Biophys Res Commun 2020; 525(1): 135-40. [http://dx.doi.org/10.1016/j.bbrc.2020.02.071] [PMID: 32081428]

[3] Wan Y, Shang J, Graham R, Baric RS, Li F. Receptor recognition by novel corona virus from Wuhan: An analysis based on decade-long structural studies of SARS. J Virol 2020; 94(7): e00127-20. [http://dx.doi.org/10.1128/JVI.00127-20] [PMID: 31996437]

[4] Ortega JT, Serrano ML, Pujol FH, Rangel HR. Role of changes in SARS-CoV-2 spike protein in the interaction with the human ACE2 receptor: An *in silico* analysis. EXCLI J 2020; 19: 410-7. [PMID: 32210742]

[5] Snyder MR, Ravi SJ. 1818, 1918, 2018: Two Centuries of Pandemics. Health Secur 2018; 16(6): 410-5. [http://dx.doi.org/10.1089/hs.2018.0083] [PMID: 30511884]

[6] Al-Halabi M, Salami A, Alnuaimi E, Kowash M, Hussein I. Assessment of paediatric dental guidelines and caries management alternatives in the post COVID-19 period. A critical review and clinical recommendations. Eur Arch Paediatr Dent 2020; 21(5): 543-56. [http://dx.doi.org/10.1007/s40368-020-00547-5] [PMID: 32557183]

[7] Su L, Ma X, Yu H, *et al.* The different clinical characteristics of corona virus disease cases between children and their families in China – the character of children with COVID-19. Emerg Microbes Infect 2020; 9(1): 707-13. [http://dx.doi.org/10.1080/22221751.2020.1744483] [PMID: 32208917]

[8] Shen Q, Guo W, Guo T, *et al.* Novel coronavirus infection in children outside of Wuhan, China. Pediatr Pulmonol 2020; 55(6): 1424-9. [http://dx.doi.org/10.1002/ppul.24762] [PMID: 32259403]

[9] Dhama K, Khan S, Tiwari R, *et al.* Coronavirus Disease 2019–COVID-19. Clin Microbiol Rev 2020; 33(4): e00028-20. [http://dx.doi.org/10.1128/CMR.00028-20] [PMID: 32580969]

[10] Meng L, Hua F, Bian Z. Coronavirus Disease 2019 (COVID-19): Emerging and Future Challenges for Dental and Oral Medicine. J Dent Res 2020; 99(5): 481-7. [http://dx.doi.org/10.1177/0022034520914246] [PMID: 32162995]

[11] Lu C, Liu X, Jia Z. 2019-nCoV transmission through the ocular surface must not be ignored. Lancet 2020; 395(10224): e39. [http://dx.doi.org/10.1016/S0140-6736(20)30313-5] [PMID: 32035510]

[12] Chung JY, Thone MN, Kwon YJ. COVID-19 vaccines: The status and perspectives in delivery points of view. Adv Drug Deliv Rev 2021; 170: 1-25. [http://dx.doi.org/10.1016/j.addr.2020.12.011] [PMID: 33359141]

[13] Ghai S. Teledentistry during COVID-19 pandemic. Diabetes Metab Syndr 2020; 14(5): 933-5.

[http://dx.doi.org/10.1016/j.dsx.2020.06.029] [PMID: 32593116]

[14] Machado RA, de Souza NL, Oliveira RM, Martelli Júnior H, Bonan PRF. Social media and telemedicine for oral diagnosis and counselling in the COVID-19 era. Oral Oncol 2020; 105: 104685. [http://dx.doi.org/10.1016/j.oraloncology.2020.104685] [PMID: 32291154]

[15] Kühnisch J, Ekstrand KR, Pretty I, *et al.* Best clinical practice guidance for management of early caries lesions in children and young adults: an EAPD policy document. Eur Arch Paediatr Dent 2016; 17(1): 3-12.
[http://dx.doi.org/10.1007/s40368-015-0218-4] [PMID: 26732946]

[16] Crystal YO, Niederman R. Evidence-Based Dentistry Update on Silver Diamine Fluoride. Dent Clin North Am 2019; 63(1): 45-68.
[http://dx.doi.org/10.1016/j.cden.2018.08.011] [PMID: 30447792]

[17] Patil NG, Yan YCH, Yan H. SARS and its effect on medical education in Hong Kong. Med Educ 2003; 37(12): 1127-8.
[http://dx.doi.org/10.1046/j.1365-2923.2003.01723.x] [PMID: 14984121]

SUBJECT INDEX

A

B

C

G

H

I

J

L

M

N

O

P

R

S

T

U

V

X

Z

www.ingramcontent.com/pod-product-compliance
Lightning Source LLC
LaVergne TN
LVHW070944210926
848482LV00002B/88